Cardiovascular Involvement in Systemic Diseases

Cardiovascular Involvement in Systemic Diseases

J. David Talley, M.D.

Professor of Internal Medicine
Director, Division of Cardiology
University of Arkansas for Medical Sciences
Chief, Cardiology Section
John L. McClellan Memorial Veterans Hospital
Little Rock, Arkansas

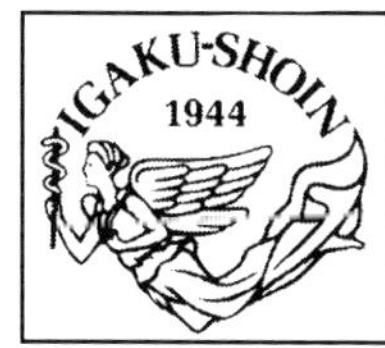

IGAKU-SHOIN New York • Tokyo

This book is dedicated to my teachers, students, and patients who have provided the pathway, stimulus, and opportunity to learn.

Published and distributed by

IGAKU-SHOIN Medical Publishers, Inc.
One Madison Avenue, New York, New York 10010

IGAKU-SHOIN Ltd.,
5-24-3 Hongo, Bunkyo-ku, Tokyo 113-91

Library of Congress Cataloging-in-Publication Data

Cardiovascular involvement in systemic diseases / [edited by] J. David Talley.
    p.   cm.—(Topics in clinical cardiology)
    Includes bibliographical references and index.
    1. Cardiological manifestations of general diseases. I. Talley J. David. II. Series.
    [DNLM: 1. Cardiovascular Diseases—etiology. 2. Cardiovascular System—physiopathology. WG 120 C2675 1996]
    RC682.C414 1996
    616.1—dc21
    DNLM/DLC
    for Library of Congress   96-45182
                                CIP

ISBN: 0-89640-317-3 (New York)
ISBN: 4-260-14317-4 (Tokyo)

Printed and bound in the U.S.A.

10 9 8 7 6 5 4 3 2 1

Preface

The field of cardiovascular diseases has exploded with the advent of invasive and interventional diagnostic and therapeutic technology. Despite refined clinical acumen and this advancement in technology, there is now a greater awareness and appreciation that diseases seldom occur in isolation. The adage, "cardiology is internal medicine, and internal medicine is cardiology" provided the stimulus to compile and edit the monograph, *Cardiovascular Involvement in Systemic Diseases*.

Cardiovascular Involvement in Systemic Diseases is a compilation of common diseases and their synergistic effects on the heart and cardiovascular system. Each section is compiled by an editor of the discipline who is an expert in the field. Each editor and author was given the charge to focus on common diseases and refined diagnostic techniques and optimal therapeutic options. In doing so, *Cardiovascular Involvement in Systemic Diseases* is of distinct value to physicians who provide primary care.

Special note should be given to the rigorous format used in each section. The symptoms and signs, diagnostic criteria and differential diagnosis of each disease are discussed. Emphasis is given to the pathogenesis and treatment options of the disease. References of historic interest and those which may serve as a springboard for additional investigation are provided. This structure allows the busy clinician to focus on areas of individual interest and concern.

I wish to thank several individuals for their influence and guidance which have been essential in the publication of *Cardiovascular Involvement in Systemic Diseases*. J. Willis Hurst, MD provided the "spark" for this monograph and Gene Kearn's diligent prodding assured that this effort would come to fruition. Finally, I appreciate my family, particularly my mother and uncles who provide the foundation; teachers, who provide the stimulus; friends, who provide the support; and my children, Graham, Nathan, and Alexis, who provide the motivation for this work.

J. David Talley, M.D.

Foreword

If anything has characterized the evolution of cardiology in my professional lifetime, which is now approaching four decades, it has been an increasing focus by cardiologists on the heart as an isolated entity. By that I mean that cardiologists have rightfully placed an extraordinary degree of emphasis on devising various ways—cardiac catheterization, nuclear cardiology, echocardiography, and PET scanning—to study unique aspects of cardiac function. Cardinal among these, obviously, have been cardiac mechanics, the coronary circulation, the conduction system, valvular function, and ways in which diseases of those various entities can be approached either non-invasively or invasively.

Indeed, the last three decades have wrought a sea of change in the way we approach ischemic heart disease, cardiomyopathies, valvular dysfunction and arrhythmias. Coronary revascularization, valvular replacement and the therapy of arrhythmias by surgical intervention or by AICD's have transformed cardiology with respect to the limitations medicine faced with these dread maladies even as recently as three decades ago.

For cardiomyopathies and congestive failure, cardiac transplantation is, at least for the present, one of our few successful modalities of therapy. Yet even here, understanding the mechanisms of cardiac remodeling at a molecular basis—for example, the involvement of the angiotensinogen gene and the renin-angiotensin system in cardiac remodeling—lends new hope to the development of medical therapies for these disorders.

But the heart is not an isolated entity. Rather, it is affected in a variety of systemic diseases. It is therefore to the particular credit of David Talley and his colleagues that they have undertaken this book, *CARDIOVASCULAR INVOLVEMENT IN SYSTEMIC DISEASES*. This compliment is even more telling if one knows David Talley as I do, since his clear passion is for interventional cardiology. Yet in *CARDIOVASCULAR INVOLVEMENT IN SYSTEMIC DISEASES*, Talley puts aside his personal passion to focus on cardiac involvement in an eclectic array of disorders including endocrinopathies, vasculidities, drug overdose, infectious diseases—which, regretfully, because of AIDS, have become commonplace—as well as renal diseases, gastrointestinal diseases, and pulmonary diseases and neoplasia, the latter two often neglected entities. Finally, Talley and his colleagues end with elegant narratives on the effects of aging, neuromuscular disease and other derangements of the heart.

On balance, I consider this book to be a singularly valuable source of information about cardiac involvement in systemic diseases, written in a way that has remarkable explanatory power for diseases where cardiac involvement is often a neglected entity. It is again a tribute to David Talley, a passionate cardiac interventionalist, as well as to his co-authors, that they have focused their attention on these important topics.

Thomas E. Andreoli, M.D.
The Nolan Professor of Internal Medicine
Professor and Chairman
Department of Internal Medicine
University of Arkansas for Medical Sciences

Contributors

Sameh R. Abul-Ezz, M.D.
Assistant Professor of Internal Medicine
Division of Nephrology
University of Arkansas for Medical Sciences
Little Rock, Arkansas

Paula J. Anderson, M.D.
Associate Professor of Internal Medicine
Division of Pulmonary and Critical Care
University of Arkansas for Medical Sciences
Little Rock, Arkansas

Robert W. Bradsher, M.D.
Professor of Internal Medicine
Vice-Chairman, Department of Internal
  Medicine
Director, Division of Infectious Diseases
University of Arkansas for Medical Sciences
Little Rock, Arkansas

Thomas D. Conley, M.D.
Assistant Professor of Internal Medicine
Division of Cardiology
University of Arkansas for Medical Sciences
Medical Director, Cardiac Catheterization
  Laboratories
John L. McClellan Memorial Veterans
  Hospital
Little Rock, Arkansas

Marcia L. Erbland, M.D.
Associate Professor of Internal Medicine
Division of Pulmonary and Critical Care
University of Arkansas for Medical Sciences
Director, Medical Intensive Care Unit
John L. McClellan Memorial Veterans
  Hospital
Little Rock, Arkansas

Sami I. Harik, M.D.
Professor of Neurology
Chairman, Department of Neurology
University of Arkansas for Medical Sciences
Little Rock, Arkansas

F. Charles Hiller, M.D.
Professor of Internal Medicine
Vice-Chairman, Department of Internal
  Medicine
Director, Division of Pulmonary and Critical
  Care
University of Arkansas for Medical Sciences
Chief, Pulmonary Section
John L. McClellan Memorial Veterans
  Hospital
Little Rock, Arkansas

Hugo E. Jasin, M.D.
Professor of Internal Medicine
Director, Division of Rheumatology and
  Clinical Immunology
University of Arkansas for Medical Sciences
Little Rock, Arkansas

Tyrone T. Lee, M.D.
Fellow in Pulmonary Diseases and Critical
  Care
Division of Pulmonary and Critical Care
University of Arkansas for Medical Sciences
Little Rock, Arkansas

Jon P. Lindemann, M.D.
Professor of Internal Medicine
Division of Cardiology
University of Arkansas for Medical Sciences
Little Rock, Arkansas

David A. Lipschitz, M.D. Ph.D.
Professor of Internal Medicine
Director, Division of Aging
University of Arkansas for Medical Sciences
Director, Geriatric Research Education and
  Clinical Center
John L. McClellan Memorial Veterans
  Hospital
Little Rock, Arkansas

Eleanor A. Lipsmeyer, M.D.
Professor of Internal Medicine
Division of Rheumatology and Clinical
  Immunology
University of Arkansas for Medical Sciences
Little Rock, Arkansas

James W. Logan, M.D.
Assistant Professor of Internal Medicine
Division of Rheumatology and Clinical
  Immunology
University of Arkansas for Medical Sciences
Little Rock, Arkansas

Laszlo J.K. Makk, M.D.
Research Fellow
Division of Gastroenterology/Hepatology
University of Louisville School of Medicine
Louisville, Kentucky

Rebecca E. Martin, M.D.
Associate Professor of Internal Medicine
Division of Infectious Diseases
University of Arkansas for Medical Sciences
Little Rock, Arkansas

Richard W. McDonnell, M.D.
Assistant Professor of Internal Medicine
Division of Infectious Diseases
University of Arkansas for Medical Sciences
Little Rock, Arkansas

Mark L. Mullens, M.D.
Fellow in Cardiovascular Disease
Division of Cardiology
University of Arkansas for Medical Sciences
Little Rock, Arkansas

Kirkland C. Nolan, M.D.
Fellow in Pulmonary Diseases and Critical
  Care
Division of Pulmonary and Critical Care
University of Arkansas for Medical Sciences
Little Rock, Arkansas

James Rish, M.D.
Fellow in Pulmonary Diseases and Critical
  Care
Division of Pulmonary and Critical Care
University of Arkansas for Medical Sciences
Little Rock, Arkansas

Stacy A. Rudnicki, M.D.
Assistant Professor of Neurology
Department of Neurology
University of Arkansas for Medical Sciences
Little Rock, Arkansas

Ellis Samols, M.D.
Chief of Staff
Las Vegas Veterans Administration Medical
  Center
Las Vegas, Nevada

J. David Talley, M.D.
Professor of Internal Medicine
Director, Division of Cardiology
University of Arkansas for Medical Sciences
Chief, Cardiology Section
John L. McClellan Memorial Veterans
  Hospital
Little Rock, Arkansas

Gary L. Templeton, M.D.
Instructor of Internal Medicine
Division of Pulmonary and Critical Care
University of Arkansas for Medical Sciences
Little Rock, Arkansas

Muthusamy Velusamy, M.D.
Fellow in Cardiovascular Disease
Division of Cardiology
University of Arkansas for Medical Sciences
Little Rock, Arkansas

Richard A. Wright, M.D.
Professor of Medicine
Chief, Division of
  Gastroenterology/Hepatology
University of Louisville School of Medicine
Louisville, Kentucky

Contents

I. Cardiovascular Involvement With Diseases of the Endocrine System **1**

Section Editor: Ellis Samols, M.D.

Diabetes Mellitus 1
J. David Talley, M.D.
Ellis Samols, M.D.

Hypothyroidism 4
Ellis Samols, M.D.

Hyperthyroidism 10
Ellis Samols, M.D.

Adrenal Insufficiency 17
J. David Talley, M.D.
Ellis Samols M.D.

Hyperaldosteronism 19
J. David Talley, M.D.
Ellis Samols M.D.

Glucocorticoid Excess 22
J. David Talley, M.D.
Ellis Samols, M.D.

Obesity 25
J. David Talley, M.D.

Pheochromocytoma 27
J. David Talley, M.D.

Acromegaly 31
J. David Talley, M.D.

II. Cardiovascular Involvement with Connective Tissue Diseases **35**

Section Editor: Hugo E. Jasin, M.D.

Systemic Lupus Erythematosus 35
Eleanor A. Lipsmeyer, M.D.

Systemic Sclerosis 39
Eleanor A. Lipsmeyer, M.D.

Ankylosing Spondylitis   42
James W. Logan, M.D.

Reiter's Syndrome   46
James W. Logan, M.D.

Rheumatoid Arthritis   48
James W. Logan, M.D.

Marfan's Syndrome   51
Hugo E. Jasin, M.D.

**III.   Cardiovascular Involvement with Excessive Use
        of Drugs and Medications**   **55**

Section Editor: J. David Talley, M.D.

Alcoholic Heart Disease   55
Thomas D. Conley, M.D.
J. David Talley, M.D.

Cigarette Smoking   60
Thomas D. Conley, M.D.
J. David Talley, M.D.

Cocaine-Related Cardiac Disorders   62
Thomas D. Conley, M.D.
J. David Talley, M.D.

Miscellaneous Drugs/Prescription Medications   66
Thomas D. Conley, M.D.
J. David Talley, M.D.

IV.   Cardiovascular Involvement with Infectious Diseases   **69**

Section Editor: Robert W. Bradsher, M.D.

Cardiac Manifestations of Human Immunodeficiency Virus   69
Rebecca E. Martin, M.D.
Richard W. McDonnell, M.D.
Robert W. Bradsher, M.D.

Spirochetal Disease   76
Rebecca E. Martin, M.D.
Richard W. McDonnell, M.D.
Robert W. Bradsher, M.D.

Sepsis   80
Rebecca E. Martin, M.D.
Richard W. McDonnell, M.D.
Robert W. Bradsher, M.D.

V.   Cardiovascular Involvement with Renal Disease   **88**

Section Editor: Sameh R. Abul-Ezz, M.D.

Left Ventricular Dysfunction   88
Sameh R. Abul-Ezz, M.D.

Ischemic Heart Disease   91
Sameh R. Abul-Ezz, M.D.

Pericarditis   96
Sameh R. Abul-Ezz, M.D.

Disorders of Potassium Balance   100
Sameh R. Abul-Ezz, M.D.

Disorders of Calcium Homeostasis   107
Sameh R. Abul-Ezz, M.D.

Disorders of Magnesium Homeostasis   113
Sameh R. Abul-Ezz, M.D.

VI.   Cardiovascular Involvement with Diseases Related to Gastrointestinal System/Nutrition   **119**

Section Editor: Richard A. Wright, M.D.

Noncardiac Chest Pain   119
Laszlo J.K. Makk, M.D.
Richard A. Wright, M.D.

Cardiac Involvement with Liver Disease   126
Laszlo J.K. Makk, M.D.
Richard A. Wright, M.D.

Nutritional Conditions That Affect the Cardiovascular System   136
Laszlo J.K. Makk, M.D.
Richard A. Wright, M.D.

VII.   Cardiovascular Involvement with Pulmonary Diseases   **139**

Section Editor: F. Charles Hiller, M.D.

Chronic Obstructive Pulmonary Disease   139
Marcia L. Erbland, M.D.

Cystic Fibrosis   143
Paula J. Anderson, M.D.

Interstitial Lung Disease   146
James Rish, M.D.

Myocardial Sarcoidosis   149
Gary L. Templeton, M.D.

Primary Pulmonary Hypertension   151
F. Charles Hiller, M.D.

Pulmonary Embolism   158
Kirkland C. Nolan, M.D.
J. David Talley, M.D.

Pulmonary Vasculitis   162
Tyrone T. Lee, M.D.

**VIII. Cardiovascular Involvement with Diseases Related
to Hematology and Oncology**   **165**

Section Editor: J. David Talley, M.D.

Amyloidosis   165
Muthu Velusamy, M.D.
J. David Talley, M.D.

Carcinoid Syndrome   168
J. David Talley, M.D.

Hemochromatosis   173
J. David Talley, M.D.

Hemoglobinopathies   177
J. David Talley, M.D.

Multiple Myeloma   180
J. David Talley, M.D.

Cardiac Toxicity Due to Chemotherapy   183
J. David Talley, M.D.

Radiation Therapy   187
Mark L. Mullens, M.D.
J. David Talley, M.D.

**IX. Cardiovascular Involvement with Diseases Related
to Aging**   **191**

Section Editor: David A. Lipschitz, M.D., Ph.D.

Effect of Age   191
David A. Lipschitz, M.D., Ph.D.

Isolated Systolic Systemic Arterial Hypertension   192
David A. Lipschitz, M.D., Ph.D.

Orthostatic Hypotension   195
David A. Lipschitz, M.D., Ph.D.

Congestive Heart Failure   197
David A. Lipschitz, M.D., Ph.D.

X. **Cardiovascular Involvement with Neuromuscular Diseases** **199**

Section Editor: Sami I. Harik, M.D.

Stroke 199
Stacy A. Rudnicki, M.D.
Sami I. Harik, M.D.

Epilepsy 200
Stacy A. Rudnicki, M.D.
Sami I. Harik, M.D.

Myotonic Dystrophy 201
Stacy A. Rudnicki, M.D.
Sami I. Harik, M.D.

Duchenne's Muscular Dystrophy 204
Stacy A. Rudnicki, M.D.
Sami I. Harik, M.D.

Becker's Muscular Dystrophy 207
Stacy A. Rudnicki, M.D.
Sami I. Harik, M.D.

Guillain-Barré Syndrome 209
Stacy A. Rudnicki, M.D.
Sami I. Harik, M.D.

Friedreich's Ataxia 213
Stacy A. Rudnicki, M.D.
Sami I. Harik, M.D.

Polymyositis and Dermatomyositis 216
Stacy A. Rudnicki, M.D.
Sami I. Harik, M.D.

Mitochondrial Myopathies 220
Stacy A. Rudnicki, M.D.
Sami I. Harik, M.D.

XI. **Cardiovascular Involvement with Special Conditions** **224**

Section Editor: Jon P. Lindemann, M.D.

Pregnancy 224
Mark L. Mullens, M.D.
J. David Talley, M.D.

Exercise 228
Jon P. Lindemann, M.D.

Electrical Shock and Lightning 232
Jon P. Lindemann, M.D.

Index **239**

Cardiovascular Involvement with Diseases of the Endocrine System

Ellis Samols, M.D.
Section Editor

Diabetes Mellitus

J. David Talley, M.D.
Ellis Samols, M.D.

PRESENTING MANIFESTATIONS

History

Patients with insulin-dependent (type I) diabetes present before the age of 30. Patients with non-insulin-dependent (type II) diabetes typically present over the age of 40. Patients with type I diabetes mellitus frequently have a relative with a similar disorder or one associated with other HLA antigen or other autoimmune diseases. In contrast, patients with type II diabetes mellitus are frequently obese and respond to therapeutic measures including a modified diet and the use of oral hypoglycemic agents.

Symptoms of type I diabetes mellitus include a history of overeating without weight gain, fatigue, weight loss, lethargy, weakness, and blurred vision. Patients with type II diabetes mellitus are frequently asymptomatic and are diagnosed because of a routine blood test demonstrating hyperglycemia. Other common symptoms include polyuria, polydipsia, polyphagia, weight loss or gain, pruritis, dry mouth, visual disturbances, fatigue, and *Candida* vaginitis or balanitis.

Physical Examination

Patients with type I diabetes mellitus present with signs of weight loss due to fat and protein breakdown as well as dehydration. In extreme conditions, patients may present with diabetic ketoacidosis and resulting manifestations due to metabolic acidosis. In contrast, patients with type II diabetes mellitus may be obese but otherwise may have a nondescript physical examination. Due to the widespread atherosclerotic peripheral vascular disease, diabetic cardiomyopathy, and hypercholesterolemia, signs referable to these abnormalities may be present.

Laboratory Evaluation

The pathognomonic laboratory test of diabetes is hyperglycemia. Diabetes is present if the fasting plasma glucose level is 140 mg/dL or more, if 2 hr after consuming 75 g of glucose it is 200 mg/dL or more, or if a random plasma glucose measurement is 200 mg/dL or more on two separate occasions.[1] Impaired glucose tolerance is defined as a normal fasting plasma glucose level less than 140 mg/dL and a 2-hr post prandial glucose level of 140–190 mg/dL.[2]

The complications of diabetes mellitus have distinctive laboratory findings, including impaired renal function as well as electrocardiographic and echocardiographic changes. Diabetic females, in particular, appear to have an increased left ventricular mass and wall thickness on echocardiography.[3]

DIAGNOSTIC CRITERIA

The pathognomonic finding of diabetes mellitus is the finding of hyperglycemia, as noted above.

DIFFERENTIAL DIAGNOSIS

The differential diagnosis of diabetes mellitus is limited and includes transient hyperglycemia seen in periods of severe stress, infection, or trauma. Additionally, salicylate intoxication may mimic diabetic ketoacidosis.

PATHOPHYSIOLOGY

There are three primary complications related to diabetes: atherosclerosis, diabetic cardiomyopathy, and systemic arterial hypertension.

Atherosclerosis

Diabetes mellitus is associated with accelerated atherosclerosis and with the development of atherosclerotic coronary and peripheral vascular disease. In general, the presence and severity of atherosclerosis are directly associated with the age of the patient and the duration of the disease. Atherosclerosis accounts for more than 75% of hospital admissions related to diabetic complications and is the major cause of death in patients with this abnormality. The risk factors for atherosclerosis and diabetes include systemic arterial hypertension, hypercholesterolemia, male gender, duration of diabetes, glycemic control, hypertension, and hypercoagulability. The mortality is directly related to the presence and number of risk factors.[4]

The basic underlying pathophysiologic abnormalities include a dysfunction of the vascular endothelium, hypercoagulability, and the development of other risk factors including systemic arterial hypertension.

Diabetic Cardiomyopathy

In 1972, Rubler and colleagues described a cardiomyopathy of patients without significant coronary artery disease.[5] Subsequent epidemiologic studies have confirmed the association.[6] The pathogenesis of the cardiomyopathy is multiple, including diminished glucose availability, high concentrations of free fatty acids, and microangiopathic changes.[7] There is also impairment of left ventricular systolic and diastolic function.

Systemic Arterial Hypertension

Raised blood pressure is a major risk factor for the development of atherosclerosis. The etiology of systemic arterial hypertension includes increased activity of the sympathetic nervous system, sodium retention, and vascular smooth muscle hypertrophy. Other causes include atherosclerosis, renal artery stenosis, glomerulonephritis, and other endocrine disorders.

NATURAL HISTORY OF THE DISEASE

If left untreated, patients with diabetes mellitus succumb to the ravages of the disease related to atherosclerosis, hypertension, and end-stage renal disease. Age-adjusted mortality rates of diabetics are comparable to those of patients without diabetes mellitus until age 40. Thereafter, there is an accelerated mortality rate in diabetic patients so that at age 55, the risk of death of a diabetic patient is approximately 10-fold that of a nondiabetic.[8]

CURRENT METHODS OF TREATMENT

Atherosclerosis

Prevention and lifestyle modification are fundamental components of the initial management of the diabetic patient. It has been shown that glycemic control reduces the risk of atherosclerosis in patients with type I diabetes mellitus.[9] Proper dietary management includes adhering to guidelines regarding fat and cholesterol intake and limiting the use of alcohol. Risk factor modifications include eliminating cigarette use. Oral hypoglycemic agents and insulin are effective in preventing or delaying the development of diabetic complications.[10]

Should atherosclerotic complications develop, there are minimal restrictions of the use of agents for control of myocardial, cerebral, or peripheral vascular ischemia. Patients with diabetes mellitus and acute myocardial infarction have excess mortality compared to nondiabetics, even those receiving thrombolytic therapy.[11] This adverse trend is seen in all age groups, and females are at higher risk than males.[12]

Diabetic Cardiomyopathy

The treatment of congestive heart failure due to diabetic cardiomyopathy is similar to that of nondiabetic patients. Angiotensin-converting enzyme inhibitors should be used carefully in patients with coexisting renal dysfunction.

Systemic Arterial Hypertension

Vigorous treatment of systemic arterial hypertension in a patient with diabetes mellitus is essential to prevent the ravages of systemic complications. Control of blood pressure has been shown to decrease the incidence of fatal and nonfatal stroke, cardiovascular death, nonfatal myocardial infarction, and major cardiovascular events.[13] While initial attempts at lifestyle modification are recommended, pharmacologic management is frequently necessary. Angiotensin-converting enzyme inhibitors and calcium channel blockers are the first-line agents. Caution must be exercised when using beta-adrenergic receptor blockers (which cause progressive left ventricular dysfunction and delay in recovering from hypoglycemic episodes), thiazide diuretics (increased cholesterol and glucose and decreased potassium), and central adrenergic agonists (exacerbation of autonomic dysfunction).[14] Excessive mortality in diabetic hypertensive patients treated with diuretics has been observed.[15]

REFERENCES

1. Report of a WHO Study Group: Diabetes mellitus. *World Health Organization Technical Report Series,* 727, 1985:1–113.
2. WHO Expert Committee on Diabetes Mellitus. Diabetes mellitus: second report. *World Health Organization Technical Report Series,* 646, 1980:1–80.

3. Galderisi M, Anderson KM, Wilson PWF, et al: Echocardiographic evidence for the existence of a distinct diabetic cardiomyopathy (the Framingham Heart Study). *Am J Cardiol* 68:85–89, 1991.

4. Samuelsson O, Hedner T, Persson B, et al: The role of diabetes mellitus and hypertriglyceridaemia as coronary risk factors in treated hypertension: 15 years of follow-up of antihypertensive treatment in middle-aged men in the Primary Prevention Trial in Göteborg, Sweden. *J Intern Med* 235: 217–227, 1994.

5. Rubler S, Dlugash J, Yuceoglu YZ, et al: New type of cardiomyopathy associated with diabetic glomerulosclerosis. *Am J Cardiol* 30:595–602, 1972.

6. Kannel WB, Hjortland M, Castelli WP: Role of diabetes in congestive heart failure: The Framingham study. *Am J Cardiol* 34:29–34, 1974.

7. van Hoeven KH, Factor SM: A comparison of the pathological spectrum of hypertensive, diabetic, and hypertensive-diabetic heart disease. *Circulation* 82:848–855, 1990.

8. Krolewski AS, Kosinski EJ, Warram JH, et al: Magnitude and determinants of coronary artery disease in juvenile-onset, insulin-dependent diabetes mellitus. *Am J Cardiol* 59:750–755, 1987.

9. The Diabetes Control and Complications Trial Research Group: The effect of intensive treatment of diabetes on the development and progression of long-term complications in insulin-dependent diabetes mellitus. *N Engl J Med* 329:977–986, 1993.

10. Wang PH, Lau J, Chalmers TC: Meta-analysis of effects of intensive blood-glucose control on late complications of type I diabetes. *Lancet* 341:1306–1309, 1993.

11. Barbash GI, White HD, Modan M, et al: Significance of diabetes mellitus in patients with acute myocardial infarction receiving thrombolytic therapy. *J Am Coll Cardiol* 22:707–713, 1993.

12. Zuanetti G, Latini R, Maggioni AP, et al: Influence of diabetes on mortality in acute myocardial infarction: Data from the GISSI-2 study. *J Am Coll Cardiol* 22:1788–1794, 1993.

13. Eschwege E, Richard JL, Thibult N, et al: Coronary heart disease mortality in relation with diabetes, blood glucose and plasma insulin levels: The Paris Prospective Study, ten years later. *Horm Metab Res Suppl Ser* 15:41–46, 1985.

14. Kaplan NM, Rosenstock J, Raskin P: A different view of treatment of hypertension in patients with diabetes mellitus. *Arch Intern Med* 147:1160–1162, 1987.

15. Warram JH, Laffel LMB, Valsania P, et al: Excess mortality associated with diuretic therapy in diabetes mellitus. *Arch Intern Med* 151:1350–1356, 1991.

Hypothyroidism

Ellis Samols, M.D.

PRESENTING MANIFESTATIONS

History

Hypothyroidism is a disorder of diverse causes resulting in inadequate secretion of thyroid hormone from the thyroid gland. In the United States, the most common cause of primary (e.g., thyroid) hypothyroidism is chronic autoimmune (Hashimoto's) thyroiditis. Other causes include ablation by radioactive iodine or surgery, external irradiation, and a thyroid gland organification defect. Central hypothyroidism includes pituitary hypothyroidism (secondary hypothyroidism) and hypothalamic hypothyroidism (tertiary hypothyroidism).

The history may be helpful in defining the cause of hypothyroidism—for example, postpartum hemorrhage with pituitary infarction (Sheehan's syndrome). However, the overwhelming majority of cases of hypothyroidism are due to primary gland failure, the major

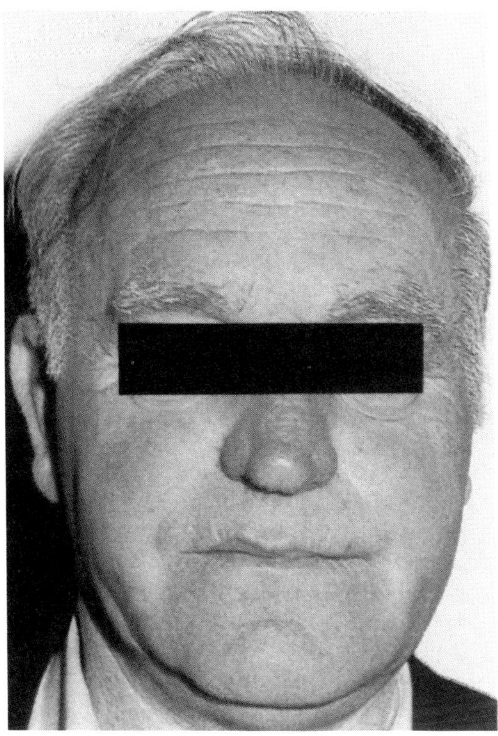

Figure 1.1. The facial appearance of a patient with hypothyroidism may show thickening of the skin on the forehead and facial puffiness. From Shapiro LM, Fox KM. *Color Atlas of Physical Signs in Cardiovascular Disease*, Chicago, IL: Year Book Medical Publishers, Inc. 1989: pg. 17. Reprinted with permission from author and publisher.

topic of this chapter. The symptoms are generally related to the duration and severity of hypothyroidism, the rapidity with which hypothyroidism occurs, and the psychological characteristics of the patient. A medical history may uncover symptoms that are not volunteered. If the diagnosis has been made, it is important to confirm it and to document pretreatment thyroid function tests. In the past, patients were treated with thyroid hormone for reasons that would not be acceptable by present criteria. Many patients on thyroid hormone are uncertain why they are taking the hormone, nor may they know whether they feel better for doing so.

Patients should be asked about the following symptoms, which may be nonspecific or subtle, especially in women over 50 years old: fatigue, weakness, sleepiness, cold intolerance, dry skin, hoarseness, constipation, joint pains or carpal tunnel syndrome, muscle cramps, mental or memory impairment, depression, menorrhagia, infertility, and weight gain associated with anorexia. Although intellectual and motor activity slow, patients may exhibit a remarkable sense of humor.

Physical Examination

Florid myxedema is relatively rare in the United States. Findings on physical examination that may suggest hypothyroidism include goiter or a small or nonpalpable thyroid, hoarseness, slow speech, deafness, cool dry skin, bradycardia, and cardiac enlargement (Figure 1.1.). Clinically, cardiac enlargement is common in primary hypothyroidism because of cardiac dilation and/or pericardial effusion. Cardiomegaly is very unusual in pituitary or hypothalamic hyperthyroidism, and heart size is normal in autoimmune diseases that cause both primary thyroid and adrenal deficiency.

In elderly persons, hypothyroidism (like hyperthyroidism) is often characterized by a paucity of signs and symptoms. The symptoms may be subtle, especially in the elderly, such as confusion, cognitive dysfunction, dementia, depression, ataxia, hair loss, and dry skin.

Laboratory Evaluation

The diagnosis of primary hypothyroidism is confirmed with a raised thyroid-stimulating hormone (TSH) measurement and a low free thyroxine (T_4) estimate (or direct measurement). It is useful to obtain antimicrosomal antibodies (antithyroid peroxidase antibody) prior to aspiration needle biopsy when the diagnosis of autoimmune chronic thyroiditis is suspected. With a low TSH level, either inappropriately normal or insufficiently elevated in the face of a low T_4 level, central hypothyroidism should be considered prior to instituting thyroid replacement therapy. The most difficult decisions involve sick hospitalized patients since serum T_4 or free T_4 and/or TSH levels may suggest hypothyroidism.

Assay of triiodothyronine (T_3) may be misleading in the diagnosis of hypothyroidism. Subclinical hypothyroidism is a laboratory diagnosis in which the patient has a normal free T_4 estimate (or direct measurement) and an elevated TSH concentration but few if any symptoms of hyperthyroidism. This entity cannot be diagnosed in a patient who is sick or recovering from an illness. As many as 15% of patients older than 65 years of age may have this syndrome. Because of the prevalence of chronic thyroiditis, as well as clinical and subclinical hypothyroidism, in older patients (>60 years), it is recommended that these patients, especially older women, be screened with a serum TSH assay.

Other laboratory tests relevant to the cardiologist (but diagnostically nonspecific) include electrocardiographic changes of bradycardia, low-voltage complexes, or flattened and inverted T-waves. Primary hypothyroidism may cause an increase in the serum cholesterol level, as well as elevated concentrations of serum creatinine kinase (at times with a mild increase in the MB band), lactic dehydrogenase, and glutamic-oxaloacetate transaminase. It is uncertain whether these skeletal and cardiac enzyme abnormalities reflect damage or impaired clearance.

DIAGNOSTIC CRITERIA

The essential criteria needed to establish a diagnosis of primary hypothyroidism are a high TSH together with a low free T_4 measurement in an ambulatory person who has not recently been sick.[1] Because of the spectrum of symptoms, some clinical justification for the diagnosis can often be found. The diagnosis of subclinical hypothyroidism (high TSH, normal free T_4) is supported by clinical or laboratory manifestations of Hashimoto's thyroiditis or Graves' disease, particularly after thyroid ablation, when subclinical hypothyroidism is usually a stage in the evolution toward clinical primary hypothyroidism.

For primary hypothyroidism, a high index of suspicion and frequent sampling of serum TSH are recommended in elderly women, patients with a prior history of any medically or surgically treated thyroid disease, patients with other autoimmune diseases, and those with unexplained depression, cognitive dysfunction, or hypercholesterolemia.

The diagnosis of secondary or tertiary hypothyroidism can be entertained in the presence of the appropriate clinical conditions, a low free T_4 measurement, and a TSH level that is normal, slightly raised, low, or undetectable. If the patient is ill and hospitalized, it may be difficult to rule out central hypothyroidism in one who is diagnosed as having sick euthyroid syndrome (i.e., the most common low T_4 variant). In rare cases, assay of reverse T_3 may be useful, suggesting central hypothyroidism if it is low, as reverse T_3 is usually raised in sick euthyroid syndrome. Theoretically, TRH stimulation should be useful for the differentiation of primary, secondary, and tertiary hypothyroidism, but in practice this interpretation has many pitfalls and requires great experience. Radioactive iodine uptake is often not diagnostic because of the very low limits of normal, and changes in thyroid pool size are confusing when a routine test is performed. Parenteral administration of exogenous TSH has been replaced by the TSH assay for the diagnosis of primary hypothyroidism.

DIFFERENTIAL DIAGNOSIS

For the cardiologist and the general internist, the differential diagnosis has changed dramatically in the past 15 years. Today the most common (and sometimes most difficult) diagnostic problem is the differentiation of sick euthyroid syndrome from central hypothyroidism, from primary clinical or subclinical hypothyroidism, and, very rarely, from T_4 toxicosis. Our group was among the first to recognize the syndrome, which we originally labeled the *CCU-TFT syndrome* because we noticed the problem most often in the coronary care unit. The term *nonthyroidal illness (NTI)* is used interchangeably with *sick euthyroid syndrome*. The nomenclature of this syndrome emphasizes that although the most common manifestation of the syndrome, a low T_4 or free T_4 level, is associated with a marked increase in mortality, thyroid hormone replacement has thus far been unable to improve survival. However, the terminology will probably change again because there may be genuine changes in thyroid function. In general, the sicker the patient, the lower the current clinical measurement of free T_4. For ease of description, it is useful to classify sick euthyroid syndrome into three variants: low, normal, and high T_4. The use of the term T_4 *variant* indicates that the changes may be seen not only in total T_4, but also very commonly in free T_4 (by commercial kits) and, less commonly, in free T_4E. These syndromes are caused by changes in the peripheral transport and conversion of T_4 or T_3 and reverse T_3, changes in the pituitary or hypothalamic regulation of TSH, and changes in thyroid function per se. Perhaps these "laboratory" syndromes that do not require treatment would be noted less frequently if laboratory tests for thyroid function were ordered only in the presence of strong clinical suspicion. However, if such a policy was adopted, the majority of sick thyrotoxic or hypothyroid older patients would not be correctly diagnosed and effective therapy would be sacrificed.

The *low T_4 variant* of sick euthyroid syndrome is common in severe illness. The S-thyroid stimulating hormone may be low, normal, or mildly raised and, during recovery, moderately raised. A normal TSH level suggests sick euthyroid syndrome, and abnormal thyroid antibody tests suggest primary thyroid disease. This variant often cannot be diagnosed with confidence until good recovery without thyroid hormone therapy is established. Claims that measurement of reverse T_3 or that a thyrotrophin releasing hormone (TRH) test is diagnostic are not valid.

The *normal T_4 variant* of sick euthyroid syndrome tends to occur in moderate or mild illness and is not usually a diagnostic problem if the TSH concentration is normal, as it frequently is. If the TSH concentration is raised during the recovery phase, the possibility of subclinical hypothyroidism can be ruled out by follow-up testing.

A *high T_4 variant* of sick euthyroid syndrome is rare, and is reported especially in elderly women who have received iodine-rich medication. Typically, the serum T_4 is elevated but the serum T_3 is normal. Differential diagnosis from T_4 toxicosis is assisted by the finding of a normal S-TSH level.

Several clinical syndromes are traditionally included in the differential diagnosis, including *nephrotic syndrome* with puffy face, hypercholesterolemia, anemia, fluid accumulation, and sick euthyroid syndrome type on thyroid function tests, but *severe hypoalbuminemia* is not caused by hypothyroidism. *Congestive cardiac failure* and *pericardial effusion* currently are less commonly caused or aggravated by hypothyroidism, but correct diagnosis is important, as therapy with thyroid hormone is needed for recovery. Diagnosis of primary hypothyroidism requires a low free T_4E level and a high TSH level. Minor diagnostic clues from the electrocardiogram, echocardiogram, and central cardiac pressures are redundant. Hypothyroid cardiac failure and/or pericardial effusion respond poorly to digitalis and diuretics and well to thyroid hormone therapy.

The differential diagnosis of pituitary hypothyroidism may be assisted by finding hyposecretion of other pituitary hormones (adrenocorticotropic, gonadotropins, growth hormone, for example). Infarction of the anterior pituitary is compatible with many years of survival and slow-growing, space-occupying tumors in the sella may be present. Hypothalamic hypothyroidism may be either transient (as in sick euthyroid syndrome) or progressive (as with tumor). Theoretically, the TSH response to TRH and the T_4 response to TSH should be helpful differentially, but the problems in assessment of TRH responses stem from pituitary thyrotrophic modification by chronic absence of TRH, which normally stimulates thyrotroph gene expression. There are other inhibitors of TRH secretion as well. Dopamine inhibits TRH secretion, so that patients on recent dopamine infusion may have a condition simulating hypothalamic hypothyroidism, while those on chronic dopamine infusion may have a condition resembling pituitary hypothyroidism. Thyrotroph responsiveness to TRH is also inhibited by glucocorticoids, alpha-1-adrenergic stimulation, somatostatin, tumor necrosis factor, and several interleukins. These complexities may explain the diagnostic problems of low T_4 and/or low TSH in the sick. On the other hand, estrogen and alpha-2-adrenergic stimulation augment pituitary responsiveness to TRH, possibly explaining some normal or high T_4 variants of sick euthyroid syndrome.

Amiodarone therapy influences thyroid function, with diagnostic consequences.[2] First, amiodarone blocks binding to thyrotroph nuclear receptors for TSH, including the TSH response. Second, the peripheral conversion of T_4 to T_3 is blocked. Third, and most important probably, is the effect of the high iodide content of amiodarone (35% by weight). Patients may develop goiter and/or hypothyroidism in the United States; thyrotoxicosis may occur in individuals who have been living in endemic iodine deficiency areas. Finally, amiodarone can stimulate a1-positive T cells, similar to the abnormality seen in Graves' disease. This confusing picture is further complicated by the long half-life of amiodarone, so that biochemical and clinical abnormalities induced by amiodarone can persist for months after its discontinuation.

PATHOPHYSIOLOGY

Deficiency of active thyroid hormone causes hypometabolism and decreased caloric consumption.[3] The heart in florid myxedema is pale and yellow (anemia and hypercarotenemia), flabby, and dilated by biventricular cardiomyopathy. Well before the stage of florid myxedema, primary hypothyroid patients exhibit reduced cardiac output, stroke volume, blood volume, and plasma volume, with a prolonged circulation time. Cardiac filling pressures in the left and right ventricles are usually normal in the absence of pericardial effusion. The isovolumetric relaxation time is prolonged, the pre-ejection period is lengthened, and the ratio of the pre-ejection period to the left ventricular ejection time is increased. These changes are the converse of the pathophysiologic effect of hyperthyroidism.

Lipid abnormalities, especially hypercholesterolemia, are known to occur in hypothyroidism. However, although it is widely assumed that hypercholesterolemia has the same atherogenic potential regardless of the cause, convincing evidence that atherosclerosis is induced or aggravated by hypothyroidism is scanty. The decrease in metabolic rate protects the heart from ischemia and angina, and thyroid ablation was a recognized treatment for intractable angina 40 years ago.

NATURAL HISTORY

The course of untreated hypothyroidism depends on the cause and the age of onset. In the untreated newborn and infant, cretinism occurs. In the untreated adult, permanent untreated hypothyroidism eventually causes myxedema and death. It is interesting that the natural history of many cases of hypothyroidism and hyperthyroidism has been reinterpreted, mainly because of the variable course of chronic autoimmune thyroiditis. Parenthetically, hyperthyroidism in Hashimoto's thyroiditis is usually temporary, and it is possible for a patient with chronic autoimmune thryroiditis to have reversible and/or repetitive hyperthyroidism and/or hypothyroidism, as well as subclinical, permanent hypothyroidism.[4] The management of patients on long-term thyroid therapy is discussed below.

CURRENT METHODS OF TREATMENT

The treatment plan for hypothyroidism will depend on the cause. However, regardless of the cause, levothyroxine is the treatment of choice for chronic hypothyroidism.[5,6,7] Preparations containing T_3, either as a mixture with T_4 or as pure synthetic T_3 (liothyronine), are not recommended for chronic therapy because regulation of T_3 oral dosage is difficult with fluctuating and often elevated T_3 concentrations and because some individuals, particularly elderly ones, are very sensitive to the adverse effect of T_3. Levothyroxine is now available in many different dosages to facilitate the attainment of a normal range of TSH in all cases of primary hypothyroidism. Serum S-TSH should be measured at least 6 weeks after any dosage adjustment to assess the adequacy of the dose. In the outpatient setting, it has been found that up to 30% of patients on T_4 replacement do not need it. These patients can be identified by clinical suspicion and the levothyroxine replacement dose can be reduced to a third of the calculated full replacement dose (e.g., 50 μg/day), measuring S-TSH after 6 weeks. If the TSH concentration is normal, there is no need for T_4 therapy; if the TSH is elevated, T_4 is indeed required.

In general, adults with primary hypothyroidism require approximately 1.7 μg per kilogram of body weight per day for full replacement. Children may require up to 4 μg/kg/day, whereas older patients may need less than 1 μg/kg/day. Full replacement therapy is usually initiated immediately in adults under 50 years of age. For older patients and for any patient with a history of cardiac disease, a lower initial dosage is indicated (0.025 to 0.05 mg levothyroxine daily), with clinical and biochemical reevaluation every 6 to 8 weeks until the S-TSH is normalized. Many older patients can be started on full replacement doses of T_4 if they have recently been treated for hyperthyroidism for only a few months. Certain medications interfere with the absorption or metabolism of levothyroxine, and appropriate spacing of dosage adjustments is recommended.

Continuing care with periodic monitoring is essential in all patients with hypothyroidism. As previously noted, patients should initially be evaluated every 6 to 8 weeks until the TSH is normalized; thereafter, monitoring may be lengthened to 6 and then 12 months. Any adjustment of dosage should be followed by reassessment after 2 to 3 months.

Subclinical hypothyroidism should always be considered for treatment, especially if thyroid autoantibodies are positive, because overt hypothyroidism often develops in such patients. Whether treated or not, patients should be evaluated at yearly intervals, particularly if treatment has been withheld.

Pituitary or hypothalamic hypothyroidism should be treated with thyroid only after treatment with hydrocortisone to avoid adrenocortical insufficiency. Aggressive or urgent therapy may be required in patients with cardiovascular disease. In these cases, partial protection by beta-adrenergic blockade, if not contraindicated, is useful. Emergency therapy may be required in hypothyroid hypothermia, in myxedema coma, and in the preparation of hypothyroid patients for surgery. Successful emergency treatment, even during surgery, may be achieved with intravenous T_4 (1 mg) together with intravenous hydrocortisone and/or propranolol.

REFERENCES

1. Surks MI, Chopra IJ, Mariash CN, et al: American Thyroid Association guidelines for use of laboratory tests in thyroid disorders. *JAMA* 263:1529–1532, 1990.

2. Khanderia V, Jaffe CA, Theisen V: Amiodarone-induced thyroid dysfunction. *Clin Pharm* 12:774–779, 1993.
3. Larsen PR, Ingbar SH: The thyroid gland. In: *Williams Textbook of Endocrinology, 8th edition.* Wilson JD, Goster DW. Philadelphia, PA; W.B. Saunders Company, 1992, pp 357–487.
4. Rapoport B: Pathophysiology of Hashimoto's thyroiditis and hypothyroidism. *Ann Rev Med* 42:91–100, 1991.
5. Mandel SJ, Brent GA, Larsen PR: Levothyroxine therapy in patients with thyroid disease. *Ann Intern Med* 119:492–502, 1993.
6. Roti E, Minelli R, Gardini E, et al: The use and misuse of thyroid hormone. *Endocr Rev* 14:401–423, 1993.
7. Singer PA, Cooper DS, Levy EG, et al: Treatment guidelines for patients with hyperthyroidism and hypothyroidism. *JAMA* 273:808–812, 1995.

Hyperthyroidism

Ellis Samols, M.D.

PRESENTING MANIFESTATIONS

History

The classical symptoms of hyperthyroidism are seen only in younger patients (with peak incidences in adolescence and then in the third and fourth decades, when the female:male ratio is a striking 6:1). Two or more of the following symptoms should be found: hyperactivity, heat intolerance, emotional lability, anxiety, sleep disturbance, palpitations, tremor, weight loss despite increased appetite, decreased menstrual flow, and thyroid enlargement. As Graves' disease is the most common cause of hyperthyroidism, patients should also be asked about photophobia, eye irritation, diplopia, or a change in visual acuity. In considering other causes of hyperthyroidism, patients should be asked about recent iodine exposure, thyroid hormone use, anterior neck pain, pregnancy, a history of goiter, and a family history of thyroid disease.

In older patients, especially those more than 60 years of age, the diagnosis of hyperthyroidism is much more readily missed, as the classical history is often muted or absent.[1] A history of fatigue, dyspnea, cardiac failure, or atrial fibrillation resistant to standard therapy is relatively common. Similarly, a physician with a high index of suspicion may find that new-onset ischemia or aggravation of existing ischemia is precipitated by hyperthyroidism. Female predominance becomes progressively less marked from the sixth to the eighth decade. The nomenclature *masked, occult,* or *apathetic hyperthyroidism* may be self-explanatory, but it tends to obscure the fact that many older patients fall into this category. *Myopathic thyrotoxicosis* describes weakness, perhaps with wasting, in proximal muscle groups, with difficulty in negotiating stairs. A syndrome of hyperthyroid-induced periodic paralysis has been described in Asians.

The duration of hyperthyroidism varies with the etiology. For example, the various forms of thyroiditis tend to be time-limited, so that thyrotoxic cardiac effects like worsening angina are usually limited to 3 to 4 months. Recurrences cause diagnostic confusion. Moreover, the cardiac manifestations of hypothyroidism may manifest in the same patients, especially during the natural course of Hashimoto's thyroiditis and after radioiodine therapy for Graves' disease.

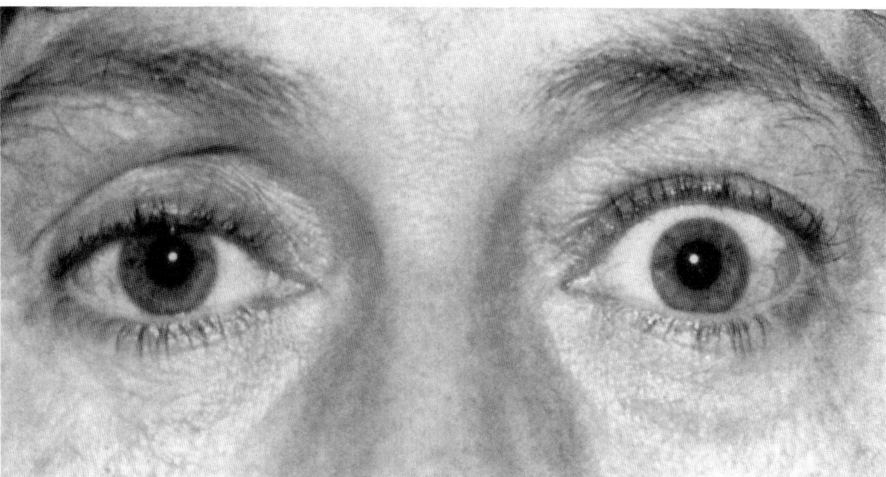

Figure 1.2. Ocular signs of hyperthyroidism are those of beta-adrenergic stimulation (retraction of the eyelids, stare and lid lag). The infiltrative opthalmopathy specific to Graves' disease causes exophthalmos, which is usually asymmetrical, as in this left eye, and is independent of the concentration of circulating thyroid hormones. From Shapiro LM, Fox KM. *Color Atlas of Physical Signs in Cardiovascular Disease*, Chicago, IL: Year Book Medical Publishers, Inc. 1989: pg. 17. Reprinted with permission from author and publisher.

Physical Examination

There is an important difference between hyperthyroidism and the extrathyroidal manifestations of Graves' disease. Increased levels of free T_4 and/or free T_3 in nonresistant subjects cause hyperthyroidism. Graves' disease is a complex of autoimmune abnormalities, with circulating antibodies which (1) stimulate the thyroid and (2) somehow may cause an ophthalmopathy and (3) rarely a dermopathy (pretibial myxedema) and/or osteopathy (resembling hypertrophic pulmonary osteoarthropathy).[2] The infiltrative ophthalmopathy (Figure 1.2) may cause chemosis and periorbital edema, proptosis (exophthalmos) which is usually asymmetrical, extraocular palsies, and the risk of corneal ulceration. Ocular signs of Graves' disease differ from those of hyperthyroidism per se. The ocular signs of hyperthyroidism are those of beta-adrenegic stimulation, that is, widened palpebral fissures, stare with infrequent blinking, and lid lag without significant exophthalmos.

Cardiovascular signs of thyrotoxicosis include resting tachycardia (>90 beats/ min in 90% of younger patients), atrial fibrillation (15–35% of older patients), systolic systemic arterial hypertension (occasionally diastolic hypertension) with increased pulse pressure, and a hyperdynamic pulse in a patient with warm, sweaty hands and a fine tremor. On physical examination, the features of a hyperdynamic heart may be present, including a hyperactive apical impulse, a loud first heart sound and a loud pulmonary component of the second heart sound, a basal midsystolic murmur, a third heart sound, and a systolic scratch or click in the second left intercostal space (Means-Lerman scratch) originating perhaps from a pleura-pericardial rub.

Laboratory Evaluation

The diagnosis of hyperthyroidism requires a suppressed supersensitive-thyroid stimulating hormone (S-TSH) except for the rare thyroid stimulating hormone (TSH)-secreting pituitary adenoma.

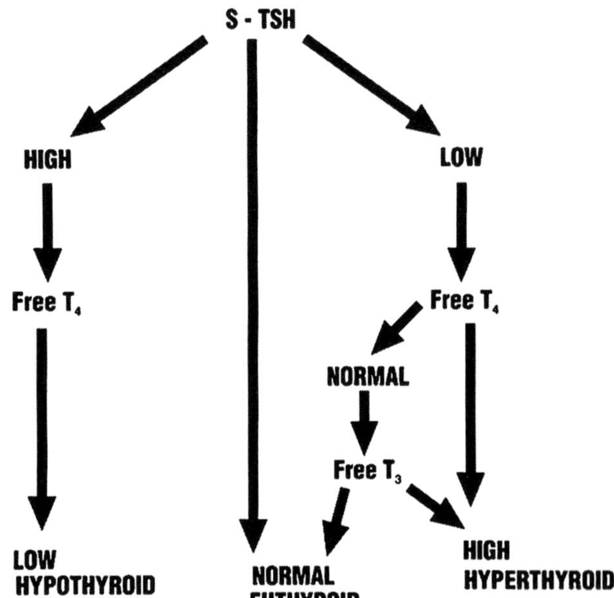

Figure 1.3. Assessment of thyroid function in ambulatory patients based on a sensitive thyroid stimulating hormone assay.

DIAGNOSTIC CRITERIA

First, the diagnosis of hyperthyroidism (versus euthyroidism or hypothyroidism) must be established; next, the cause of the hyperthyroidism must be sought. (Figure 1.3) With the supersensitive TSH assay, it is now necessary to demonstrate a suppressed TSH level in all cases of hyperthyroidism, except for TSH-secreting tumors (e.g., a rare pituitary macroadenoma). If the S-TSH level is low (<0.1 μm/ml), either the free T_4 or the free T_3 (measured directly or estimated) must be raised. The cause of the hyperthyroidism is diagnosed on the basis of the clinical presentation, the TSH levels, thyroid uptake and scan, and a variety of tests for thyroid autoantibodies.

Graves' disease is characterized by an enlarged (>85% cases) gland with a smooth, juicy texture. The enlargement may be missed in the elderly. A true arterial thyroid bruit is sometimes heard. Radioactive iodine uptake (I-123 or, in the elderly, the less expensive I-131) is increased, and the scan shows an enlarged gland with uniform uptake. Extrathyroidal infiltrative lesions may be diagnostic of Graves' disease but do not assess thyroid function. Thyroid-stimulating or -inhibiting immunoglobulins are similarly suggestive of Graves' disease but do not measure thyroid function, which is the critical element from the cardiac point of view.

TSH-secreting tumors produce a Graves' disease-like uniform uptake in an enlarged gland, but the increase in TSH concentration is diagnostic.

Iodine-induced hyperthyroidism usually occurs after exposure to large amounts of iodide (Jod-Basedow effect) in euthyroid patients in endemic iodine deficiency areas and in euthyroid patients with multinodular goiter. Because many of the latter patients are elderly, the radiologic contrast medium used should be neutralized (some advocate) by 7–10 days of pre- and postcatheterization propylthiouracil. The Jod-Basedow phenomenon requires a careful history, as radioactive iodine uptake is variable.

Toxic adenoma, now called a single nodule in *nodular toxic goiter*, may favor T_3 toxicosis. The diagnostic scan shows a "hot" spot accompanied by suppression of uptake by the remaining thyroid. *Toxic multinodular goiter* and hyperthyroidism show multiple areas of high, normal, and poor uptake. *Hashimoto's thyroiditis* is the most common diagnostic problem, as this autoimmune disease is more common than Graves' disease. The clinical features may include, at different times in the same patient, euthyroidism, hyperthyroidism, and hypothyroidism. The finding of a very high microsomal antibody titer is most helpful diagnostically.

Iatrogenic excessive thyroid intake, whether deliberate or accidental "hamburger toxicosis," metastatic thyroid follicular cancer, and struma ovarii induce a reduced radioactive iodine uptake by a small thyroid, with whole body scans demonstrating extrathyroidal functioning tumor.

The diagnosis of T_3, T_4, or T_4–T_3 toxicosis is not too helpful in establishing the cause of hyperthyroidism. The important point is that in addition to its association with nodular toxic goiter, T_3 toxicosis occurs in Graves' disease, particularly at its early stage or with recurrence, reinforcing the admonition to measure free T_3 in all patients with suspected hyperthyroidism in whom the estimated free T_4 is normal. T_4 toxicosis is usually seen in elderly and ill patients, with a clear elevation of estimated free T_4, a normal level of estimated free T_3, and suppressed TSH.

DIFFERENTIAL DIAGNOSIS

Anxiety, irritability, tremor, and sleep disturbance are features of thyrotoxicosis; therefore, the differential diagnosis of psychological or psychiatric anxiety states must be considered. Clinically, the warm hands in thyrotoxicosis compared with the cold, clammy hands in some anxiety states may be helpful in making the differential diagnosis, but in the final analysis, thyroid function tests are crucial.

Noncardiac presentations may involve the differential diagnosis of myasthenia gravis, hypokalemic periodic paralysis, sprue, metastatic carcinoma, and retro-orbital tumor.

A cardiac differential diagnosis should rule out hyperthyroidism in all cases of cardiac failure, ischemia, and atrial fibrillation. Suspicion of clinical thyrotoxicosis is aroused by a rapid onset of, or a poor response to, therapy in patients with failure, ischemia, and/or atrial fibrillation and by the finding of high-output failure. Specific lab tests including a determination of free T_4 and, if necessary, T_3, as well as a supersensitive TSH assay, are indispensable. The most common reason for the cardiologist to notice abnormal thyroid function tests is the sick euthyroid syndrome. However, the high T_4 variant is the least common manifestation of sick euthyroid syndrome, and a suppressed S-TSH strongly favors hyperthyroidism.

PATHOPHYSIOLOGY

Active thyroid hormone changes cardiac function both directly (by binding to intracellular receptors) and indirectly (by stimulating the sympathetic nervous system).[3] The direct effect is demonstrated because nerve blockade (sympathetic and parasympathetic) only partially reverses the tachycardia and the augmented myocardial contractility in experimental thyrotoxicosis induced by feeding thyroid hormone. The indirect sympathetic stimulation is predominantly beta-adrenergic. The direct effect is mediated by a change in intracellular protein synthesis that occurs when thyroid hormone binds to several intracellular nuclear complexes in cardiac cells, thereby activating specific chromosomal regulatory sites. This activation influences genomic expression for myosin type, and could contribute to other increases in cardiac cellular metabolic rate by increasing the activity of the sodium pump and increasing the number of slow calcium channels in cardiac cells.

The direct and indirect stimulation by thyroid hormone is due to a positive chronotrope and inotrope, respectively. There is an increase in the size of the left ventricle, with no change in either end-diastolic pressure or sarcomere length. Thyrotoxic tachycardia may result from an increased rate of diastolic depolarization and/or a decreased duration of action potential in the sinoatrial node cells. The remarkable tendency toward atrial fibrillation could result from a shortened refractory period in atrial cells.

Hyperthyroidism can induce congestive cardiac failure experimentally in animals and pathophysiologically in children. Also, hyperthyroid patients may have angina in the presence of normal coronary arteries. Abnormal left ventricular function during exercise is not reversed by beta-adrenergic blockage but is reversed by treatment of hyperthyroidism. Current opinion, based on clinical experience, is that while it is possible for thyrotoxicosis to overtax the normal heart, the vast majority of patients with hyperthyroid heart failure and/or myocardial ischemia have underlying cardiac and/or coronary vascular disease. As hyperthyroidism is common and its causes tend to be familial or geographic, it is not surprising to encounter an increased frequency of hyperthyroidism in a variety of syndromes. From a cardiovascular standpoint, these syndromes include familial hypertrophic cardiomyopathy and mitral valve prolapse.

NATURAL HISTORY OF THE DISEASE

The natural history of hyperthyroidism obviously depends on the cause. Nevertheless, the most common causes of noniatrogenic hyperthyroidism, Graves' disease, toxic adenoma, toxic multinodular goiter, and autoimmune thyroiditis are often characterized by cyclic phases of exacerbation and remission. As Graves' disease may evolve into a chronic thyroiditis with hyperthyroidism, this possibility becomes a factor in evaluating different therapies.

All causes of hyperthyroidism may produce complications in older patients with underlying cardiovascular disease, and death may ensue from cardiac failure or myocardial infarction if the hyperthyroidism is not specifically treated. In either young or old untreated patients, a syndrome called *thyroid storm* can occur, precipitated by a surgical emergency or an additional unrelated illness, usually sepsis.[4] When therapy for the hyperthyroidism is inadequate or absent, the prognosis is poor.

Toxic nodular goiter (Plummer's disease) is more common than Graves' disease in elderly patients. Hyperthyroidism may be caused by multiple hyperfunctioning nodules (toxic multinodular goiter) or, less commonly, by a single hyperfunctioning nodule (toxic adenoma). Hyperfunction may continue progressively or may be aborted spontaneously or made cyclical by intra-adenoma hemorrhage and/or necrosis. Hyperfunctioning nodules, whether single or multiple, are very rarely malignant. Toxic multinodular goiter occurs in long-standing, previously nontoxic "simple" goiter and is therefore usually a disease of the elderly, predominantly with a cardiovascular presentation and/or weakness and wasting.

Subactue thyroiditis, usually painful, may cause a transient hyperthyroidism. Chronic painless thyroiditis also tends to cause transient (2–5 months) hyperthyroidism, but these hyperthyroid episodes may be repetitive. Hyperthyroid Hashimoto's thyroiditis, also called *Hashitoxicosis*, predisposes the patient to eventual hypothyroidism, especially if ablative treatment by surgery or radioiodine is inappropriately performed.

CURRENT METHODS OF TREATMENT

Graves' hyperthyroidism is initially treated with the objective of lowering serum concentrations of free T_4 and T_3 to the normal range. As the serum TSH may remain suppressed for several months after the T_4 and T_3 levels have normalized, a serum TSH alone is not sufficient for evaluation until the patient has clearly stabilized over a prolonged treatment period. Radioactive iodine therapy (I-131) is the most popular treatment in the United States; antithyroid drugs and/or surgery are effective alternatives. The patient should be an active participant in the decision on the type of therapy and should therefore have a clear understanding of the indications, implications, and costs of all forms of therapy, including risks, benefits, and side effects.

None of these three therapies are indicated in patients with hyperthyroidism and a low radioactive iodine uptake; these patients usually have thyroiditis, which is best managed by beta-adrenergic blockade. In thyroiditis the increased circulating thyroid hormone is derived from inflammatory destruction of preexisting thyroglobulin of thyroid follicles, a process which should not respond to antithyroid drugs (ATD), which block hormone synthesis. Thyroid ablation by surgery or I-131 strongly risks permanent hypothyroidism in patients whose thyroiditis generally resolves spontaneously.

Antithyroid drugs, with daily propylthiouracil (100–200 mg every 6–8 hr) or methimazole (10–20 mg every 6–8 hr) is usually adequate initially. ATD is continued at an adjusted dosage for 6 months to 2 years or more as primary therapy for Graves' disease until remission is induced or occurs, or as preparative therapy before (and sometimes after) I-131 therapy or surgery. A combination of ATD and levothyroxine has been preferred by some physicians for the past 40 years. Today it is again popular to avoid frequent adjustment of the ATD dosage and perhaps to decrease the severity of ophthalmopathy.

Adverse effects of ATD include rash, pruritis, arthralgias, and, very rarely, hepatic cholestasis and necrosis (both with methimazole). It may be wise to record white blood cell counts before initiating ATD therapy to obtain a baseline which is commonly mildly leukopenic in Graves' disease. The most serious reaction to propylthiouracil and methimazole is agranulocytosis (0.3% of patients). Patients who develop fever, rash, jaundice, arthralgia, or oropharyngitis should promptly discontinue the medication and have appropriate lab studies.

Stable iodine (2 drops saturated potassium iodine tid or ipodate, 1 g/day orally) may be useful in addition to ATD in patients with severe cardiac disease, as release of thyroid hormone is more rapidly inhibited than can occur by inhibition of synthesis. Treatment with lithium carbonate has a similar rationale; remember that either iodine or lithium alone may inhibit release incompletely or transiently.

Radioactive iodine therapy is safe and does not cause cancer or infertility. Pregnancy and breast-feeding are contraindications. Usage of I-131 therapy in patients <20 years old is controversial but common in the United States. In patients with Graves' disease or toxic nodular goiter who are elderly or have cardiovascular disease, a relatively large dose of I-131 is logical in order to avoid recurrence or incomplete treatment. Radiation thyroiditis should be anticipated (usually at 7–10 days) and avoided because the thyroiditis may cause thyrotoxic crisis in the elderly or sick and may aggravate problems in patients with underlying heart disease. Pretreatment with ATD is useful to deplete stored thyroglobulin, thereby reducing radiation-induced hyperthyroidism before and after I-131 therapy to facilitate uptake and retention of I-131. Although propranolol should be used cautiously, keeping in mind cardiac complications, beta blockade may be helpful if cardiac failure is aggravated by tachycardia. Propranolol without ATD is not recommended.

Surgical subtotal thyroidectomy is infrequently performed in Graves' disease unless it is regarded as necessary in the very young, the pregnant, or patients subject to potential pressure effects by substernal radiation thyroiditis.[7] Although I-131 is frequently used in the treatment of toxic nodular goiter, surgery is appropriate in those who prefer surgery, in children and adolescents, in patients with large goiters and/or tracheal or esophageal pressure, and when there is a suspicion of malignancy. Surgery should be performed only by an experienced physician and only after careful medical preparation. Patients should know that potential complications include hypoparathyroidism and injury to the recurrent laryngeal nerve.

Adjunctive therapy for symptoms is best provided by beta-adrenergic blockade (e.g., propranolol or nadolol). Patients unable to tolerate beta blockade may be treated with calcium channel blockers like diltiazem.

Therapy for cardiac failure is conventional, but supranormal doses of digitalis will usually be required, with careful observation for digitalis toxicity when euthyroidism is approached. Because congestive failure and/or atrial fibrillation are resistant to conventional doses of cardiac glycosides, digitalis toxicity may develop with a dose that has little cardiac therapeutic effect. Beta-adrenergic blockers, which are used cautiously in cardiac failure, are especially useful to slow the ventricular rate in atrial fibrillation because beta blockade acts synergistically with cardiac glycosides to increase the refractoriness of the atrioventricular conduction system. This therapeutic combination often avoids the adverse effects of either agent alone at a higher dosage. Beta-adrenergic blockade improves many peripheral manifestations of thyrotoxicosis, including tachycardia, palpitations, tremor, restlessness, muscle weakness, and heat intolerance. It also inhibits the conversion of T_4 to biologically active T_3 in peripheral tissues.

Continuing care is often required for a few years, and a follow-up plan is necessary. Patients treated with ATD should be seen at monthly intervals until euthyroidism is achieved, when the ATD dose can often be reduced. Thereafter, they should be monitored every 3–4 months to ensure that clinical biochemical euthyroidism is continuing. After ATD therapy is stopped, monitoring at monthly intervals for the first 3 months can be followed by increasing intervals for the first year. Evaluation yearly for the next 3 years can be followed by evaluation at increasing intervals thereafter. Patients treated with I-131 should be monitored at similar intervals, with a special early check for radiation thyroiditis if indicated. Hypothyroidism may occur either at 6–12 months or at any interval for life. A minimal annual follow-up is advised for euthyroid patients. Once hypothyroidism develops, the endpoint of replacement therapy is a normal free T_4E and TSH level. Once patients are on a stable dose of levothyroxine, annual serum TSH testing is now regarded as adequate monitoring if clinical euthyroidism is maintained.[8] Similar principles apply to follow-up after surgery.

Special therapeutic problems such as hyperthyroidism associated with pregnancy, Graves' ophthalmopathy, and thyroid storm deserve a specialist's assistance therapeutically, as the patient's life or eyesight may be threatened. Iatrogenic hyperthyroidism is probably the most common form of hyperthyroidism in the United States. Some patients, especially the elderly, cannot tolerate the standard doses of thyroid hormone (by old or even new criteria) and develop symptoms of hyperthyroidism. If the S-TSH is suppressed, levothyroxine therapy should be withheld for 1 week and restarted at a lower does. Often the patient has no symptoms despite elevated T_4 and/or suppression of S-TSH. Currently there is no agreed-upon term to describe the combination of high T_4 and low TSH in the absence of symptoms, as subclinical hyperthyroidism is supposed to be restricted to the combination of no symptoms, normal estimates of free T_4 and T_3, and suppressed TSH in the absence of other causes of TSH suppression, such as glucocorticoid use, severe illness, and pituitary dysfunction. From the therapeutic point of view, patients who are hyperthyroid, even in the absence of symptoms, usually need treatment. This general principle applies to all forms of hyperthyroidism, including Graves' disease, toxic nodular goiter, TNG, and the most common form of subclinical hyperthyroidism, overreplacement of thyroid hormone. The long-term effects of overreplacement have significant public health implications, particularly in postmenopausal women, encouraging osteoporosis and leading to increased bone fractures.[9] Overreplacement may also have cardiac consequences. Today correct levothyroxine replacement is judged by achieving a S-TSH concentration in the normal range, so that the dose of levothyroxine replacement is reduced if TSH is suppressed. Conditions requiring suppressed TSH, such as differentiated thyroid cancer and possibly hypofunctional thyroid nodules, are exceptions to this general principle. Thyroid hormone dependency with hyperthyroidism is a neglected problem, and is more frequent than is generally appreciated. These women enjoy the stimulating effect of T_4, and/or the greater ease of weight control and/or some possible antidepressive effect, and may resist requests to decrease the dosage of levothyroxine even in the presence of unwanted cardiac manifestations.

REFERENCES

1. Sawin CT: Thyroid dysfunction in older persons. *Adv Intern Med* 37:223–248, 1991.
2. Burch HB, Wartofsky L: Graves' ophthalmopathy: current concepts regarding pathogenesis and management. *Endocr Rev* 14:747–793, 1993.
3. Larsen PR, Ingbal SH: The thyroid gland. In: *Williams Textbook of Endocrinology, 8th ed.* Wilson JD, Foster DW (eds) Philadelphia, PA: W.B. Saunders 1992;357–487.

4. Gavin LA: Thyroid crises. *Med Clin North Am* 75:179–193, 1991.

5. Cooper DS: Antithyroid drugs. *N Engl J Med* 311:1353–1362, 1984.

6. Hennemann G, Krenning EP, Sankaranarayanan K: Place of radioactive iodine in treatment of thyrotoxicosis. *Lancet* 325:1369–1372, 1986.

7. Patwardhan NA, Movont M, Rao S, et al: Surgery still has a role in Graves' hyperthyroidism. *Surgery* 114:1108–1113, 1993.

8. Mandel SJ, Brent GA, Larsen PR: Levothyroxine therapy in patients with thyroid disease. *Ann Intern Med* 119:492–502, 1993.

9. Stall GM, Harris S, Sokoll LJ, Dawson-Hughes B: Accelerated bone loss in hypothyroid patients overtreated with L-thyroxine. *Ann Intern Med* 113:265–269, 1990.

Adrenal Insufficiency

J. David Talley, M.D.
Ellis Samols, M.D.

PRESENTING MANIFESTATIONS

History

Patients with aldosterone insufficiency (insufficient glucocorticoids and/or mineralocorticoids) present with symptoms of weakness, syncope, skin or mucosal pigmentation, weight loss, anorexia, nausea, or vomiting. The patient may have a history of tuberculosis, lymphoma, or human immunodeficiency virus or may present with manifestations of polyglandular autoimmune endocrinopathy.[1,2]

Physical Examination

Generalized brownish hyperpigmentation of the skin and mucous membranes is an almost universal finding in patients with adrenal insufficiency. (Figure 1.4) The systemic arterial blood pressure is low.[3] Orthostatic hypotension is a frequent finding.

Laboratory Evaluation

Adrenal insufficiency is suggested by the presence of hyperkalemia, hyponatremia, and hypercalcemia. The cardiac silhouette is small on chest x-ray, and an echocardiogram may show findings consistent with mitral valve prolapse. The electrocardiogram may show sinus bradycardia, low voltage, inverted T waves, and a prolonged QT interval.[4]

DIAGNOSTIC CRITERIA

The diagnosis of adrenal insufficiency is suggested by finding low serum levels of cortisone and aldosterone and elevated levels of adrenocorticotropin and plasma renin.[5] The diagnosis is confirmed by finding an inadequate functional reserve of the adrenal glands when measuring the response to cosyntropin (1-24 adrenocorticotropin hormone). A level below 20 µg/dL is consistent with the diagnosis.

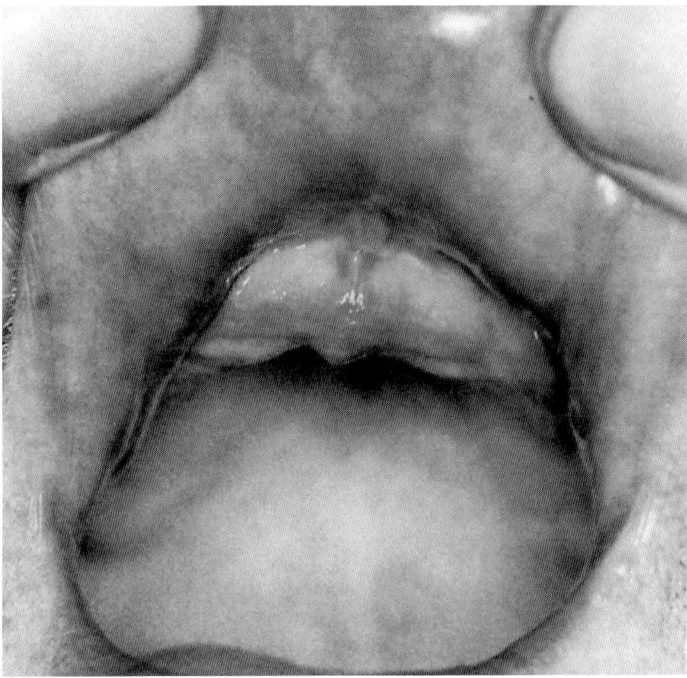

Figure 1.4. Patients with adrenal insufficiency may show signs of generalized hyperpigmentation, here of the buccal mucosa. From Shapiro LM, Fox KM. *Color Atlas of Physical Signs in Cardiovascular Disease*, Chicago, IL: Year Book Medical Publishers, Inc. 1989: pg. 28. Reprinted with permission from author and publisher.

DIFFERENTIAL DIAGNOSIS

Adrenal insufficiency is usually idiopathic and related to primary destruction of the adrenal glands. Rarely, it may be part of polyglandular failure. Secondary adrenal insufficiency is classically described as being due to tuberculosis, but it may also be seen with other infiltrative entities such as viral infections or tumors.

PATHOPHYSIOLOGY

Adrenal insufficiency may develop because of failure of the hypothalamus to produce adequate levels of corticotrophin-releasing hormone or failure of the pituitary to secrete enough adrenocorticotropin. The adrenal cortex may also be unresponsive to adequate levels of adrenocorticotropin or corticotropin-releasing hormone due to autoimmune involvement of other endocrine glands.

Congestive heart failure has been reported.[6,7]

NATURAL HISTORY

Patients with adrenal insufficiency are treated with glucocorticoids and mineralocorticoids. If left untreated, adrenal insufficiency may progress to fatal adrenal failure.

CURRENT METHODS OF TREATMENT

Most patients with adrenal insufficiency require small doses of steroid replacement. The average daily oral dose of cortisone acetate is 25–37.5 mg. Fludrocortisone, a mineralocorticoid, is given in a dose of 0.1 mg on alternate days.[3]

The electrocardiographic findings described above and echocardiographic findings of mitral valve prolapse resolve with steroid replacement.[8,9]

REFERENCES

1. Eisenbarth GS, Wilson PW, Ward F, et al: The polyglandular failure syndrome: Disease inheritance, HLA type, and immune function: Studies in patients and families. *Ann Intern Med* 91:528–533, 1979.
2. Membreno L, Irony I, Klein R, et al: Adrenocortical function in acquired immunodeficiency syndrome. *J Clin Endocrinol Metab* 65:482–487, 1987.
3. De Rosa G, Corsello SM, Cecchini L, et al: A clinical study of Addison's disease. *Exp Clin Endocrinol* 90:232–242, 1987.
4. Surawicz B, Mangiardi ML: Electrocardiogram in endocrine and metabolic disorders. In Rios JC (ed): *Clinical Electrocardiographic Correlations*. Philadelphia, FA Davis, 1977, pp 243.
5. Oelkers W, Diederich S, Bähr V: Diagnosis and therapy surveillance in Addison's disease: Rapid adrenocorticotropin (ACTH) test and measurement of plasma ACTH, renin activity, and aldosterone. *J Clin Endocrinol Metab* 75:259–264, 1992.
6. Knowlton AI, Baer L: Cardiac failure in Addison's disease. *Am J Med* 74:829–836, 1983.
7. Dorin RI, Kearns PJ: High output circulatory failure in acute adrenal insufficiency. *Crit Care Med* 16:296–297, 1988.
8. Lavis VR, Mueller SD, Willerson JT: Endocrine disorders and the Heart. In Willerson JT, Cohn JN (eds): *Cardiovascular Medicine*. New York, Churchill Livingtone, 1995, pp 1609–1610.
9. Williams GH, Braunwald E: Endocrine and nutritional disorders and heart disease. In Brawnwald E (ed): *Heart Disease: A Textbook of Cardiovascular Medicine*, ed 4. Philadelphia, WB Saunders, 1992, pp 1838–1839.

Hyperaldosteronism

J. David Talley, M.D.
Ellis Samols, M.D.

PRESENTING MANIFESTATIONS

History

A patient with hyperaldosteronism may present with symptoms consistent with hypokalemia, including nocturia, polyuria, proximal muscle weakness, ventricular arrhythmias, intermittent paralysis, and parasthesia. The patient may also have a history of difficult-to-control systemic arterial hypertension with intermittent headache.

Physical Examination

The typical age of presentation is 30 to 50 years. A 3:1 female:male predominance is seen with aldosterone-secreting adenomas. Both genders are equally affected by bilateral adrenal hyperplasia. Careful examination of the cardiovascular system may show evidence of enhanced sympathetic tone with systemic arterial hypertension and tachycardia.[1] Secondary manifestations of long-standing severe systemic arterial hypertension, including retinopathy and left ventricular hypertrophy, may be seen. Hypokalemic alkalosis may cause Trousseau's (muscle spasm due to nerve compression) or Chvostek's (spasm of the facial muscles) signs. Edema is unusual without associated heart failure.

Laboratory Evaluation

Hyperaldosteronism is characterized by hypokalemia, borderline hypernatremia and a depressed renin concentration, and a high level of aldosterone. Hypokalemic changes may be seen on the electrocardiogram.

DIAGNOSTIC CRITERIA

The diagnosis of primary aldosteronism is confirmed by finding elevated levels of aldosterone that are increased relative to sodium excretion. A key diagnostic feature is the failure of the aldosterone concentration to be suppressed normally following volume expansion with the infusion of 2L of normal saline over a period of 4 hr.[2]

DIFFERENTIAL DIAGNOSIS

The numerous causes of hypokalemia should be considered in establishing this diagnosis. (See section VIII, pg 104.)

PATHOPHYSIOLOGY

Systemic arterial hypertension is seldom due to hyperaldosteronism. In the general population of patients with elevated blood pressure, it is the etiology in less than 2%. In selected hypertensives, especially those with severe elevation of blood pressure, the incidence may be as high as 10%.[3]

With primary aldosteronism (Conn's syndrome), the primary defect is excessive secretion of aldosterone either from an adrenal adenoma (approximately 60%) or from bilateral adrenal hyperplasia (approximately 25%).[4] Adrenal adenomas are usually benign (less than 1% are malignant) and less than 3 cm in diameter. Bilateral adrenal hyperplasia is characterized as focal or diffuse hyperplasia of the zona glomerulosa layer of the adrenal cortex. Excessive secretion of aldosterone causes reabsorption of sodium, with excretion of potassium and hydrogen ions.

The systemic arterial hypertension seen with hyperaldosteronism is both systolic and diastolic, severe, and resistant to treatment. Bravo and associates noted that the mean blood pressure of 25 patients with primary aldosteronism was 186/118 despite treatment with a diuretic, sympatholytic, and vasodilator.[5]

NATURAL HISTORY OF THE DISEASE

Untreated primary aldosteronism is associated with severe vascular complications. Beevers and colleagues reported nearly a 25% incidence of stroke, myocardial infarction, dissecting aortic aneurysm, or claudication over a 6-year follow-up period.[6]

CURRENT METHODS OF TREATMENT

Management of Excessive Aldosterone Secretion

Pharmacotherapy

Medical therapy may be the primary therapy for patients with bilateral adrenal hyperplasia or adjunctive therapy for patients in whom surgery has not been curative. Potassium-sparing medications (spironolactone, triamterene, amiloride) which block the effect of aldosterone at the distal tubule are the medications of choice.

Surgery

Patients with primary aldosteronism may be cured with surgical removal of the aldosteronoma. Potassium-sparing medications should be used for several months to normalize the blood pressure and eliminate the metabolic abnormalities prior to surgery. A unilateral posterior retroperitoneal surgical incision is standard.[7]

Management of Cardiovascular Symptoms

Caution must be exercised when using digitalis preparations in patients with congestive heart failure due to the adverse effects seen with hypokalemia. The combination of an angiotensin-converting enzyme inhibitor and a potassium-sparing diuretic should be avoided due to the possibility of inducing hyperkalemia. Direct vasodilators, such as calcium channel blockers, are second-line agents for the treatment of severe hypertension.[8]

REFERENCES

1. Tarazi RC, Ibrahim MM, Bravo EL: Hemodynamic characteristics of primary aldosteronism. *N Engl J Med* 289:1330–1335, 1973.
2. Arteaga E, Klein R, Biglieri EG: Use of the saline infusion test to diagnose the cause of primary aldosteronism. *Am J Med* 79:722–728, 1985.
3. Grim CE, Weinberger MH, Higgins JT, et al: Diagnosis of secondary forms of hypertension: A comprehensive protocol. *JAMA* 237:1331–1335, 1977.
4. Conn JW: Primary aldosteronism: A new clinical entity. *Trans Assoc Am Physicians* 68:215–233, 1955.
5. Bravo EL, Fouad-Tarazi FM, Tarazi RC, et al: Clinical implications of primary aldosteronism with resistant hypertension. *Hypertension* 11:I-207–I-211, 1988.
6. Beevers DG, Brown JJ, Ferriss JB, et al: Renal abnormalities and vascular complications in primary hyperaldosteronism. Evidence on tertiary hyperaldosteronism. *Q J Med* 45:401–410, 1976.
7. Grant CS, Carpenter P, van Heerden JA, et al: Primary aldosteronism: Clinical management. *Arch Surg* 119:585–590, 1984.
8. Nadler JL, Hsueh W, Horton R: Therapeutic effect of calcium channel blockade in primary aldosteronism. *J Clin Endocrinol Metab* 60:896–899, 1985.

Glucocorticoid Excess

J. David Talley, M.D.
Ellis Samols, M.D.

PRESENTING MANIFESTATIONS

History

Patients with glucocorticoid excess present with symptoms of weight gain, fatigue, proximal muscle group weakness, cranial baldness, facial hirsutism, easy bruisability, and poor wound healing. Depression and emotional changes may also be seen.

Physical Examination

Patients with excess cortisol production may have purplish abdominal striae, peripheral edema, systemic arterial hypertension, and bruises (Figure 1.5). Areas of abnormal fat deposition produce characteristic physical features, including moon facies, centripetal obesity, buffalo hump, and truncal obesity. Generalized muscle weakness may be present. Severe osteoporosis may cause kyphosis.[1]

Laboratory Evaluation

Cushing's syndrome is due to excess cortisol production by the adrenal glands. Therefore, measurement of total cortisol excretion (obtained with a 24-hr urine free cortisol measurement) and cortisol suppression (the dexamethasone suppression test) are commonly used diagnostic modalities. Overnight 1-mg dexamethasone suppression, with an early morning plasma cortisol level greater than 10 μg/dL, suggests Cushing's' syndrome. A plasma cortisol level suppressed below 5 μg/dL is seen in normal patients.[2]

Other metabolic abnormalities include hyperglycemia, glycosuria, hypokalemia, and hypochloremia. Spinal x-rays may show osteoporosis.

Cardiovascular tests show changes consistent with systemic arterial hypertension or hypocalcemia. On electrocardiography, the PR interval may be short, the QRS voltage prominent, and the T wave negative. Asymmetric septal hypertrophy is seen on echocardiography.[3]

DIAGNOSTIC CRITERIA

A high index of suspicion is necessary to consider the possibility of glucocorticoid excess syndrome. Appropriate clinical findings and laboratory tests (elevated 24-hr urine free cortisol excretion and an abnormal overnight dexamethasone suppression test) confirm the diagnosis.

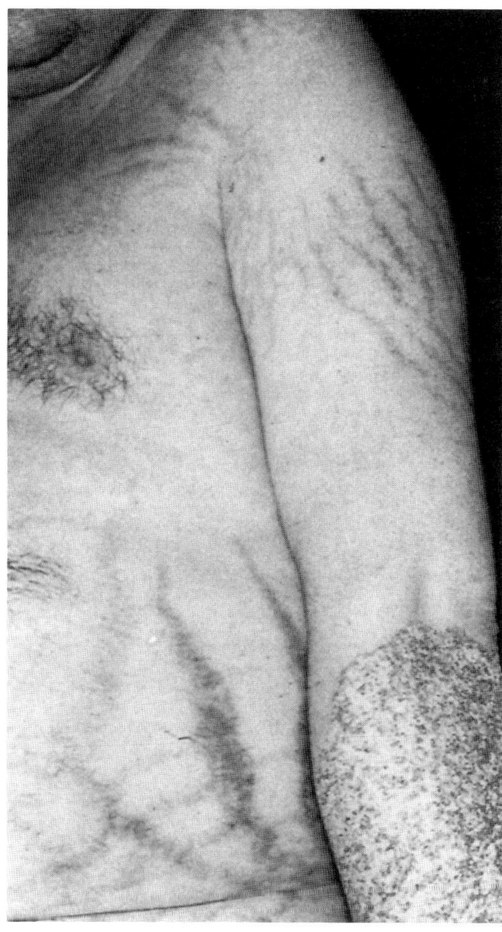

Figure 1.5. A patient with glucocorticoid excess with typical features of truncal obesity and multiple pigmented striae. (From Shapiro LM, Fox KM. *Color Atlas of Physical Signs in Cardiovascular Disease.* Chicago, Year Book Medical, 1989, p 15. Reprinted with permission from author and publisher.)

DIFFERENTIAL DIAGNOSIS

A differential diagnosis of excess glucocorticoid syndrome involves localization of the site of corticotropin production. Cushing's disease (pituitary corticotropin excess) is characterized by inappropriately high levels of corticotropin and may be stimulated by the use of metyrapone. Adrenal adenomas or carcinomas are characterized by low levels of corticotropin. Plasma corticotropin is markedly elevated with ectopic tumor production.

PATHOPHYSIOLOGY

Glucocorticoid excess syndrome was initially described by Cushing in 1932.[4] The excessive secretion of corticotropin leads to adrenal cortical hyperplasia. Excess levels of cortisol have systemic manifestations. Pituitary excess cortisol production is seen in females nine times more commonly than in males and is unusual in children. Adrenal adenomas or carcinomas are seen with equal frequency in both genders. Adrenal carcinoma is commonly seen in patients in their 30s and 40s. Ectopic corticotropin production is seen in males 10 times more commonly than in females.

The cardiovascular symptoms are related to systemic arterial hypertension and atherosclerosis. The development of systemic arterial hypertension in patients with glucocorticoid excess syndromes is related to an abnormality of salt and water balance, volume shifts, and enhanced responsiveness to catecholamines and adrenergic agents.

Atherosclerosis is common and is due to the multiple risk factors in these patients. Hyperglycemia, hyperlipidemia, and systemic arterial hypertension predispose the patient to premature development of atherosclerosis. Cardiovascular manifestations of Cushing's syndrome account for nearly one-half of untreated patients.

NATURAL HISTORY OF THE DISEASE

Patients with pituitary glucocorticoid excess have a 5-year mortality rate of 50%. Death is due to complications related to diabetes mellitus, systemic arterial hypertension, and infection. Morbidity is related to osteoporosis with compression fractures.[5]

CURRENT METHODS OF TREATMENT

Treatment is related to the site of excess corticotropin production. Transsphenoidal hypophysectomy is the preferred approach for patients with excessive pituitary corticotropin production. In experienced centers, this procedure achieves a complete remission in approximately 75% of patients.[6,7]

Patients with adrenal adenomas or carcinomas are referred for total adrenalectomy.[8] Adrenal carcinomas are nearly always fatal within 3 years of diagnosis. Patients with unresectable malignant disease may be treated with mitotane, ketoconazole, RU 486, metyrapone, mitotane, or aminoglutethimide.[9–11]

REFERENCES

1. Gabrilove JL, Krakoff LR: Diagnosis and pathophysiology of Cushing's syndrome. *Compr Ther* 12:17–21, 1986.
2. Kaye TB, Crapo L: The Cushing syndrome: An update on diagnostic tests. *Ann Intern Med* 112:434–444, 1990.
3. Sugihara N, Shimizu M, Kita Y, et al: Cardiac characteristics and postoperative courses in Cushing's syndrome. *Am J Cardiol* 69:1475–1480, 1992.
4. Cushing H: The basophil adenomas of the pituitary body and their clinical manifestations (pituitary basophilism). *Bull Johns Hopkins Hosp* 50:137–195, 1932.
5. Plotz CM, Knowlton AI, Ragan C: The natural history of Cushing's syndrome. *Am J Med* 13:597–614, 1952.
6. Tindall GT, Herring CJ, Clark RV, et al: Cushing's disease; Results of transsphenoidal microsurgery with emphasis on surgical failures. *J Neurosurg* 72:363–369, 1990.
7. Mampalam TJ, Tyrrell JB, Wilson CB: Transsphenoidal microsurgery for Cushing's disease: A report of 216 cases. *Ann Intern Med* 109:487–493, 1988.
8. Bennett AH, Cain JP, Dluhy RG, et al: Surgical treatment of adrenocortical hyperplasia: 20-year experience. *J Urol* 109:321–324, 1973.

9. Luton JP, Mahoudeau JA, Bouchard PH, et al: Treatment of Cushing's disease by O,p'DDD: Survey of 62 cases. *N Engl J Med* 300:459–464, 1979.

10. Neiman LK, Chrousos GP, Kellner C, et al: Successful treatment of Cushing's syndrome with the glucocorticoid antagonist RU 486. *J Clin Endocrinol Metab* 61:536–540, 1985.

11. Oelkers W, Bähr V, Hensen J, et al: Primary adrenocortical micronodular adenomatosis causing Cushing's syndrome. Effect of ketoconazole on steroid production and in vitro performance of adrenal cells. *Acta Endocrinol (Copenh)* 113:370–377, 1986.

Obesity

J. David Talley, M.D.

PRESENTING MANIFESTATIONS

History

Physical Examination

Besides excess body weight, obese patients may have systemic arterial hypertension and signs consistent with congestive heart failure and hypoventilation.

Laboratory Evaluation

Metabolic abnormalities include hyperlipidemia and diabetes mellitus. Obese patients have a 25–50% larger cardiac silhouette on chest x-ray than do normotensive subjects.[1] There may also be evidence of congestive heart failure. The electrocardiogram may show myocardial ischemia, injury, or infarction.

DIAGNOSTIC CRITERIA

Obesity is defined in terms of the body mass index. The body mass index is weight in kilograms divided by the square of the height in meters. Normal body mass index is between 19 and 25. Patients with a body mass index between 25 and 29 are considered moderately overweight, and patients with an index greater than 29 are considered severely overweight.[2]

DIFFERENTIAL DIAGNOSIS

The differential diagnosis of obesity is presented in Table 1.1.

PATHOPHYSIOLOGY

Obesity is causally linked to several cardiovascular syndromes including atherosclerosis, systemic arterial hypertension, and congestive heart failure. There is conflicting evidence regarding obesity as a risk factor for the development of atherosclerosis.[3,4] Several recent reports

TABLE 1.1. Causes of Obesity

Primary endocrine	*Hypothalamic-pituitary*	*Possible genetic*
Hyperinsulinemia	Tumors or inflammatory lesions of the hypo-thalamus or pituitary	Lawrence-Moon-Biedl syndrome
Glucocorticoid excess		Hyperostosis frontails interna
Primary hypogonadism	Trauma or surgical injury to the brain	Alstrom's syndrome
Primary hypothyroidism	Pseudotumor cerebri	Pseudohypoparathyroidism
Polycystic ovarian syndrome	Empty ssella syndrome	Down's syndrome
		Familial obesity

Modified from DiGirolamo M. Obesity. In: Hurst JW (ed.), *Medicine for the practicing physician, 3rd edition.* Boston, MA, Butterworth-Heinemann. 1992;603–606. Reprinted with permission from author and publisher.

have noted an association of fat distribution and coronary artery disease. These studies have shown that truncal or abdominal fatness, assessed by either skinfolds or circumference, is related to coronary artery disease.[5–7]

There is a well-established association between obesity and the development of systemic arterial hypertension. In the Framingham Study, obese patients had an eightfold increased risk of developing systemic arterial hypertension compared to normotensive subjects.[8]

The increased metabolic demand imposed by excessive accumulation of adipose tissue is met by high cardiac output due to increased stroke volume. Obese patients also have an expanded plasma volume. The combination of high stroke volume and expanded plasma volume results in increased myocardial wall stress, which is compensated for by myocardial dilation.[9]

NATURAL HISTORY

Obese patients have accelerated total mortality and mortality related to cardiovascular causes. The survival curves for total and cardiovascular causes resemble a U shape, with accelerated mortality related to a body mass index greater than 30. Patients with a body mass index greater than 35 have approximately 35% excess total mortality.[10] Cardiovascular mortality increases 2% per kilogram of body weight from a body mass index greater than 23.[11]

CURRENT METHODS OF TREATMENT

Behavioral Modification

Several techniques of behavioral modification, including a balanced diet, yield encouraging results. A successful dietery program needs continued reinforcement and encouragement. The importance of exercise should not be underestimated. Exercise decreases elevated insulin levels and improves carbohydrate tolerance. It also decreases systemic arterial hypertension and hyperlipoproteinemia.[12]

Pharmacotherapy

Drug therapy is an important mainstay in the management of patients with obesity. Anorectic agents produce a significant short-term weight loss; however, they have long-term adverse effects.

Surgical Therapy

End-stage obesity syndrome may be treated with surgery. Surgical reduction of the stomach is a useful therapeutic option in many patients.

REFERENCES

1. Woodard CB, Quinones MA, Alexander JK: Pathogenesis of myocardial dysfunction in extreme obesity (abstract). *Circulation* 57 and 58:II-230, 1978.
2. *Nutrition and Your Health: Dietary Guidelines for Americans.* Washington, DC: U.S. Department of Agriculture and U.S. Department of Health and Human Services, 1995, 1–43.
3. Barrett-Connor EL: Obesity, atherosclerosis, and coronary artery disease. *Ann Intern Med* 103:1010–1019, 1985.
4. Manson JE, Colditz GA, Stampfer MJ, et al: A prospective study of obesity and risk of coronary heart disease in women. *N Engl J Med* 322:882–889, 1990.
5. Higgins M, Kannel W, Garrison R, et al: Hazards of obesity—the Framingham experience. *Acta Med Scand* 723:23–36, 1988.
6. Donahue RP, Abbott RD, Bloom E, et al: Central obesity and coronary heart disease in men. *Lancet* 1:821–824, 1987.
7. Ducimetiere P, Richard J, Cambien F: The pattern of subcutaneous fat distribution in middle-aged men and the risk of coronary heart disease: The Paris Prospective Study. *Int J Obesity* 10:229–240, 1986.
8. Kannel WB, Brand N, Skinner JJ, Jr, et al: The relation of adiposity to blood pressure and development of hypertension: The Framingham study. *Ann Intern Med* 67:48–59, 1967.
9. Messerli FH, Christie B, DeCarvalho JRG, et al: Obesity and essential hypertension: Hemodynamics, intravascular volume, sodium excretion, and plasma renin activity. *Arch Intern Med* 141:81–85, 1981.
10. Waaler HT: Height, weight, and mortality: The Norwegian experience. *Acta Med Scand* 679:1–56, 1983.
11. Larsson B: Obesity, fat distribution and cardiovascular disease. *Intern J Obesity* 15. 53–57, 1991.
12. Reisin E, Abel R, Modan M, et al: Effect of weight loss without salt restriction on the reduction of blood pressure in overweight hypertensive patients. *N Engl J Med* 298:1–6, 1978.

Pheochromocytoma

J. David Talley, M.D.

PRESENTING MANIFESTATIONS

History

The five H's are a useful mnemonic when considering the diagnosis of pheochromocytoma: hypertension, hypermetabolism, headache, hyperhidrosis, and hyperglycemia. Other presenting manifestations of pheochromocytoma are listed in Table 1.2. Systemic arterial hypertension is most common; it is usually sustained but may be intermittent. Postural hypotension is occasionally reported.

Approximately 10% of patients with pheochromocytoma have a family history of the tumor.[1] Pheochromocytomas may occur as part of several endocrine abnormalities. The mul-

TABLE 1.2. Symptoms and Signs of Pheochromocytoma

Common Features	Percent	Less Common Features	Percent
Hypertension	>98	Visual disturbance	3–21
Intermittent hypertension	2–50	Constipation	0–13
Sustained hypertension	50–60	Paresthesia/pain in arms	0–13
Paroxysms superimposed	~50	Flushing	~18
Headache	72–92	Acrocyanosis	~3
Fever	≤66	Dyspnea	11–19
Sweating	60–70	Dizziness	3–11
Palpitations ± tachycardia	51–73	Convulsions (grand mal)	3–5
Nervousness	35–40	Bradycardia	3–8
Weight loss	40–70	Warmth ± heat intolerance	13–15
Fundoscopic changes	50–70	Palpable mass in abdomen	10–14
Pallor	28–60	Tightness in throat	~8
Chest/abdominal pain	28–60		
Nausea ± vomiting	26–43		
Weakness, fatigue	15–38		

From Kaplan, NM: Adrenal Diseases: Pheochromocytoma. In: Kaplan NM (ed), *Clinical Hypertension*. 4th edition, Baltimore, MD, Williams and Wilkins, 1986, p 381.

tiple endocrine neoplasia (MEN II) complex includes pheochromocytoma and medullary carcinoma of the thyroid. MEN type IIa (Sipple syndrome) includes hyperparathyroidism. Type IIb (or type III, mucosal neuroma syndrome) includes marfanoid habitus, multiple mucosal neuromas of the tongue, lips, gastrointestinal tract, or conjunctivas, without parathyroid disease.[2,3] Pheochromocytoma is also seen in patients with von Recklinghausen's disease, tuberous sclerosis, Sturg-Weber syndrome, and von Hipple-Lindau disease.[4]

Physical Examination

While systemic arterial hypertension is the most consistent finding on physical examination, other signs of catecholamine excess are also seen. These include tachycardia, diaphoresis, and a hyperactive heart.

Laboratory Evaluation

Patients with pheochromocytoma have a plasma catecholamine (epinephrine and norepinephrine) level above than 2000 pg/ml. A level below 500 pg/ml rules out the probability of a pheochromocytoma. A concentration between 500–2000 pg/ml requires the use of additional pharmacologic tests. Failure to reduce epinephrine and norepinephrine 3 hr after administration of 0.3 mg clonidine (the clonidine suppression test) to less than 500 μm/dL suggests the presence of a pheochromocytoma.[5] A 24-hr urine collection for metanephrines (normetanephrine and metanephrine; the products of o-methylation enzymatic metabolism) has a high sensitivity for the presence of a pheochromocytoma.[6]

The electrocardiogram may show tachycardia and signs of left ventricular hypertrophy. Systolic anterior motion of the mitral value may be seen on the echocardiogram during periods of catecholamine excess.[7]

DIAGNOSTIC CRITERIA

Suggestive symptomatology coupled with a plasma catecholamine level above 2000 pg/ml confirms the diagnosis of a pheochromocytoma.

DIFFERENTIAL DIAGNOSIS

Multiple conditions may mimic the presence of a pheochromocytoma (Table 1.3). Importantly, anxiety and abrupt withdraw of alpha- or beta-adrenergic blocking medications used in the treatment of systemic arterial hypertension must be considered.

PATHOPHYSIOLOGY

Pheochromocytoma is a tumor of primitive neural crest cells. These cells produce excessive catecholamines, which result in characteristic cardiovascular effects reflecting the balance between alpha- and beta-adrenergic receptor stimulation. Norepinephrine is a potent alpha agonist which increases systolic blood pressure. Epinephrine, a beta agonist, is a positive

TABLE 1.3. Differential Diagnosis of Pheochromocytoma

Cardiovascular
    Hyperdynamic, labile hypertension
    Paroxysmal tachycardia
    Angina, coronary insufficiency
    Acute pulmonary edema
    Eclampsia
    Hypertensive crisis during or after surgery
    Hypertensive crisis with monoamine oxidase inhibitors
    Rebound after abrupt discontinuation of clonidine and other
        antihypertensives

Psychoneurologic
    Anxiety with hyperventilation
    Migraine and cluster headaches
    Brain tumor
    Stroke
    Diencephalic seizures
    Porphyria
    Lead poisoning
    Familial dysautonomia
    Acrodynia
    Autonomic hyperreflexia, as with quadriplegia

Endocrinologic
    Menopause
    Thyrotoxicosis
    Diabetes mellitus
    Hypoglycemia
    Carcinoid
    Mastocytosis

Factitious
    Ingestion of sympathomimetics

From Kaplan NM. Adrenal Diseases: Pheochromocytoma. In: Kaplan NM (ed), *Clinical Hypertension*, 4th edition, Baltimore, MD, Williams and Wilkins, 1986, p 381. Reprinted with permission from author and publisher.

chronotrope and vasodilator. Therefore the systolic blood pressure rises, while the diastolic blood pressure remains stable or falls slightly.

Myocarditis, focal necrosis with infiltration of inflammatory cells, perivascular inflammation, and contraction band necrosis may be seen on endomyocardial biopsy or at autopsy.[8] A catecholamine-induced dilated cardiomyopathy with congestive heart failure has been reported.[9,10]

NATURAL HISTORY

Pheochromocytoma is fatal without treatment. Mortality and morbidity are related to severe systemic arterial hypertension, cerebral hemorrhage, congestive heart failure, and arrhythmias with sudden death.[11] A minority of deaths are due to malignant disease from other tumors.

METHODS OF TREATMENT

Surgical removal is the treatment of choice. The perioperative mortality rate is less than 5%.[12] Hypertension is cured in approximately 80% of patients with complete tumor removal. Alpha-adrenergic blockage is used preoperatively to control systemic arterial hypertension and restore normal plasma volume. After alpha blockade is completely established, beta-adrenergic blocking agents may be added to block epinephrine-induced tachycardia and arrhythmias. Beta blockade must be used with caution due to the possibility of unsuppressed alpha-adrenergic action.

Pheochromocytomas which cannot be removed or which recur may be medically managed. Systemic arterial hypertension can be controlled with alpha-adrenergic blocking medications. Alpha-methy-para-tyrosine (metyrosine) inhibits tyrosine hydroxylase, the enzyme which hydroxylates tyrosine to dopa. This medication decreases total catecholamine levels by 80%. Radiotherapy may be used and is occasionally successful. Partial remissions may be induced by the chemotherapeutic combination of cyclophosphamide, vincristine, and dacarbazine.[13]

REFERENCES

1. Glowniak JV, Shapiro B, Sisson JC, et al: Familial extra-adrenal pheochromocytoma: A new syndrome. *Arch Intern Med* 145:257–261, 1985.
2. Steiner AL, Goodman AD, Powers SR: Study of a kindred with pheochromocytoma, medullary thyroid carcinoma, hyperparathyroidism and Cushing's disease: Multiple endocrine neoplasia, type 2. *Medicine* 47:371–409, 1968.
3. Khairi MRA, Dexter RN, Burzynski NJ, et al: Mucosal neuroma, pheochromocytoma and medullary thyroid carcinoma: Multiple endocrine neoplasia type 3. *Medicine* 54:89– 112, 1975.
4. Havik RJ, Cahow CE, Kinder BK: Advances in the diagnosis and treatment of pheochromocytoma. *Arch Surg* 123:626–630, 1988.
5. Bravo EL, Tarazi RC, Fouad FM, et al: Clonidine-suppression test: A useful aid in the diagnosis of pheochromocytoma. *N Engl J Med* 305:623–626, 1981.
6. Manu P, Runge LA: Biochemical screening for pheochromocytoma: Superiority of urinary metanephrines measurements. *Am J Epidemiol* 120:788–790, 1984.
7. Shub C, Cueto-Garcia L, Sheps SG, et al: Echocardiographic findings in pheochromocytoma. *Am J Cardiol* 57:971–975, 1986.

8. Van Vliet PD, Burchell HB, Titus JL: Focal myocarditis associated with pheochromocytoma. *N Engl J Med* 274:1102–1108, 1966.

9. Imperato-McGinley J, Gautier T, Ehlers K, et al: Reversibility of catecholamine-induced dilated cardiomyopathy in a child with a pheochromocytoma. *N Engl J Med* 316: 793–796, 1987.

10. Scott I, Parkes R, Cameron DP: Pheochromocytoma and cardiomyopathy. *Med J Aust* 148:94–96, 1988.

11. Scardigli K, Biller J, Brooks MH, et al: Pontine hemorrhage in a patient with pheochromocytoma. *Arch Intern Med* 145:343–344, 1985.

12. Deoreo GA Jr, Stewart BH, Tarazi RC, et al: Preoperative blood transfusion in the safe surgical management of pheochromocytoma. A review of 46 cases. *J Urol* 111:715– 721, 1974.

13. Averbuch SD, Steakley CS, Young RC, et al: Malignant pheochromocytoma: Effective treatment with a combination of cyclophosphamide, vincristine, and dacarbazine. *Ann Intern Med* 109: 267–273, 1988.

Acromegaly

J. David Talley, M.D.

PRESENTING MANIFESTATIONS

History

The peak incidence occurs in the early to mid 40s.[1] Patients may present with neurologic symptoms including paresthesias, muscle weakness, carpel tunnel syndrome, or headache. Additional symptoms include malocclusion of the teeth, sweating, and arthralgia. Menstrual irregularity is seen in females. Cardiovascular symptoms are the cause of the presentation in approximately 4%.[2]

Acromegaly is usually seen in isolation. However, it may occur as a part of the multiple endocrine neoplasm (MEN) type I syndrome, which includes hyperparathyroidism and islet cell tumors of the pancreas. Acromegaly is also part of a multisystemic tumor syndrome consisting of pigmented skin lesions, cardiac myxomas, and endocrine tumors with an autosomal dominant inheritance pattern (Carney complex).[3] Finally, acromegaly may be part of the empty sella turcica syndrome, which consists of a variety of endocrine and neurologic abnormalities.[4]

Physical Examination

Objective findings related to acromegaly are due to the growth of the pituitary gland itself or consist of excessive bone and soft tissue growth. Mass effects of the pituitary tumor may cause headache and visual disturbances. Pituitary compression may also decrease the secretion of other pituitary hormones, resulting in secondary panhypopituitarism.

The excessive secretion of growth hormone causes longitudinal bone growth in children. In adults, bones and soft tissues thicken. The size of the lips, tongue (macroglossia), hands, feet, and skull is out of proportion to that of other body parts. Skin tags (acrochordon) and a barrel chest may be present. Excessive hair growth (hypertrichosis) and diaphoresis (hyperhidrosis) may also be seen. Adenomatous colonic polyps are seen in one-half of patients with acromegaly, and nearly 10% of these are malignant.[4]

Laboratory Abnormalities

Patients with acromegaly have impaired glucose tolerance and excessive levels of insulin, leading to hyperglycemia. They may also have other metabolic abnormalities, including glycosuria, hyperphosphotemia, and hypercalcemia. Cardiomegaly may be seen on the electrocardiogram or chest x-ray.

DIAGNOSTIC CRITERIA

The diagnosis of acromegaly depends on finding an elevated level of insulin-like growth factor-1 or failure to suppress growth hormone after ingesting a glucose load. Growth hormone is measured 1 hour after consuming 100 g of oral glucose. An elevated growth hormone level greater than 10 µg/L in combination with objective findings confirms the diagnosis.[6] The enlarged pituitary gland may also be imaged with computer tomography or magnetic resonance imaging.

DIFFERENTIAL DIAGNOSIS

Excessive secretion of growth hormone is most commonly due to an isolated pituitary tumor. Infrequently, it may be part of the constellation of other endocrine abnormalities seen in MEN syndrome, Carney complex, or empty sella turcica syndrome.

PATHOPHYSIOLOGY

Acromegaly was initially described in 1886.[7] The annual incidence of acromegaly is 3–4 per million patients, with a total incidence of 50–70 cases per million. Acromegaly is most commonly due to excess growth hormone secretion from a pituitary adenoma, but excessive secretion may also be due to tumors outside the pituitary. Less commonly, acromegaly is due to excess growth-hormone-releasing hormone secretion from the hypothalamus, although ectopic sources have also been described. Finally, patients with acromegalic features who have a normal level of growth hormone have been described (acromegaloidism).[8]

The excessive secretion of growth hormone causes several cardiovascular abnormalities, including systemic arterial hypertension, dysrhythmias, and cardiac hypertrophy. Systemic arterial hypertension occurs in one-third of patients, is mild, is associated with the duration of the disease, and improves with treatment. The elevated blood pressure is due in part to extracellular fluid expansion.[9]

Cardiac hypertrophy and interstitial fibrosis cause systolic and diastolic dysfunction, with resulting congestive heart failure in approximately 20% of patients with acromegaly. The development of this cardiomyopathy may be a manifestation of systemic arterial hypertension or atherosclerosis. However, symptoms of congestive heart failure without evidence of hypertensive cardiovascular disease point to a distinct clinical entity, acromegalic cardiomyopathy. Histologic features include cellular hypertrophy, patchy fibrosis, and myofibrillar degeneration.[10]

Arrhythmias may be seen in patients with acromegaly. These arrhythmias may be secondary to degenerative and inflammatory changes seen in the sinoatrial and atrioventricular nodes.[11]

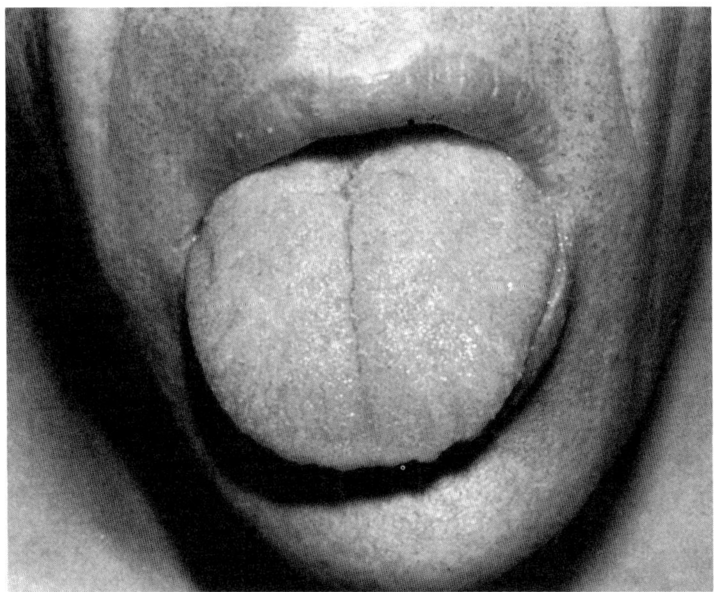

Figure 1.6. Macroglossia is a common physical manifestation of acromegaly. From Shapiro LM, Fox KM. *Color Atlas of Physical Signs in Cardiovascular Disease,* Chicago, Il, Year Book Medical Publishers, Inc, 1989, p 27. Reprinted with permission of author and publisher.

NATURAL HISTORY

The death rate of patients with acromegaly is twice that of the general population. The excess mortality is related to cardiovascular disease in males and to malignancy in females, and an equal proportion of mortality in both males and females is related to respiratory and cerebral vascular disease.[12]

CURRENT METHODS OF TREATMENT

Management of Excessive Secretion of Growth Hormone

Pharmacotherapy

Bromocriptine and octreotide can be used as primary or adjunctive therapy. Bromocriptine suppresses the secretion of growth hormone by binding pituitary dopamine receptors. Octreotide is a somatostatin analogue. These agents are used preoperatively to shrink the pituitary adenoma or adjunctively for patients in whom irradiation and surgery have not been curative.[13,14] These agents may restore normal blood pressure in hypertensive patients.

Radiation

Both cobalt and proton-beam radiation have been used in acromegalic patients. Irradiation is effective, but beneficial results require prolonged treatment. Concerns regarding the long-term sequelae of radiation, the prolonged course of treatment required, and panhypopituitarism have led to infrequent use of this form of therapy.

Surgery

The treatment of choice of pituitary acromegaly is transsphenoidal hypophysectomy. The cure rate is approximately 75%, and this treatment is more successful with small tumors. Mortality is less than 1%, and the complication rate is less than 5%.[15]

Management of Cardiovascular Symptoms

Most patients with acromegaly have a normal response to standard medical therapy of systemic arterial hypertension and congestive heart failure. Some patients with systemic arterial hypertension are particularly volume sensitive; therefore, caution is necessary when using diuretics. Patients with acromegalic cardiomyopathy are particularly resistant to standard forms of treatment of congestive heart failure. Cardiac transplantation has been described in patients with refractory congestive heart failure.[16]

REFERENCES

1. Alexander L, Appleton D, Hall R, et al: Epidemiology of acromegaly in the Newcastle region. *Clin Endocrinol (Oxf)* 12:71–79, 1980

2. Molitch ME: Clinical manifestations of acromegaly. *Endocrinol Metab Clin North Am* 21:597–614, 1992.

3. Carney JA, Gordon H, Carpenter PC, et al: The complex of myxomas, spotty pigmentation, and endocrine overactivity. *Medicine* 64:270–283, 1985.

4. Gallardo E, Schächter D, Caceres E, et al: The empty sella: Results of treatment of 76 successive cases and high frequency of endocrine and neurological disturbances. *Clin Endocrinol* 37:529–533, 1992.

5. Ituarte EA, Petrini J, Hershman JM: Acromegaly and colon cancer. *Ann Intern Med* 101:627–628, 1984.

6. Earll JM, Sparks LL, Forsham PH: Glucose suppression of serum growth hormone in the diagnosis of acromegaly. *JAMA* 201:134–136, 1967.

7. Marie PP: Sur deux cas d'acromégalie: Hypertrophie singulière non congénitale des extrémitiés supérieures, inférieures et céphalique. *Rev Med* 6:297–333, 1886.

8. Ashcraft MW, Hartzband PI, Van Herle AJ, et al: A unique growth factor in patients with acromegaloidism. *J Clin Endocrinol Metab* 57:272–276, 1983.

9. Moore TJ, Thein-Wai W, Dluhy RG, et al: Abnormal adrenal and vascular responses to angiotension II and an angiotensin antagonist in acromegaly. *J Clin Endocrinol Metab* 51:215–222, 1980.

10. Lie JT, Grossman SJ: Pathology of the heart in acromegaly: anatomic findings in 27 autopsied patients. *Am Heart J* 100:41–52, 1980.

11. Rossi L, Thiene G, Caregaro L, et al: Dysrhythmias and sudden death in acromegalic heart disease: A clinicopathologic study. *Chest* 72:495–498, 1977.

12. Wright AD, Hill DM, Lowy C, et al: Mortality in acromegaly. *Q J Med* 39:1–16, 1970.

13. Rau H, Althoff P-H, Schmidt K, et al: Bromocriptine treatment over 12 years in acromegaly: Effect on growth hormone and prolactin secretion. *Acta Endocrinol* 126:247–252, 1992.

14. Vance ML, Harris AG: Long-term treatment of 189 acromegalic patients with the somatostatin analog octreotide: Results of the international multicenter acromegaly study group. *Arch Intern Med* 151:1573–1578, 1991.

15. Tindall GT, Barrow DL. Acromegaly. In: *Disorders of the Pituitary.* Tindall GT, Barrow DL (eds). St. Louis, CV Mosby, 1986, pg 203–229.

16. Albat B, Leclercq F, Serr I, et al: Heart transplantation for terminal congestive heart failure in an acromegalic patient. *Eur Heart J* 14:1572–1575, 1993.

— II —
Cardiovascular Involvement with Connective Tissue Diseases

Hugo E. Jasin, M.D.
Section Editor

Systemic Lupus Erythematosus

Eleanor A. Lipsmeyer, M.D.

PRESENTING MANIFESTATIONS

History

Systemic lupus erythematosus (SLE) affects mostly young females in the second to fourth decade (female:male ratio: 3:1). Most patients have joint pain with or without objective arthritis. Skin changes are common and may be related to sun exposure.

Patients describe positional precordial pain, pleuritic change, or dyspnea. Renal disease with hematuria or nephrotic syndrome is common and occurs in approximately 50% of patients. Central nervous system involvement may present with seizures, coma, stroke, or psychosis. Diffuse lymphadenopathy, splenomegaly, and fever may occur.

Physical Examination

Joint involvement is usually symmetrical; ulnar deviation of the digits without erosive changes (Jaccoud's deformity) may be present. Skin lesions may be extensive. The classic "butterfly rash," an erythematous malar rash, may be present. Pleuritic or pericardial rubs, congestive heart failure, arrhythmias, or conduction defects may develop.

Laboratory Evaluation

Patients may present with the anemia of chronic disease. Hemolytic anemia with a positive direct Coombs' test, leukocytopenia, lymphopenia, and thrombocytopenia may be present. The urinalysis may show red blood cells and red blood cell casts, as well as significant proteinuria. The acute phase reactants are usually elevated; however, the C-reactive protein are rarely elevated. A positive test for antinuclear antibody (ANA) is the hallmark of the disease and is present in over 90% of patients with SLE. Antibodies directed against double-stranded DNA or Sm (Smith antigen) are virtually diagnostic of SLE. These reflect disease activity but do not predict organ involvement.[1] Immune complexes may be present, and complement components (CH50, C3, and C4) may be decreased.[1]

DIAGNOSTIC CRITERIA

The diagnostic criteria for the classification of SLE[2] were devised in 1982. Eleven criteria were defined, and four or more of them must be present for the purpose of classifying patients (Table 2.1).

DIFFERENTIAL DIAGNOSIS

SLE must be differentiated from other collagen vascular diseases, including rheumatoid arthritis, progressive systemic sclerosis, and mixed connective tissue disease, an "overlap disease."

PATHOPHYSIOLOGY

Widespread immunologic abnormalities of T and B lymphocytes in SLE result in the production of a variety of autoantibodies. Immune complexes of antigens and autoantibodies are deposited in the vessel walls of joints and renal glomeruli, where they activate complement and cause inflammatory disease. In addition, autoantibodies may react directly with an organ or cell to cause localized damage. Skin, joints, serosal surfaces, and vascular basement membranes may be damaged.

NATURAL HISTORY OF THE DISEASE

Pericarditis

Pericarditis is the most common cardiac manifestation of SLE and may be present in 50% of patients. Pericarditis may be asymptomatic or may cause anterior chest pain. Generally, the disease is mild and bothersome, but in some cases cardiac tamponade occurs and must be treated urgently.[3] Pericardial fluid is usually exudative and may contain immune complexes. On histologic examination, pericarditis is fibrinous or fibrotic, with acute or chronic inflammatory infiltrates and vascular proliferation. SLE pericarditis must be differentiated from uremic or infectious causes.

Myocarditis

Myocarditis has been reported in 8–25% of patients with SLE; however, it usually presents as myocardial wall dysfunction rather than florid myocarditis. If there is associated anti-ribonucleoprotein (anti-RNP) antibody, active myocarditis may accompany skeletal myositis. Eleva-

TABLE 2.1. Criteria for Classification of SLE

1. Photosensitivity	7. Renal disorder
2. Malar rash	8. Neurologic or psychiatric disorder
3. Discoid skin lesions	9. Hematologic abnormalities
4. Mucosal ulcers	10. Positive antinuclear antibody
5. Arthralgia or nondeforming arthritis	11. Immunologic abnormality
6. Polyserositis	False-positive VDRL, + lupus erythematosus preparation or antibody to double-stranded DNA or Sm antigen

Modified from Tan EM, Cohen AS, Fries JF, et al: The 1982 revised criteria for the classification of systemic lupus erythematosus. *Arthritis Rheum* 25:1271–1277, 1982. Reprinted with permission of author and publisher.

tion of the cardiac (MB) fraction of creatine kinase may occur. In a study of left ventricular function, 28 patients with lupus and 20 healthy volunteers were studied for 5 years. The increases in left ventricular mass index, mean wall thickness, and end-systolic volume and the decreases in ejection fraction were found to be related to the presence of hypertension or coronary artery disease,[4] and not to SLE alone.

Studies using M-mode and two-dimensional echocardiography have shown pericardial abnormalities in mitral valve leaflet thickening, aortic valve thickening, and, rarely, mitral annular calcification, correlated with the duration but not with the severity of the disease. In some patients with SLE, valvular abnormalities detected by two-dimensional echocardiography were not seen on M-mode echocardiography; therefore, the former is the preferred test in these patients.[5]

Valvular Disease

Libman and Sacks first described the cardiac abnormalities associated with SLE in 1924.[6] They recognized noninfectious verrucous vegetations in areas of proliferating and degenerating tissue located at valve margins, on chordae tendineae, on papillary muscles, and on endocardium. The occurrence of valvular disease in SLE is rare. Recently, however, there has been a relative increase in valvular disease attributed to SLE. A wide variety of valvular lesions may be seen: thinning of the aortic valve leaflets with perforations of the cusps producing aortic insufficiency; thrombotic deposits on the aortic valve causing aortic stenosis; calcified verrucae and sudden rupture of the chordae tendineae (Figure 2.1) causing mitral valve incompetence; occlusive vegetations in the mitral valve causing mitral stenosis; necrotizing mitral valvulitis; annular dilatation and elongation of the chordae tendineae causing tricuspid regurgitation; and calcified interventricular and interatrial multilobulated masses causing both valvular stenosis and regurgitation.[7]

Antiphospholipid Antibody Syndrome (APS)

Antibodies which react with phospholipid are associated with a clinical syndrome of recurrent thromboses, thrombocytopenia, and spontaneous abortion. APS occurs predominantly in females with no other clinical syndrome, but a subset of SLE patients (~25%) may also have this autoantibody. Three markers are present for APS: a biologic false-positive test for syphilis, lupus anticoagulant, and antibodies to cardiolipins and other phospholipids. Patients with APS develop thrombotic, noninflammatory, vaso-occlusive complications. Arterial thromboses are more common than venous thromboses. Patients with APS and lupus have an increased incidence of valvular heart disease,[8] valvular vegetations, mural thrombi, and embolic central nervous system vascular events. There is a higher incidence of aortic than of mitral valvular lesions. The presence of APS may be a marker for more rapid valvular disease progression and for a higher incidence of thromboembolic complications after valve replacement.

Coronary Artery Disease (CAD)

Atherosclerotic heart disease or vasculitis may cause myocardial infarction in patients with SLE. Coronary arteritis is diagnosed when coronary angiography demonstrates saccules or aneurysms without obstruction in the vessels which supply the involved area.[9] Since the prognosis of SLE has improved in recent years, there has been an increasing proportionate mortality rate over the past decade from atherosclerotic coronary artery disease (CAD), probably associated with protracted use of corticosteroids.[10] The risk factors for CAD in SLE appear to be the age at diagnosis of SLE, duration of prednisone use, need for antihypertensive treatment, maximum cholesterol level, and obesity. There appeared to be no relationship with smoking, diabetes, family history of CAD, race, or sex.

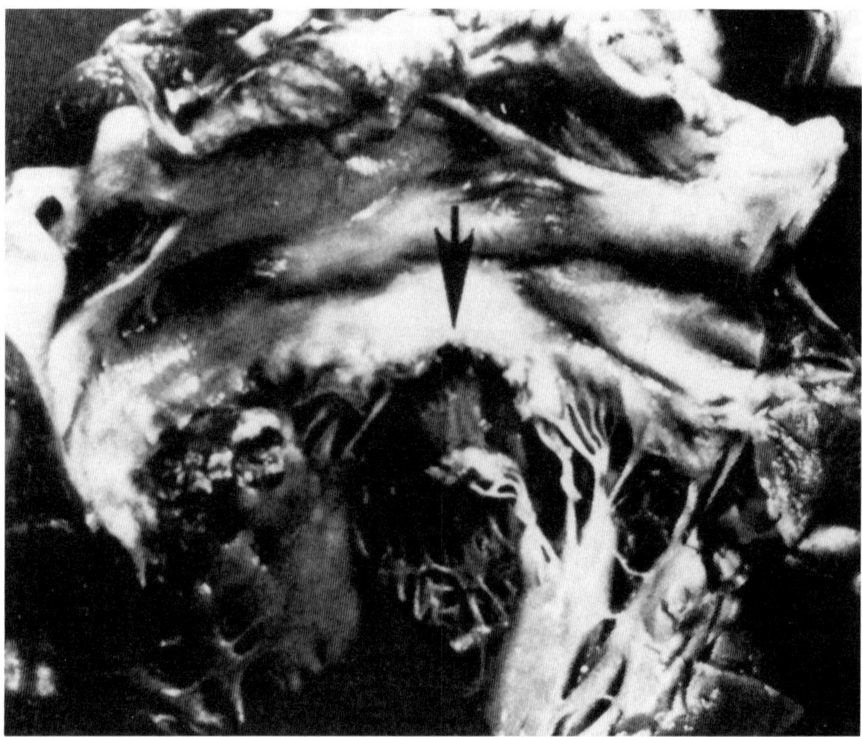

Figure 2.1.   Rupture of mitral valve leaflet with vegetations in SLE. Arrow indicates site of rupture on anterior leaflet. Reprinted from Straaton, KV, Chatham WW, Reveille FD, et al. Clinically significant valvular heart disease in systemic Lupus erythematous. *Am J Med.* 85:645–650, 1988. Reprinted with permission of author and publisher.

Conduction Defects

Conduction defects in adults with SLE are usually associated with myocarditis. First-degree heart block is usually transient; second- or third-degree blocks are rare. Congenital complete heart block occurring in infants is believed to be the result of transplacental passage of maternal antibody to Ro(SS-A) and/or La(SS-B).[11] The same mechanism is thought to be responsible for the manifestations of neonatal lupus syndrome; although skin rash and cytopenias are transient, heart block generally is irreversible. Generally, the mother is clinically asymptomatic, and her serologic state is not recognized until her infant is shown to have heart block.

CURRENT METHODS OF TREATMENT

Treatment of the cardiac manifestations of SLE is determined by the clinical presentation. Pericarditis is initially treated with nonsteroidal anti-inflammatory agents; if these fail, high-dose corticosteroids are given. Symptomatic pericardial effusion requires either pericardiocentesis or placement of a pericardial window. Myocarditis is treated with high doses of corticosteroids and occasionally with cytotoxic drugs. Valvular disease, CAD, and congestive heart failure are treated with the usual modalities. The treatment for APS remains controversial.[8] Patients who have no clinical symptoms should be observed but not treated. Heparinization and conversion to prolonged warfarin treatment are indicated in patients with venous or arterial thrombosis. The role of corticosteroids in the treatment of this syndrome is unknown.

Treatment for congenital complete heart block remains controversial, but intrauterine treatment with dexamethasone has been used.[12] When complete heart block is present in the infant at delivery, a permanent pacemaker must be placed.

REFERENCES

1. Lloyd W, Schur PH: Immune complexes, complement, and anti-DNA in exacerbations of systemic lupus erythematosus (SLE). *Medicine* 60:208–217, 1981.
2. Tan EM, Cohen AS, Fries JF, et al: The 1982 revised criteria for the classification of systemic lupus erythematosus. *Arthritis Rheum* 25:1271–1277, 1982.
3. Kahl LE: The spectrum of pericardial tamponade in systemic lupus erythematosus: Report of ten patients. *Arthritis Rheum* 35:1343–1349, 1992.
4. Winslow TM, Ossipov MA, Fazio GP, et al: The left ventricle in systemic lupus erythematosus: Initial observations and a five-year follow-up in a university medical center population. *Am Heart J* 125:1117–1129, 1993.
5. Klinkhoff AV, Thompson CR, Reid GD, et al: M-mode and two-dimensional echocardiographic abnormalities in systemic lupus erythematosus. *JAMA* 243:3273–3277, 1985.
6. Libman E, Sacks B: A hitherto undescribed form of valvular and mural endocarditis. *Arch Intern Med* 33:701–709, 1924.
7. Straaton KV, Chatham WW, Reveille JD, et al: Clinically significant valvular heart disease in systemic lupus erythematosus. *Am J Med* 85:645–650, 1988.
8. Bowles CA: Vasculopathy associated with the antiphospholipid antibody syndrome. *Rheum Dis Clin North Am* 16:471–490, 1990.
9. Heibel RH, O'Toole JD, Curtiss EL, et al: Coronary arteritis in systemic lupus erythematous. *Chest* 69:700–703, 1976.
10. Petri M, Perez-Gutthann S, Spence D, et al: Risk factors for coronary artery disease in patients with systemic lupus erythematosus. *Am J Med* 93:513–519, 1992.
11 Buyon JP, Winchester R: Congenital complete heart block: A human model of passively acquired autoimmune injury. *Arthritis Rheum* 33:609–614, 1990
12. Carreira PE, Gutierrez-Larraya F, Gomez-Reino JJ: Successful intrauterine therapy with dexamethasone for fetal myocarditis and heart block in a woman with systemic lupus erythematosus. *J Rheum* 20:1204–1207, 1990.

Systemic Sclerosis

Eleanor A. Lipsmeyer, M.D.

PRESENTING MANIFESTATIONS

History

Systemic sclerosis is a connective tissue disease in which there is abnormal thickening and fibrosis of the skin. Two groups of patients may be distinguished by their degree of involvement: those with progressive systemic sclerosis (SSc, scleroderma) and limited systemic sclerosis (LSSc). Most patients who have SSc present with Raynaud's phenomenon. Symmetric swelling of the fingers and hands may be followed by tightening and induration of the skin.

Joints and tendons may be painful, and the patient may complain of muscle tenderness and weakness. Dysphagia is common, with gastroesophageal reflux. Dyspnea and congestive heart failure may occur because of cardiac or renal abnormalities.

Physical Examination

Examination of the patient may show blanching or cyanosis of the fingers or toes. The skin of the hands may be taut, shiny, and hidebound, and tightening of the facial skin may occur. Polyarthritis is rare but diffuse joint pain is common. Friction rubs over moving tendons may accompany tenosynovitis. Flexion contractures are common in severe disease. Patients with pulmonary involvement or heart failure may have bibasilar or diffuse crackles. Chronic hypoxemia or right ventricular overload may become apparent later in the disease.

Laboratory Evaluation

These conditions are marked by fairly specific immunologic tests. Antinuclear antibody (ANA) is usually positive in both forms; SSc usually has either a speckled or a nucleolar pattern. In addition, patients with SSc may have antibody against topoisomerase I (SCL-70). Patients with LSSc have anticentromere antibody (ACA), and a discrete speckled pattern on routine ANA.[1,2] Earlier visceral involvement with increased morbidity and mortality is seen in patients with SSc. Patients with LSSc have a smaller incidence or later occurrence of visceral involvement, usually in the second to fifth decades of the illness. Up to 40% of the patients with LSSc may develop pulmonary hypertension.

DIAGNOSTIC CRITERIA

The criteria developed for SSc include the major criterion of skin thickening proximal to the metacarpal-pharyngeal joints and the minor criteria of sclerodactyly, loss of tissue from the finger pad, and bibasilar pulmonary fibrosis. The diagnosis of SSc may be made if the patient has one major or two minor criteria.[3] LSSc is also known as *CREST syndrome* (calcinosis, Raynaud's phenomenon, esophageal dysmotility, sclerodactyly, and telangiectasia).

DIFFERENTIAL DIAGNOSIS

There may be some confusion with other collagen vascular diseases. Early on, the disease may be difficult to differentiate from "overlap syndrome" or mixed connective tissue disease. It is important to remember that many females may have Raynaud's phenomenon with or without associated primary pulmonary hypertension.

PATHOPHYSIOLOGY

Abnormal vascular reactivity is thought to be the origin of the visceral changes seen in both forms of systemic sclerosis. The underlying vascular lesion in SSc is characterized by endothelial abnormalities and a proliferative change in the vascular endothelium. The intimal lesions are seen in arteries, arterioles, and capillaries; they may be seen externally in the periungual capillary bed as enlarged capillaries with areas of avascularity.[4] It is thought that fibrosis may be secondary to the vascular lesion.

NATURAL HISTORY OF THE DISEASE

Pericardial involvement may occur, but clinical symptoms are rare. At autopsy, 35% of patients have pericardial effusions, but only 10–15% are symptomatic. Pericardial tamponade has been described rarely in SSc and in LSSc.

Myocardial involvement occurs more frequently in patients with SSc than in those with LSSc. The most common lesion is contraction band fibrosis, which occurs in 30–50% of patients. It is thought to be the result of repeated ischemic episodes followed by reperfusion. It appears to be unrelated to true CAD and probably represents small artery spasm within the myocardium. Fibrosis is distributed throughout the myocardium and differs from true atherosclerotic disease in its lack of subendocardial involvement and the preponderance of left ventricular disease. Cardiopulmonary function studies have shown that abnormalities of myocardial perfusion are common. Patients usually have normal cardiac angiography; thus, the abnormalities of myocardial perfusion may be due to a disturbance of the microcirculation of the heart.

Myocardial function is also abnormal in patients with scleroderma without clinically evident cardiac disease.[5] When myocardial perfusion is investigated while the hands are cooled, a perfusion defect on thallium-201 scintigraphy is seen. This change does not occur in control patients with chest pain and normal coronary angiograms. This mechanism may be responsible for the contraction band fibrosis. The prognostic implications of cardiac arrhythmias in systemic sclerosis were studied by Kostis et al.[6] They found supraventricular tachyarrhythmias and ventricular tachycardia to be common, and more pronounced in patients with other evidence of cardiac, pulmonary, and renal involvement. Arrhythmias are associated with increased mortality.

The cardiac manifestations of LSSc are distinct from those of SSc.[7] Both diseases have abnormalities of thallium perfusion, but the defects in LSSc are significantly smaller. Left ventricular function abnormalities are minor, seen only during exercise, and unrelated to thallium perfusion defects. Approximately one-third of the patients with LSSc have abnormal resting right ventricular function associated with a decrease in pulmonary diffusing capacity. Left ventricular function is impaired in SSc; patients with LSSc demonstrate right ventricular dysfunction primarily related to pulmonary vascular involvement and pulmonary hypertension.

CURRENT METHODS OF TREATMENT

Treatment of the myocardial abnormalities of SSc is very difficult. When the effect of nifedipine on myocardial perfusion and metabolism was studied,[8] there was an increase in myocardial perfusion associated with modification in energy metabolism thought to result from the anti-ischemic effect. Nifedipine was used to study pulmonary and systemic hemodynamics in patients with pulmonary hypertension associated with various collagen diseases.[9] Oral nifedipine produced an acute, sustained reduction in pulmonary vascular resistance in patients with pulmonary hypertension associated with SSc and LSSc. Another study of nifedipine and prazosin in LSSc found a favorable response to the oral administration of these drugs, but the authors warned of the risk of nonselective pulmonary and systemic vasodilatory effects. They suggested that these drugs be started with close hemodynamic monitoring.[10]

Further studies of nifedipine and captopril in SSc[11] demonstrated that patients with SSc fall into two groups. One group had a disease of shorter duration which responded poorly to nifedipine and captopril. The second group, with abnormal baseline elevations in pulmonary vascular resistance and borderline pulmonary arterial hypertension, had significant decreases in pulmonary vascular resistance and pulmonary mean pressures in response to nifedipine but not to captopril. Sfikakis et al.[12] demonstrated that nifedipine significantly improved the diffusing capacity of the lung in patients with SSc who had no evidence of cardiac disease or pulmonary hypertension.

REFERENCES

1. Steen VD, Powell DL, Medsger TA Jr: Clinical correlations and prognosis based on serum autoantibodies in patients with systemic sclerosis. *Arthritis Rheum* 31:196–203, 1988.

2. Weiner ES, Earnshaw WC, Senecal JL, et al: Clinical associations of anti-centromere antibodies and antibodies to topoisomerase I: A study of 355 patients. *Arthritis Rheum* 31:378–385, 1988.

3. Masi AT, Rodnan GP, Medsger TA Jr, et al: Preliminary criteria for the classification of systemic sclerosis (scleroderma). *Arthritis Rheum* 23:581–590, 1980.

4. LeRoy EC: A brief overview of the pathogenesis of scleroderma (systemic sclerosis). *Ann Rheum Dis* 51:286–288, 1992.

5. Alexander EL, Firestein GS, Weiss JL, et al: Reversible cold-induced abnormalities in myocardial perfusion and function in systemic sclerosis. *Ann Intern Med* 105:661–668, 1986.

6. Kostis JB, Seibold JR, Turkevich D, et al: Prognostic importance of cardiac arrhythmias in systemic sclerosis. *Am J Med* 84:1007–1015, 1988.

7. Follansbee WP, Curtiss EI, Medsger TA Jr, et al: Myocardial function and perfusion in the CREST syndrome variant of progressive systemic sclerosis: Exercise radionuclide evaluation and comparison with diffuse scleroderma. *Am J Med* 77:489–496, 1984.

8. Duboc D, Kahan A, Maziere B, et al: The effect of nifedipine on myocardial perfusion and metabolism in systemic sclerosis. *Arthritis Rheum* 34:198–203, 1991.

9. Alpert MA, Pressly TA, Mukerji V, et al: Acute and long-term effects of nifedipine on pulmonary and systemic hemodynamics in patients with pulmonary hypertension associated with diffuse systemic sclerosis, the CREST syndrome and mixed connective tissue disease. *Am J Cardiol* 68:1687–1691, 1991.

10. Glikson M, Pollack A, Dresner-Feigin R, et al: Nifedipine and prazosin in the management of pulmonary hypertension in CREST syndrome. *Chest* 98:759–761, 1990.

11. Sfikakis PP, Kyriakidis MK, Vergos CG, et al: Cardiopulmonary hemodynamics in systemic sclerosis and response to nifedipine and captopril. *Am J Med* 90:541–546, 1991.

12. Sfikakis PP, Kyriakidis MK, Vergos CG, et al: Diffusing capacity of the lung and nifedipine in systemic sclerosis. *Arthritis Rheum* 33:1634–1639, 1990.

Ankylosing Spondylitis

James W. Logan, M.D.

PRESENTING MANIFESTATIONS

History

Ankylosing spondylitis (AS) is a chronic inflammatory arthritis of axial joints, particularly the sacroiliac joints. It is more common in men than in women, and its peak period of onset is puberty. Extra-articular manifestations commonly include enthesitis and anterior uveitis. Pulmonary disease is usually seen after 10–15 years of disease and is most commonly restrictive lung disease. Many patients have ascending involvement of the lumbar, thoracic, and cervical spines with ankylosis and severe kyphosis in extreme cases.[1]

Physical Examination

Stiffness, stooped posture, and diminished spinal motion are common. Asymmetric tenderness or swelling of peripheral joints may be seen. Although sacroiliitis is a hallmark of the disease, there are no satisfactory methods to determine its presence.[1] Spinal motion evaluation is important in the diagnosis and management of AS patients.[2]

Laboratory Evaluation

The HLAB-27 antigen is present in over 90% of patients in most studies whether the population prevalence of HLAB-27 is high or low. In general, blacks have a lower prevalence of HLAB-27 than whites; however, the highest figures are noted in Asians and Native Americans. Other laboratory studies are nonspecific.[1]

Radiographic studies of the spine and sacroiliac joints are important. Sacroiliitis is symmetric but may be unilateral early in the course of the disease. Spinal changes begin with squaring of vertebral bodies and the formation of syndesmophytes. In severe cases, bamboo spine may form.[1]

DIAGNOSTIC CRITERIA

The diagnosis is made clinically based on the following criteria, along with radiographic changes: (1) limitation of lumbar spine motion in anterior flexion, lateral flexion, and extension; (2) pain at the thoracolumbar junction or lumbar spine; and (3) limitation of chest expansion to 2.5 cm or less measured at the level of the fourth intercostal space. Radiographic criteria are graded from 0 to 4 according to the severity of sacroiliac joint changes

DIFFERENTIAL DIAGNOSIS

Patients with AS commonly have aortic insufficiency and conduction disturbances. From 5% to 10% have cardiac disease prior to the development of musculoskeletal symptoms or radiographic changes in the spine. Rheumatoid arthritis may present in a similar fashion if peripheral joint disease is widespread. In the rare cases in which rheumatoid arthritis is associated with valvular disease, the mitral valve is involved more often than the aortic valve or the subaortic region. Syphilis causes aortic dilatation and aortic insufficiency much like that of AS. There is no difference in the lesions histologically; however, syphilis spares the aortic wall posterior to the sinuses of Valsalva and will not extend below the aortic valve or involve the mitral valve, as in AS. Marfan's syndrome causes thinning of the aortic wall but does not involve the aortic valve directly, although the resultant dilation of the aortic root causes aortic regurgitation. (Figure 2.2) Reiter's syndrome has a similar cardiac lesion but a different clinical history.[3]

PATHOPHYSIOLOGY

Clinically, significant heart disease is noted in up to 50% of patients with AS. Cardiac manifestations may precede musculoskeletal manifestations by months to years in some

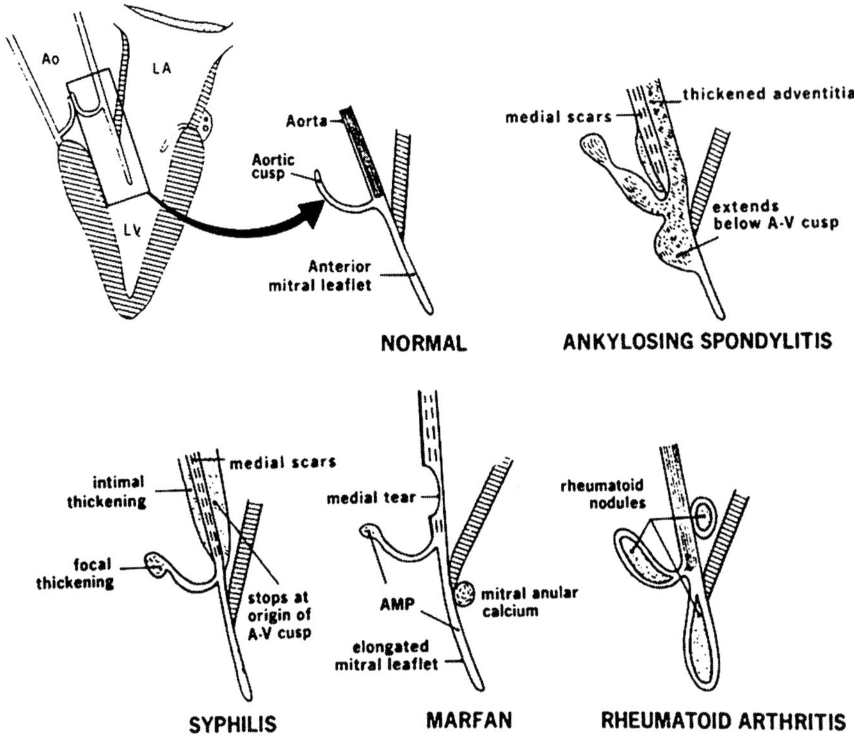

Figure 2.2. Rupture of mitral valve leaflet with vegetations in SLE. Arrow indicates site of rupture on anterior leaflet. From Bulkley BH, Roberts WG, Ankylosing spondylitis and aortic regurgitation. *Circulation* 48:1014–1027, 1973. Reprinted with permission from author and publisher.

patients.[4,5] Aortic insufficiency and conduction disturbances are the most common manifestations. Interestingly, the aortic and valvular lesions are relatively distinct. Necropsy studies show dilation of the ascending aorta and sinuses of Valsalva. Adventitial scarring between aortic valve cusps and the anterior mitral valve leaflet causes a characteristic subaortic bump, which may be seen angiographically or on echocardiography.[6] Adventitial scarring may affect the membranous ventricular septum. Valvular cusps may be shortened and thickened by fibrous tissue. Fibrous aortic wall thickening behind the commissures causes cusps to sag toward the left ventricle. Histologically, the aorta is thickened primarily from adventitial scarring and intimal proliferation, with relative sparing of the media. There are collections of lymphocytes and plasma cells surrounding the vasa vasorum.

Aortic adventitial scarring extends to the subvalvular region and ventricular septum.[3] The subaortic bump may affect the base of the anterior leaflet but is believed to cause only mild mitral regurgitation. Fibrosis may extend to involve the entire anterior mitral valve leaflet and occasionally causes significant mitral regurgitation.[7] Adventitial scarring may cause conduction disturbances most commonly affecting the region of the atrioventricular (AV) node.[5,8]

NATURAL HISTORY OF THE DISEASE

The incidence of valvular disease, conduction disturbance, and cardiomyopathy increases with the duration of the disease, as well as with peripheral joint involvement. Aortic insufficiency occurs in 5–20% of patients in most series.[3,5,9] Conduction disturbances also increase relative to the involvement of peripheral joint inflammation and the duration of the disease. Conduction disturbances are reported in 1–33% of AS patients.[3,5]

The most common disturbances involve AV node conduction. These include a prolonged P-R interval, as well as second- and third-degree AV block. Bundle branch blocks, fascicular blocks, and Wolf-Parkinson-White syndrome have also been reported.[5,10]

The course of aortic valve disease is gradual. In one study the 50% survival time from the onset of free aortic regurgitation was 7 years. Mitral regurgitation rarely becomes significant enough to cause clinical disease.[9]

CURRENT METHODS OF TREATMENT

There is no cure for AS. Patients with peripheral joint manifestations are treated with non-steroidal anti-inflammatory agents and physical therapy for maintenance of posture and function. Extra-articular manifestations such as episcleritis are occasionally treated with corticosteroids. Recent studies indicate that treatment with sulfasalazine in early cases associated with profuse peripheral joint inflammation may be of benefit. Occasional patients with complete heart block may respond to immunosuppressants.[5] All patients with valvular disease should have prophylaxis against bacterial endocarditis.

If angina develops, screening for conduction disturbance is important prior to starting treatment with beta blockers or calcium channel blockers.[5]

REFERENCES

1. Wollheim FA: Ankylosing spondylitis. In: Kelley WN, Harris ED Jr., Sledge CB, (eds). *Textbook of Rheumatology,* ed 4. Philadelphia, PA, WB Saunders, 1993, p 943.
2. Macrae IF, Wright V: Measurement of back movement. *Ann Rheum Dis* 28:584–588, 1969.
3. Bulkley BH, Roberts WC: Ankylosing spondylitis and aortic regurgitation. *Circulation* 48:1014–1027, 1973.
4. Kinsella TD, Johnson LG, Sutherland RI: Cardiovascular manifestations of ankylosing spondylitis. *CMA J* 111:1309–1311, 1974.
5. O'Neil TW: The heart in ankylosing spondylitis. *Ann Rheum Dis* 51:705–706, 1992.
6. O'Neil TW, King G, Graham IM, et al: Echocardiographic abnormalities in ankylosing spondylitis. *Ann Rheum Dis* 51:652–654, 1992.
7. Roberts WC, Hollingsworth JF, Bulkey BH, et al: Combined mitral and aortic regurgitation in ankylosing spondylitis. *Am J Med* 56:237–243, 1974.
8. Bergfeldt C, Vallin H, Edhag O: Complete heart block in HLAB-27 associated disease. Electrophysiological and clinical characteristics. *Br Heart J* 51:184–188, 1984.
9. Graham DC, Smythe HA: The carditis and aortitis of ankylosing spondylitis. *Bull Rheum Dis* 9:1711–1714, 1958.
10. Bergfeldt L, Edhag O, Vallin H: Cardiac conduction disturbances, an underestimated manifestation in ankylosing spondylitis. *Acta Med Science* 212:217–223, 1982.

Reiter's Syndrome

James W. Logan, M.D.

PRESENTING MANIFESTATIONS

History

Reiter's syndrome (RS) is a clinical triad of arthritis, nongonococcal urethritis, and conjunctivitis. It is considered a reactive arthritis related to gastrointestinal or genitourinary pathogens. There is also a strong relationship with HLA-B27 and with the male sex. In most series, 80% of white patients were HLA-B27 positive compared to 9% of controls. Symptoms usually begin within 1–3 weeks of an episode of urethritis or dysentery. The knees, ankles, and feet are most commonly affected in an asymmetric pattern. Conjunctivitis occurs early and is found in most patients.[1]

Physical Examination

Musculoskeletal findings consist of low-grade inflammation in an asymmetric pattern, most commonly in the lower extremities. The knees may exhibit large effusions, but the predominant targets are tendon insertions on bone (enthesitis). There may be a uniformly swollen toe or finger, the so-called sausage digit. Many patients have severe pain and swelling of the heels and Achilles insertions.

Conjunctivitis occurs in about 35–40% of cases. Uveitis is usually unilateral and may be severe. Mucosal lesions occur in up to 23% of patients, most commonly due to *Shigella* infection or postvenereal arthritis. These are shallow, painless ulcers of the glans penis and urethral meatus (circinate balanitis). Keratoderma blennorrhagicum, a hyperkeratotic lesion resembling pustular psoriasis, is found on the soles but also may involve the toes, scrotum, penis, palms, trunk, or scalp. Oral ulcers are usually transient and are often painless.[2]

Laboratory Evaluation

There is no specific laboratory abnormality. HLA-B27 is positive in about 80% of white patients and in about 50% of black patients.[1] Indices of inflammation are usually elevated.

DIAGNOSTIC CRITERIA

Clinically useful features for making the diagnosis of RS include preceding or current urethritis or diarrhea; conjunctivitis or unilateral iritis; sausage finger or toe; symptomatic lower extremity oligoarthritis; low back pain and sacroiliac tenderness; heel pain and swelling; positive HLA-B27; negative rheumatoid factor; and radiologic signs of periostitis, bone spurs, tendinous ossification, and asymmetric saroiliitis.[1]

DIFFERENTIAL DIAGNOSIS

Consideration of the same disease processes noted in AS is necessary. In addition, since both AS and RS have a similar pattern of peripheral arthritis, mucosal lesions with valvular heart disease, and conduction disturbances, subacute bacterial endocarditis and collagen vascular disease should be considered.

PATHOPHYSIOLOGY

RS is a reactive arthritis usually following an episode of cystitis, urethritis, or dysentery. The commonly associated organisms are *Chlamydia, Shigella, Salmonella, Campylobacter,* and *Yersinia.* In certain populations there is a strong association with the HLA-B27 gene. In whites, the association is as high as 80–90%; in blacks it is weak.[2,3] Cardiac disease in RS is much less common than in AS. RS patients with cardiac disease were noted to have fibrosis and chronic inflammatory infiltrates histologically identical to those described in AS and syphilis.[4]

NATURAL HISTORY OF THE DISEASE

Approximately 12% of patients have clinically significant cardiac disease which is mostly manifested by myocarditis, pericarditis, and conduction disturbances. Valvular disease develops in 10–15% of patients with chronic RS, with aortic regurgitation as the most common manifestation.

Patients have a slow progression of valvular heart disease as well as cardiomyopathy.[2,3] There are rare cases of acute aortic insufficiency in both AS and RS.[3] Proximal aortitis and a subaortic bump may be seen in RS and AS patients with aortic regurgitation. Coronary artery stenosis at the ostia is a rare association with aortitis.[5]

TREATMENT

The treatment and precautions are similar to those of AS.

REFERENCES

1. Fan TF, Yu DTY: Reiter's syndrome. In: Kelley WN, Harris ED Jr., Sledge CB (eds) *Textbook of Rheumatology,* ed 4. Philadelphia, PA, WB Saunders, 1993, p 961.
2. Misukiewicz P, Carlson R, Rowan C, et al: Acute aortic insufficiency in a patient with presumed Reiter's syndrome. *Ann Rheum Dis* 51:686–687, 1992.
3. Neu LT, Reider R, Mack R: Cardiac involvement in Reiter's disease. A report of a case with review of the literature. *Ann Intern Med* 53:215–219, 1960.
4. Good A: Reiter's disease. A review with special attention to cardiovascular and neurologic sequelae. *Semin Arthritis Rheum* 3:253–286, 1974.
5. Hoogland Y, Alexander EP, Patterson R, et al: Coronary artery stenosis in Reiter's syndrome: A complication of aortitis. *J Rheum* 21:757–759, 1966.

Rheumatoid Arthritis

James W. Logan, M.D.

PRESENTING MANIFESTATIONS

History

Rheumatoid arthritis (RA) is a common disease. Its incidence in the general population is about 1%. There are three general patterns of onset. Insidious onset is the most common. Symptoms develop over several weeks to many months in 55–70% of RA cases. They consist of arthralgia and stiffness in a symmetric pattern. Systemic symptoms such as fever, malaise, and weight loss may be present. The acute onset pattern may be seen in 8–15% of RA patients. Symptoms occur over the course of a few days. Intermediate onset is noted in 15–20% of cases. Symptoms develop over days to weeks, and systemic symptoms are not as severe as in the acute onset pattern.[1]

Physical Examination

Objective evidence of synovitis in multiple joints is usually present. Indications are erythema, warmth, or tenderness over the affected joints. The most common joints are the proximal interphalangeal, metacarpophalangeal, carpal, and metatarsophalangeal, as well as the ankles and knees. Persistent inflammation may cause deformity. Metacarpophalangeal joints may sublux and cause ulnar deviation of the digits. A similar deformity may affect the feet and other involved joints. Subcutaneous nodules may form over extensor surfaces of the forearms and hands. Extra-articular manifestations may include parotid gland enlargement with conjunctival and mucosal dryness in Sjögren's syndrome. Nonspecific lymphadenopathy may be seen. Peripheral neuropathy, palpable purpura, or skin ulcers are associated with rheumatoid vasculitis. Splenic enlargement is noted in 6.5% of patients.[1]

Laboratory Evaluation

Laboratory testing commonly shows leukocytosis, thrombocytosis, and mild anemia (Hgb 10.0 g/dl). The Westergren erythrocyte sedimentation rate is usually greater than 30 mm/hr. Rheumatoid factor is positive in over 90% of cases, and antinuclear factor is positive in low titer in 20%. Alpha-1 and alpha-2 globulins are elevated, and serum complement is either normal or elevated. Synovial fluid (SF) is usually straw colored, but occasionally it may be bloody. The SF leukocyte count may range from 5000 to 30,000, with polymorphonuclear cells predominating.[1]

DIAGNOSTIC CRITERIA

The most recent clinical criteria for the diagnosis of RA include (1) at least three painful limb joints and (2) swelling, limitation of motion, subluxation, or ankylosis of at least three limb joints. This should also include involvement of a hand, a wrist, or a foot and symmetry of at least one joint pain. These findings should include at least one of the following: (1) radiographic changes of marginal joint erosions or (2) serum positive for rheumatoid factor.[1]

DIFFERENTIAL DIAGNOSIS

A number of diseases mimic RA. Many are rare, but the more common conditions to consider are ankylosing spondylitis, gout, calcium pyrophosphate dihydrate deposition disease, chronic fatigue syndrome, collagen vascular disease, fibromyalgia syndrome, glucocorticoid withdrawal syndrome, infectious arthritis, osteoarthritis, Parkinson's disease, polymyalgia rheumatica, and giant cell arteritis.[1] However, symmetric joint involvement of more than 6 weeks' duration in a patient over 40 years old strongly suggests the diagnosis of RA.

PATHOPHYSIOLOGY

Clinically inapparent cardiac disease is detected in 50–65% of patients with RA. Many have nonspecific subacute inflammatory lesions with healing and fibrosis. The pericardium is affected most often (29%), followed by the myocardium (19%), endocardium (6%), and valves (5–10%).[2–5] A granuloma, pathologically identical to subcutaneous nodules, may form in any region of the heart or aorta.[2,3] Granulomatous lesions are noted in 1–3% of cases of rheumatoid heart disease. These patients tend to have high titers of rheumatoid factor, as well as visceral involvement or peripheral neuropathy.[4]

Pericarditis is the most common cardiac manifestation of RA. This was reported in up to 50% of patients in necropsy studies.[1–3] Pericardial effusion can be detected by echocardiography in up to 31% of patients with RA.[1] Most of the time, pericarditis is not detected clinically. Prakesh et al.[6] performed a prospective echocardiographic study on 16 RA patients who were asymptomatic and detected pericardial effusion in 7 of them. Most patients with pericarditis had disease of longer duration and more disability from arthritis. All patients with pericarditis had electrocardiographic changes. Most of these changes were abnormal ST segments, T waves, or evidence of left ventricular hypertrophy without underlying hypertension diabetes or coronary artery disease.[3,4] Pathologic examination of such patients shows localized areas of chronic inflammation, fibrosis, and healing. Inflammatory cells are mainly lymphocytes with few plasma cells.[5] Clinically significant pericarditis with large effusions, granuloma formation, acute pericarditis, and rare cases of tamponade have been reported.[3,7,8] Immunologic studies on pericardial fluid show similarities to synovial fluid in RA patients. Immune complex formation occurs in greater concentration than in serum. There is diminished whole hemolytic complement activity localized to pericardial fluid. This points to an intense localized inflammatory reaction similar to synovitis.[9]

Nonspecific myocarditis was reported in 20% of RA patients in necropsy studies.[2,4,5] Most patients had evidence of pericarditis or endocardial disease as well. There was focal infiltration of lymphocytes, plasma cells, and histiocytes. However, most patients did not have clinically apparent myocarditis.[2,5] Diffuse myocarditis has been reported in 1% of RA patients and may be fatal.

Endocardial disease occurs in approximately 6% of RA patients.[5] Lesions commonly consist of focal lymphocytic and mononuclear cell infiltration with fibrosis which may occur throughout the endocardium but frequently involve the base of the aortic valve and the aortic and mitral valve rings. Calcification of the valvular cusps and rings may be observed by echocardiography. Echocardiographic studies have shown some prospective evidence of abnormal mitral valve and left ventricular function. One study noted abnormality of the anterior leaflet in 25% of asymptomatic RA patients, manifested by a diminished diastolic slope (E to F) and a shortened mitral valve excursion.[6] Another study noted a subtle left ventricular diastolic abnormality in 26% of RA patients.[8]

Inflammatory lesions of coronary arteries were noted in 20% of RA patients. Most exhibited nonspecific inflammation; 3% had granulomas involving vessels and the myocardium.[4,5]

Histologic examination shows lymphocytic infiltration, edema, fibrosis, and mild proliferation of the intima of small arteries.[5]

Rheumatoid granulomas may form throughout the heart and have been observed in 2–3% of RA patients. These lesions may cause clinically apparent disease. Histologically, there is a central necrotic area with an intermediate zone of palisading histiocytes and fibroblasts, with an outer layer of chronic inflammatory cells. Granulomas have been associated with obliterative pericarditis, myocarditis with ventricular hypertrophy, and congestive heart failure and destructive valvulitis affecting the base of the mitral valve, aortic valve, and tricuspid valve in order of occurrence.[2,4,5]

NATURAL HISTORY OF THE DISEASE

Even with the high incidence of cardiac disease reported in RA (50–60%), only a minority of patients develop clinical manifestations. Many cases are clinically indistinguishable from atherosclerotic disease. RA patients have a significant incidence of calcific aortic stenosis with sclerotic change in valve bases and rings. Calcification of the mitral valve is also reported. Clinically significant valvular disease is apparent in 5–10% of RA patients, usually after 10 years of arthritis with destructive lesions.[5]

Pericarditis is a well-known manifestation of RA. In spite of the high incidence reported at necropsy and with echocardiography, clinically significant pericarditis causing tamponade or heart failure is rare and is usually seen in patients with severe erosive arthritis, other extra-articular manifestations, or a duration of RA longer than 10 years.[2,5]

Arrhythmia may occur in rheumatoid heart disease. Supraventricular tachycardia followed by ventricular arrhythmia is the most common form. The electrocardiogram shows AV block with occasional bundle branch blocks. Granulomas have been associated with second-degree and complete heart block in a few severe cases. The incidence of atherosclerotic heart disease is similar to that of the general population. There is less hypertensive cardiomyopathy.[2,5]

CURRENT METHODS OF TREATMENT

Early control of inflammatory disease is important. In most patients this includes nonsteroidal anti-inflammatory agents, corticosteroids, and disease-modifying agents such as gold, methotrexate, penicillamine, or hydroxychloroquine (Plaquenil). Patients with severe vasculitis may require alkylating agents.[1] There have been case reports of the use of colchicine in the setting of recurrent pericarditis.[10]

There have been isolated reports of accelerated granulomatous disease and severe pericarditis with methotrexate use.[7] Severe valvular or myocardial disease is treated by conventional methods. Severe pericarditis may require pericardial drainage or, rarely, pericardiectomy.[1]

REFERENCES

1. Harris ED Jr: Clinical features of rheumatoid arthritis. In Kelley WN, Harris ED Jr., Sledge CB (eds) *Textbook of Rheumatology*, ed 4. Philadelphia, WB Saunders, 1993, p 874.
2. Cruickshank B: Heart lesions in rheumatoid disease. *J Pathol Bacteriol* 75:223–240, 1958.
3. Bonfiglio T, Atwater EC: Heart disease in patients with seropositive rheumatoid arthritis. *Arch Intern Med* 124:714–719, 1969.

4. Wentraub AM, Zvaifler NJ: The occurrence of valvular and myocardial disease in patients with chronic joint deformity. *Am J Med* 35:145–162, 1963.

5. Lebowitz WB: The heart in rheumatoid arthritis. *Ann Intern Med* 58:102–123, 1963.

6. Prakash R, Atassi A, Poske R, et al: Prevalence of pericardial effusion and mitral-valve involvement in patients with rheumatoid arthritis without cardiac symptoms. *N Engl J Med* 289:597–600, 1973.

7. Abu-Shakra M, Nicol P, Urowitz MB: Accelerated nodulosis, pleural effusion and pericardial tamponade during methotrexate therapy. *J Rheum* 21:934–937, 1994.

8. Maione S, Valentini G, Giunta A, et al: Cardiac involvement in rheumatoid arthritis: An echocardiographic study. *Cardiology* 83:234–239, 1993.

9. Halla JT, Schrohenloher RE, Koopman WJ: Local immune responses in certain extra-articular manifestations of rheumatoid arthritis. *Ann Rheum Dis* 51:698–701, 1992.

10. Fernandez-Muixi J, Vidal F, Bardaji A, et al: Recurrent pericarditis and cardiac tamponade in rheumatoid arthritis: effectiveness of colchicine. *Br J Rheum* 33:596–597, 1994.

Marfan's Syndrome

Hugo E. Jasin, M.D.

PRESENTING MANIFESTATIONS

Marfan's syndrome is an autosomal dominant, inheritable disease of the connective tissues characterized by tall stature, arachnodactyly, dislocation of the lens (ectopic lentis) and dilatation of the ascending aorta with aortic regurgitation (Table 2.2). The phenotypic expression of the various features is quite variable, ranging from widespread abnormalities involving the musculoskeletal system, cardiovascular system, and eyes to the forme fruste, with only mild manifestations involving only one of two systems.[1–3]

The affected patients are tall due to disproportionately long legs. The arm span is abnormally wide; a span greater than 1.03 times the height is considered abnormal. In addition, the upper:lower segment ratio measured from the top of the symphysis pubis to the floor and subtracted from the stature to obtain the upper segment is abnormally low in most patients with Marfan's syndrome. Arachnodactyly is also a common manifestation of the disease. This is best shown by wrapping the opposite wrist with fingers I and V, resulting in overlap of these two fingers due to a combination of long digits and thin wrists. Other common manifestations include a high, narrow palate, a small mandible, and a prominent brow. The most common abnormality involving the chest is a combination of pectus excavatum and pectus carinatum resulting in thoracic deformity. Progressive scoliosis due to developmental abnormalities of the vertebrae is also seen frequently. Joint laxity is also common and is responsible for a positive "thumb sign" in which the thumb, when apposed to the palm, extends beyond the ulnar border of the hand.

A prominent feature in patients with this syndrome is ectopia lentis, or dislocation of the lens. About 60% of patients have some degree of lens displacement by 4 years of age.

In a majority of cases, the first physician contact of the patient with Marfan's syndrome is due to cardiovascular abnormalities, which are also responsible for most of the premature deaths in affected patients.[4] The main cardiac abnormalities include mitral, tricuspid, and aortic valve prolapse and conduction abnormalities. Mitral valve prolapse is the most frequent cardiac lesion, with clinical features indistinguishable from those seen in the general population. However, a higher proportion of patients with Marfan's syndrome progress to mitral

TABLE 2.2. Clinical Manifestations of Marfan's Syndrome

Pectus excavatum/carinatun	Dolichostenomelia
Tall stature	Arachnodactyly
Spinal deformities	Recurrent hernia
Ectopia lentis*	Dilatation of the ascending aorta*
Aortic dissection*	Abdominal aortic aneurism
Aortic regurgitation	Floppy mitral valve
Mitral valve prolapse	Mitral annulus calcification
Mitral regurgitation	Dural ectasia*

*Major manifestation.

regurgitation; the valve leaflet redundancy appears more pronounced, as detected by echocardiography; and calcification of the mitral annulus is more common than in patients with isolated prolapse. The aortic valve is thin, with a myxomatous appearance. The cups are often stretched by the expanding sinuses of Valsalva. Aortic regurgitation is due to progressive dilatation of the upper attachment of the cusps at the sinotubular ridge, not to stretching of the aortic annulus (Figure 2.3).[5] Occasionally, aortic leaks may be secondary to cusp collapse, aortic dissection, or endocarditis. Even at birth, the patients may show dilatation of the sinuses of Valsalva detectable by echocardiography. As a rule, children with significant dilatation are more likely to develop clinically significant aortic root aneurysms sooner than other patients with Marfan's syndrome. In general, three distinct clinical presentations may be seen: (1) chronic aortic regurgitation, (2) aortic dissection, and (3) isolated mitral regurgitation. Aortic dissection and aortic rupture occur more frequently in adult males with aortic dilatation of more than 6 cm.

DIAGNOSTIC CRITERIA

The diagnostic criteria are based solely on the phenotype and family history. If a first-degree relative is affected, the patient should have at least two systems involved and one major manifestation (Table 2.2). If there is no family history, the proband should have involvement of the skeleton and two other systems, as well as at least one major manifestation. Plasma amino acid analysis should be performed in the absence of piridoxine supplementation to rule out homocystinuria.

DIFFERENTIAL DIAGNOSIS

Phenotypic expression of Marfan's syndrome represents a continuum, from patients showing florid manifestations of the disease to normal individuals with a spidery appearance or an isolated floppy mitral valve or aortic annulus dilation. Several congenital disorders may mimic the marfanoid appearance, particularly homocystinuria. The latter, however, is an autosomal recessive disorder which, in addition to expressing the skeletal abnormalities and ectopia lentis, is associated with mental retardation and vascular thrombosis. Genetic analysis of the fibrillin gene is not yet available for routine testing.

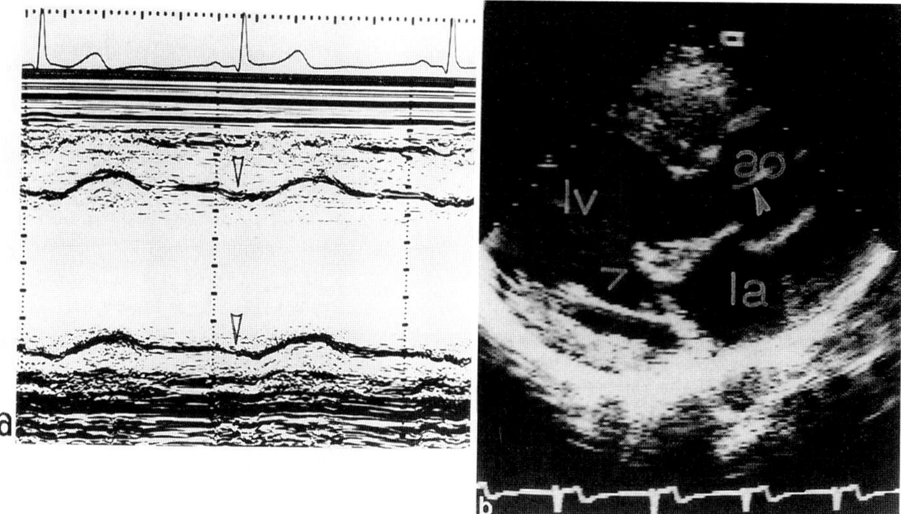

Figure 2.3. The aortic root in the Marfan syndrome as viewed by echocardiography. A: An M-mode view, in which the scale is divided into centimeters (between the large dots) and the arrowheads point to the anterior surfaces of the anterior and posterior walls of the aortic root; the diameter at end-diastolic (at the Q wave of the ECG) is 58 mm, well above the upper limit of normal for this adult of 37 mm. b: A cross-sectional, parasternal long-axis view. The open arrowhead points to a redundant anterior mitral valve leaflet, and the closed arrowhead to the aortic valve, here closed in diastole. The aortic root surrounding the aortic valve measures 41 mm (the dots along each edge of the sector are 1 cm apart). Reproduced from Pyeritz RE: The Marfan Syndrome. In Royce PM, Steinmann BU: *Connective Tissue and its Heritable Disorders.* New York, Wiley-Liss 1993, p43. Copyright 1993, Wyley-Liss. Reprinted by permission of author and John Wiley & Sons, Inc.

PATHOPHYSIOLOGY

Recent studies have shown that patients with Marfan's syndrome are affected with point mutations in the fibrillin gene located on chromosome 15.[7] This genetic abnormality leads to a major decrease in protein deposition in most connective tissues.[8] Fibrillin is a component of the microfibrils associated with elastic tissue. The deficiency leads to significant tissue weakening, resulting in stretching and thinning of the organs subjected to hemodynamic stress. The aorta and AV valves appear thin and translucent on gross inspection. Histologic examination shows fragmentation and disarray of the elastic fibers of the medial layer, a decrease in the number of muscle cells, and separation of the remaining muscle fibers by pools of collagen and mucopolysaccharides.[5] There is no evidence of necrosis, so the term *cystic medial necrosis* is a misnomer. These changes are not specific for Marfan's syndrome; they are also seen in aortas subjected to abnormal stresses.

NATURAL HISTORY OF THE DISEASE

The average life span of patients with Marfan's syndrome has not been established with certainty in view of the difficulty of making a definite diagnosis in individuals without the full-blown phenotype. However, retrospective studies have shown that both men and women have a life expectancy about two-thirds that of the population, with the survival curves dipping unfavorably in infancy. When the cause of death is known, over 90% are found to have died of cardiac causes: aortic dissection, aortic regurgitation, and congestive heart failure. Although the cardiovascular abnormalities are usually progressive, there is wide variation among patients. Aortic regurgitation in adults is rarely present when the aortic diameter is less than 40 mm, and it is always apparent when the aortic diameter surpasses 60 mm. Aortic dissection and rupture usually occur when the diameter reaches 50–55 mm; it begins in the ascending aorta and may involve the whole length of the artery. Occasionally, retrograde dissection occurs, which indicates a poor prognosis because of interference with the coronary circulation and rupture into the pericardium with tamponade.[4]

CURRENT METHODS OF TREATMENT

The main goal of treatment of the cardiovascular manifestations of Marfan's syndrome is the prevention of aortic root dilatation, since aortic regurgitation and dissection are the major causes of death. Progression of the aortic root abnormality should be followed with serial echocardiography. Dissection is best detected by magnetic resonance imaging. The mainstay of treatment includes restriction of physically activity, the administration of cardioselective beta-blocking agents,[9] and reparative surgery.[10] Pregnancy carries an increased risk of aortic dissection, particularly in the third trimester and in labor and delivery. Surgical replacement of the aortic valve is usually recommended when the sinuses dilate to 55–60 mm in diameter.[11]

REFERENCES

1. Marfan A-B: Un cas de déformation congénitale des quatre membres plus prononcée aux extrémités caractérisée par l'allongement des os avec un certain degré d'amincissement. *Bull Mém Soc Méd Hôp Paris* 13:220–226, 1896.

2. McKusick VA: The Marfan syndrome. In *Heritable Disorders of Connective Tissue* ed 4. St. Louis, MO, CV Mosby, 1972, p61.

3. Pyeritz RE: The Marfan Syndrome. In Royce PM, Steinmann BU, (eds): *Connective Tissue and its Heritable Disorders*. New York, NY, Wiley-Liss 1993, p43.

4. Marsalese DL, Moodie DS, Vacante M, et al: Marfan's syndrome: Natural history and long-term follow up of cardiovascular involvement. *J Am Coll Cardiol* 14:422–428, 1989.

5. Roberts WC, Honig HS: The spectrum of cardiovascular disease in Marfan syndrome: A clinico-morphologic study of 18 necropsy patients and comparison to 151 previously reported necropsy patients. *Am Heart J* 104:115–135, 1982.

6. Beighton P, de Paepe A, Danks D, et al: International nosology of heritable disorders of connective tissue., Berlin, 1986. *Am J Med Genet* 29:581–594, 1988.

7. Dietz HC, Pyeritz RE, Hall BD, et al: The Marfan syndrome locus: Confirmation of assignment to chromosome 15 and identification of tightly linked markers at 15q15-q21.3. *Genomics* 9:355–361, 1991.

8. Dietz HC, Cutting GR, Pyeritz RE, et al: Defects in the fibrillin gene cause the Marfan syndrome; linkage evidence and identification of a missense mutation. *Nature* 352:337–339, 1991.

9. Shores J, Berger KR, Murphy EA, Pyeritz RE: Progression of aortic root dilatation and the benefit of long-term beta-adrenergic blockade in Marfan's syndrome. *New Engl J Med* 330:1335–1341, 1994.

10. Gott VL, Cameron DE, Reitz BA, Pyeritz RE: Current diagnosis and prescription for the Marfan syndrome: aortic root and valve replacement. *Ann Thorac Surg* 55:1057–1064, 1993.

11. McDonald GR, Schaff HV, Pyeritz RE, et al: Surgical management of patients with the Marfan syndrome and dilatation of the ascending aorta. *J Thorac Cardiovasc Surg* 81:180–186, 1981.

— III —
Cardiovascular Involvement with Excessive Use of Drugs and Medications

J. David Talley, M.D.
Section Editor

Alcoholic Heart Disease

Thomas D. Conley, M.D.
J. David Talley, M.D.

PRESENTING MANIFESTATIONS

History

Patients with alcoholic heart disease present with weakness, easy fatigability, breathlessness, nocturnal dyspnea, palpitations, and a reduced exercise capacity. With careful questioning, a history of long-standing, excessive alcohol use may be elicited, though it may be difficult to obtain.

Physical Examination

In symptomatic patients, there is often elevated jugular venous pressure with evidence of right heart failure. Pulmonary crackles, tachycardia, a third and/or fourth heart sound, murmurs of mitral or tricuspid regurgitation, and peripheral edema may be present.

Laboratory Evaluation

Chest radiography may show cardiomegaly and signs of acute or chronic pulmonary congestion. The electrocardiogram may be normal or may show nonspecific abnormalities, including reduced or absent septal Q waves and poor R-wave progression. Evidence of left ventricular hypertrophy or enlargement and left atrial enlargement may be present. Left anterior fascicular block and left or right bundle branch blocks are seen in a minority of patients. Echocardiography may show dilatation of the cardiac chambers, with poor systolic function and mitral or tricuspid regurgitation.

DIAGNOSTIC CRITERIA

No definitive criteria exist for the diagnosis of alcoholic cardiomyopathy. The diagnosis should be considered in a patient who presents with signs and symptoms of a congestive cardiomy-

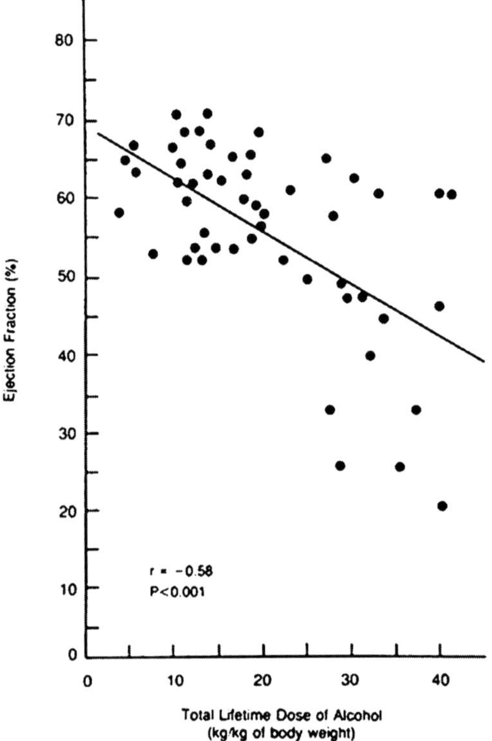

Figure 3.1. There is a progressive decline in left ventricular ejection fraction with the total lifetime dose of alcohol (kg/kg) consumed. From Urbano-Marquez A, Estruch R, Navarro-Lopez, et al. The effects of alcoholism on skeletal and cardiac muscle. *N Engl J Med* 320:409–415, 1989, Massachusetts Medical Society. Reprinted with permission from author and publisher.

opathy in whom no other etiology can be established and who has a history of prolonged, excessive alcohol consumption. To illustrate, it has been shown that a third of asymptomatic patients who consume more than the equivalent in a 70-kg man of 7 oz of 86-proof whiskey per day for 20 years have abnormal ejection fractions (Figure 3.1). In such patients with ejection fractions less than 0.50, endomyocardial biopsy has revealed abnormalities within the endocardium, interstitium, and myocytes. There may be endocardial thickening, focal or diffuse interstitial fibrosis, myocytolysis, and hypertrophy of myocytes. Fibrosis has been correlated with the severity and extent of symptoms. Electron microscopy shows interstitial fibrosis, enlarged mitochondria, disorganization of cristae, and formation of myelin bodies. The sarcoplasmic reticulum may be dilated, and large vacuoles containing glycogen have been seen.[1]

DIFFERENTIAL DIAGNOSIS

Nutritional and vitamin deficiencies and toxic additives are linked to the development of cardiomyopathy. Thiamine deficiency (beriberi) cardiomyopathy can produce a dilated cardiomyopathy similar to alcoholic cardiomyopathy. This cardiomyopathy is characterized by high, not low, cardiac output. Lead and cobalt toxicity can also produce similar pathologic findings.

PATHOPHYSIOLOGY

The use of alcohol is widespread throughout the world; it has been estimated that up to two-thirds of the adult population use alcohol to some extent. In many societies, a substantial minority of those who use alcohol are chronic alcoholics. It is not surprising, then, that alcoholic heart disease is relatively common and represents an entity that most clinicians will encounter in their practice. Usually, alcohol's impact on the cardiovascular system can be categorized by its effects on (1) cardiac mechanical function (i.e., alcoholic cardiomyopathy), (2) cardiac rhythm, (3) blood pressure, and (4) lipid metabolism/atherosclerosis.

In its later stages, alcoholic cardiomyopathy manifests as a congestive cardiomyopathy, but substantial evidence exists that early in the disease, before the development of symptoms, alcohol produces significant cardiac effects. Acutely, in healthy, nonalcoholic males, ingestion of alcohol results in decreased left ventricular diastolic dimensions, end-systolic wall stress, and systemic vascular resistance, but also in a reduction of load-independent measures of left ventricular contractility. Such observations suggest that acute ethanol ingestion has a myocardial depressant effect.[2] Similar alterations in left ventricular function due to acute ethanol ingestion have been shown in patients after myocardial infarction and in patients with class III–IV congestive heart failure.[3,4] Chronically, while still in the early preclinical stage, asymptomatic patients may have left ventricular hypertrophy, reduced compliance, and either normal or abnormal contractile function. For example, asymptomatic patients with biopsy-proven fatty liver and a history of excessive alcohol use have abnormal left ventricular contractility and an abnormal increase in left ventricular filling pressure without a corresponding increase in stroke output.[5] Asymptomatic chronic alcoholics may also have abnormalities of cardiac anatomy on echocardiography (increases in left ventricular mass, diastolic chamber size, wall thickness, and left atrial dimensions) and abnormalities of left ventricular function on radionuclide gated heart scans (subnormal left ventricular ejection fraction).[6,7] In its advanced stage, alcoholic cardiomyopathy may result in left ventricular dilatation with reduced contractile function.

The "holiday heart" syndrome is the occurrence of arrhythmias following bouts of heavy drinking and was so named because of the typical weekend or holiday presentation, with a seasonal peak around the New Year celebrations, when liquor sales also peak.[8] In alcoholics with an arrhythmia requiring hospitalization, the arrhythmias observed are, in descending order of frequency, atrial fibrillation, atrial flutter and isolated premature ventricular complexes, junctional tachycardia, isolated premature atrial complexes, paroxysmal atrial tachycardia, and ventricular tachycardia. Bundle branch aberrancy is seen occasionally but often occurs at rapid ventricular rates. Concomitant electrolyte abnormalities may be seen but are not necessary for the development of such arrhythmias. The mechanisms by which alcohol predisposes one to arrhythmias are incompletely understood. Electrocardiographically, one can show increases in PR intervals, QRS duration, and corrected QT intervals in alcoholics either with or without arrhythmias.[9] However, no significant abnormalities have been found by signal-averaged electrocardiography in asymptomatic alcoholics either during abstinence or after a bout of heavy drinking.[10] On the other hand, dogs chronically fed ethanol have a reduced ventricular fibrillation threshold that declines further with an acute infusion of ethanol. Despite their cause, arrhythmias are common in patients who use excessive amounts of alcohol either acutely or chronically and usually respond to standard therapy.

Many studies have reported the association of arterial hypertension and significant alcohol consumption. In one such study, moderate alcohol ingestion (defined as two or fewer drinks per day) affects blood pressure. However, both men and women who took three or more drinks per day had higher systolic and diastolic blood pressures and had a notably higher incidence of pressures ≥160/95 mm Hg. This effect was independent of age, sex, race, cigarette smoking, coffee use, a history of former heavy drinking, education level, and adiposity.[11] There is ample evidence to suggest that a restriction of alcohol consumption may result

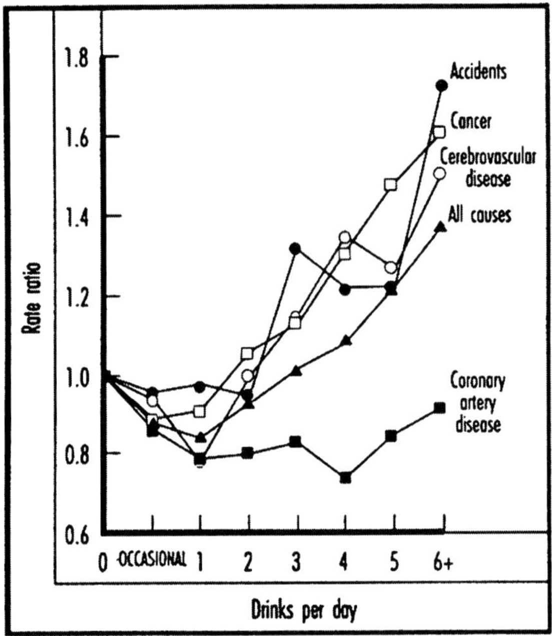

Figure 3.2. There is a "U-shape" relationship between the quantity of alcohol consumed and the death rates from accidents, cancer, cerebrovascular and coronary artery diseases. With permission from publisher and author, Folts JD, Demrow HS, Slane PR, et al. Moderate alcohol consumption, CAD, and myocardial ischemia. *J Myocardial Ischemia* 6:33–40, 1994. Reprinted with permission from author and publisher.

in significant reduction in blood pressure. The implications of such an intervention are even more profound in patients with left ventricular dysfunction, who are probably less tolerant of an increased afterload.

Despite its effects on left ventricular function, cardiac rhythm, and blood pressure, not all the effects of alcohol on the cardiovascular system are deleterious. In recent years, much attention has been focused on the effects of alcohol on serum lipids and atherosclerosis. In fact, there is a U-shaped relationship between alcohol consumption and mortality from both cardiovascular and noncardiovascular causes (Figure 3.2). Compared with nondrinkers, people who consume fewer than two drinks per day have a reduction in all cause and in coronary mortality—benefits lost with heavier consumption. This epidemiologic observation has an angiographic correlate. In a group of men undergoing coronary angiography, moderate drinkers had less coronary artery disease than teetotalers, light drinkers, or heavy drinkers.[12] This reduction in coronary disease may occur through three major mechanisms. Consumption of alcoholic beverages results in an increase in high-density lipoprotein (HDL) levels, a reduction in platelet activation, and an inhibition of low-density lipoprotein (LDL) oxidation. Many studies have noted an increase in HDL levels in people who consume alcoholic beverages, and it has been estimated that approximately 50% of the reduction in coronary mortality from alcohol may be due to increased HDL levels. Because of their central role in atherogenesis and coronary thrombosis, factors that affect platelet activity can be expected to have a favorable impact on coronary artery disease. In an animal model, high-dose pure ethanol inhibits platelet activity and coronary thrombosis. Such effects occur, however, at blood levels that would result in intoxication.[13] Nevertheless, red wine, given intravenously or orally in doses equivalent to two glasses of wine in an adult, can produce similar results. It has been concluded that red wine is a more effective antiplatelet agent than ethanol. A proposed explanation for this difference has invoked the presence of several biologically active compounds contained in red wine, some of which have been shown independently to inhibit platelet aggregation in vitro and in vivo. Lastly, alcohol, specifically wine, has been suggested to affect coronary disease through the potential antioxidant effects of some of its constituents. Oxidized LDL is more atherogenic than native LDL, and certain components of wine have been shown in vitro to inhibit LDL oxidation. The extent to which these effects have a clinical impact is not completely known.

NATURAL HISTORY OF THE DISEASE

The natural history of alcoholic cardiomyopathy is largely dependent upon the persistence of further alcohol use. In patients who abstain, symptoms and signs of cardiac dysfunction may resolve, radiographic and echocardiographic evidence of cardiomyopathy may disappear, and the outlook may be quite favorable. Improvement, however, is related to the degree of myocardial damage present when the patient begins to abstain.

CURRENT METHODS OF TREATMENT

For those in whom symptoms persist, treatment is the same as for other forms of cardiomyopathy and includes the use of diuretics, angiotensin-converting enzyme inhibitors, and digoxin. In those who continue to drink, further myocardial damage, arrhythmias, intractable heart failure, and death result. In one study, over half of such patients were dead in 4 years compared with only 9% of those who abstained.[14]

REFERENCES

1. Urbano-Marquez A, Estruch R, Navarro-Lopez F, et al: The effects of alcoholism on skeletal and cardiac muscle. *N Engl J Med* 320:409–415, 1989.
2. Lang RM, Borow KM, Neumann A, et al: Adverse cardiac effects of acute alcohol ingestion in young adults. *Ann Intern Med* 102:742–747, 1985.
3. Gould L, Gopalaswamy C, Yang D, et al: Effect of oral alcohol on left ventricular ejection fraction, volumes, and segmental wall motion in normals and in patients with recent myocardial infarction. *Clin Cardiol* 8:576–582, 1985.
4. Greenberg BH, Schutz R, Grunkemeier GL, et al: Acute effects of alcohol in patients with congestive heart failure. *Ann Intern Med* 97:171–175, 1982.
5. Regan TJ, Levinson GE, Oldewurtel HA, et al: Ventricular function in noncardiacs with alcoholic fatty liver: Role of ethanol in the production of cardiomyopathy. *J Clin Invest* 48:397–407, 1969.
6. Matthews EC, Gardin JM, Henry WL, et al: Echocardiographic abnormalities in chronic alcoholics with and without overt congestive heart failure. *Am J Cardiol* 47:570–578, 1981.
7. Read R, Bell J, Batey R: Cardiac function assessed by gated heart pool studies in an alcohol clinic population: A preliminary study. *Alcohol Clin Exp Res* 8:467–469, 1984.
8. Ettinger PO, Wu CF, De La Cruz C, et al: Arrhythmias and the "holiday heart": Alcohol-associated cardiac rhythm disorders. *Am Heart J* 95:555–562, 1978.
9. Yokoyama A, Ishii H, Takagi T, et al: Prolonged QT interval in alcoholic autonomic nervous dysfunction. *Alcohol Clin Exp Res* 16:1090–1092, 1992.
10. Koskinen P, Kupari M: Signal-averaged electrocardiography in asymptomatic alcoholics. *Am J Cardiol* 71:254 255, 1993.
11. Klatsky AL, Friedman GD, Siegelaub AB, et al: Alcohol consumption and blood pressure. Kaiser-Permanente multiphasic health examination data. *N Engl J Med* 296:1194–1200, 1977.

12. Handa K, Sasaki J, Saku K, et al: Alcohol consumption, serum lipids and severity of angiographically determined coronary artery disease. *Am J Cardiol* 65:287–289, 1990.

13. Folts JD, Demrow HS, Slane PR, et al: Moderate alcohol consumption, CAD, and myocardial ischemia. *J Myocard Ischemia* 6:33–40, 1994.

14. Demakis JG, Rahimtoola SH, Sutton GC, et al: The natural course of alcoholic cardiomyopathy. *Ann Intern Med* 80:293–297, 1974.

Cigarette Smoking

Thomas D. Conley, M.D.
J. David Talley, M.D.

PRESENTING MANIFESTATIONS

History

The effects of smoking on the cardiovascular system are extensive. The use of cigarettes is associated with ischemic heart disease, ischemic cardiomyopathy, coronary artery vasoconstriction, and cor pulmonale from chronic lung disease. As such, patients who smoke may present with stable or unstable angina, acute myocardial infarction, and left- and right-sided congestive heart failure. They may complain of chest pain, palpitations, dyspnea at rest or with exertion, peripheral edema, and abdominal distention.

Physical Examination

Patients may have tachycardia, hypertension (e.g., during ischemia) or hypotension (e.g., in low-output syndromes), elevated jugular venous pressure, pulmonary crackles, a third and/or fourth heart sound, peripheral edema, and evidence of right heart failure (e.g., hepatomegaly and ascites).

Laboratory Evaluation

Serum tests are not noteworthy in patients who present with cardiac complications related to cigarette smoking, except as they pertain to distinct clinical entities (e.g., elevated creatine kinase in myocardial infarction). The electrocardiogram may show signs of left or right ventricular and atrial enlargement, right axis deviation, and arrhythmias including premature atrial complexes, atrial fibrillation, and multifocal atrial tachycardia. The chest x-ray may show a small, midline heart with evidence of chronic pulmonary disease, prominence of the hilar vessels, and obliteration of the anterior air space on a lateral view or cardiomegaly with evidence of acute and chronic pulmonary venous congestion. Echocardiography may show enlargement of both atria and ventricles; abnormalities of myocardial thickness, systolic function and diastolic function; valvular regurgitation; and evidence of pulmonary hypertension.

DIAGNOSTIC CRITERIA

No criteria exist for the diagnosis of heart disease specifically related to cigarette smoking. Smoking is a coexistent risk factor for commonly seen entities, and the usual methods employed for diagnosing ischemic heart disease, cardiomyopathy, and other such conditions suffice.

DIFFERENTIAL DIAGNOSIS

There is no distinct differential diagnosis for heart disease specifically related to cigarette smoking. Because cigarette smoking is usually such a strong contributor to cardiac disease, its etiologic importance should not be underestimated.

PATHOPHYSIOLOGY

The mechanisms by which cigarettes affect the heart have been postulated to include (1) an increase in sympathetic nervous system stimulation by nicotine, (2) displacement of oxygen from hemoglobin by carbon monoxide, (3) increased platelet adhesiveness, (4) induction of an immunologic reaction against the vessel wall by some constituent of smoke, and (5) an unfavorable effect on serum lipids. Epidemiologically, cigarette smoking is an independent risk factor for the development of coronary artery disease, resulting in more than a doubling of risk. There is a direct association between atherosclerosis and the number of cigarettes smoked, and this effect is amplified by coexistent risk factors.[1] Data from the Multiple Risk Factor Intervention Trial suggest that smokers with cholesterol and blood pressure levels in the highest quintile have coronary heart disease death rates 20 times those of nonsmokers with cholesterol and blood pressure levels in the lowest quintile.[2]

Acutely, cigarette smoking results in increased coronary vasomotor tone during dipyridamole-induced hyperemia. It has been speculated that this effect results in lower ischemic thresholds in smokers with coronary artery disease and may contribute to an increased risk of sudden cardiac death.[3] Evidence suggests that cigarette smoking is associated with endothelial dysfunction. Intracoronary administration of acetylcholine results in dilatation of normal coronary arteries. However, in smokers with angiographically normal coronary arteries, intracoronary acetylcholine causes coronary artery constriction, although such vessels dilate normally in response to isosorbide dinitrate.[4]

Besides its effects on coronary syndromes, smoking acutely and chronically results in changes in cardiovascular hemodynamics. In chronic smokers, smoking of one cigarette produces an increase in heart rate, a prolongation of the isovolumic relaxation time, a reduction in early diastolic flow, and an increase in late diastolic flow resulting in an increase in the atrial contribution to ventricular filling.[5] Other echocardiographic abnormalities predictive of increased resting myocardial oxygen consumption may be shown in smokers.[6] Thus, cigarette smoking affects left ventricular function independently of its role as a risk factor for atherosclerosis.

NATURAL HISTORY OF THE DISEASE

As indicated above, the natural history of heart disease related to cigarette smoking is one of progressive cardiac decompensation. The clinical course of patients who continue to smoke is punctuated by repeated episodes of myocardial ischemia and ventricular dysfunction. In the Coronary Artery Surgery Study, among those who smoked at the baseline, continued smoking produced an increase in the relative risk of death 1.73 times that of controls at 10 years.[7]

After 10 years, smokers were less likely to be angina free, more likely to be unemployed, more limited in their activity, and more likely to be admitted to a hospital.

CURRENT METHODS OF TREATMENT

The increased risk of cardiovascular disease related to cigarette smoking diminishes with cessation of smoking. The risk of developing atherosclerosis, in particular, diminishes significantly with smoking cessation. Abstinence should be considered one of the most important forms of treatment of cigarette-related heart disease. Otherwise, standard therapy for the cardiac complications of cigarette smoking should be employed.

REFERENCES

1. Witteman JC, Groggee DE, Valkenbury HA, et al: Cigarette smoking and the development and progression of aortic atherosclerosis. A 9-year population-based follow-up study in women. *Circulation* 88(5 Pt 1):2156–2162, 1993.
2. Neaton JD, Wentworth D: Serum cholesterol, blood pressure, cigarette smoking, and death from coronary heart disease. Overall findings and differences by age for 316,099 white men. Multiple Risk Factor Intervention Trial Research Group. *Arch Intern Med* 152:56–64, 1992.
3. Czernin J, Sun K, Brunken R, et al: Effect of acute and long-term smoking on myocardial blood flow and flow reserve. *Circulation* 91:2891–2897, 1995.
4. Nitenberg A, Antony I, Foult JM: Acetylcholine-induced coronary vasoconstriction in young, heavy smokers with normal coronary arteriographic findings. *Am J Med* 95:71–77, 1993.
5. Stork R, Eichstadt G, Mockel M, et al: Changes of diastolic function induced by cigarette smoking: An echocardiographic study in patients with coronary artery disease. *Clin Cardiol* 15:80–86, 1992.
6. Gidding SS, Xie X, Liu K, et al: Cardiac function in smokers and nonsmokers: The CARDIA study. The Coronary Artery Risk Development in Young Adults Study. *J Am Coll Cardiol* 26:211–216, 1995.
7. Cavender JB, Rogers WJ, Fisher LD, et al: Effects of smoking on survival and morbidity in patients randomized to medical or surgical therapy in the Coronary Artery Surgery Study (CASS): 10-year follow-up. CASS investigators. *J Am Coll Cardiol* 20:287–294, 1992.

Cocaine-Related Cardiac Disorders

Thomas D. Conley, M.D.
J. David Talley, M.D.

PRESENTING MANIFESTATIONS

History

The most important cardiovascular complications of cocaine use include myocardial ischemia/infarction, cardiomyopathy/myocarditis, arrhythmias, and endocarditis. The most frequent complaints related to the use of cocaine are cardiopulmonary (chest pain, dyspnea, palpitations), neurologic (dizziness, headache, paresthesias, tremor), and psychiatric (anxiety, psychosis, confusion, and suicidal behavior).[1] Most patients have only minor complications and require neither hospitalization nor intensive medical therapy; however, serious, life-threatening, and sometimes fatal complications occur. Of these, by far the most serious ones are myocardial ischemia and infarction. Most patients with cocaine-induced myocardial infarction are relatively young males (in the fourth decade of life), and infarction may occur after first-time use. The onset of symptoms may occur minutes to hours after ingestion, is unrelated to the route of ingestion, and may occur in the presence of angiographically normal coronary arteries.

Physical Examination

Tachycardia and hypertension are common, but the pulse may be normal or reduced. Patients may have an altered sensorium. In the presence of endocarditis, fever, tachycardia, a murmur, and classic cutaneous stigmata of endocarditis may be seen.

Laboratory Evaluation

Serum blood tests are often unremarkable, although elevations of creatine kinase may be seen in myocardial infarction. Bacteremia may be seen in the presence of endocarditis. As with other forms of drug-related endocarditis, isolation of staphylococci is relatively more common. Electrocardiography may show evidence of myocardial ischemia, injury, or infarction. Arrhythmias are common and include sinus tachycardia, premature atrial and ventricular complexes, supraventricular and ventricular tachycardia, ventricular fibrillation, conduction delays, and heart block. Echocardiography may show reduced left ventricular systolic function, particularly after chronic exposure, or evidence of endocarditis. Coronary arteriography may show atherosclerosis and partial or complete coronary occlusion with thrombus, but even in the presence of myocardial infarction, the coronary arteries may be angiographically normal.

DIAGNOSTIC CRITERIA

The strongest evidence implicating cocaine as the cause of cardiovascular pathology is the finding of cocaine or its metabolites in the blood or urine. Although this does not definitively establish the cause and effect, in the appropriate clinical setting, such a finding is highly suggestive and provides sufficient evidence to plan therapy.

DIFFERENTIAL DIAGNOSIS

The differential diagnosis of cocaine-induced cardiac abnormalities includes the usual causes of cardiomyopathy, arrhythmias and ischemic coronary syndromes, but ingestion of other cardiac stimulants should also be considered (e.g., amphetamines; see below), as should the concomitant use of other cardiac toxins (e.g., alcohol).

PATHOPHYSIOLOGY

Cocaine is usually injected intravenously or insufflated nasally; crack is smoked and derives its name from the popping sound made when heated. The onset of action of these drugs is rapid, peaks in minutes, and may last for up to 90 min. The cardiac complications of cocaine use are due to its pharmacologic properties of adrenergic stimulation, sodium channel blockade, and platelet activation/thrombosis (Figure 3.3).

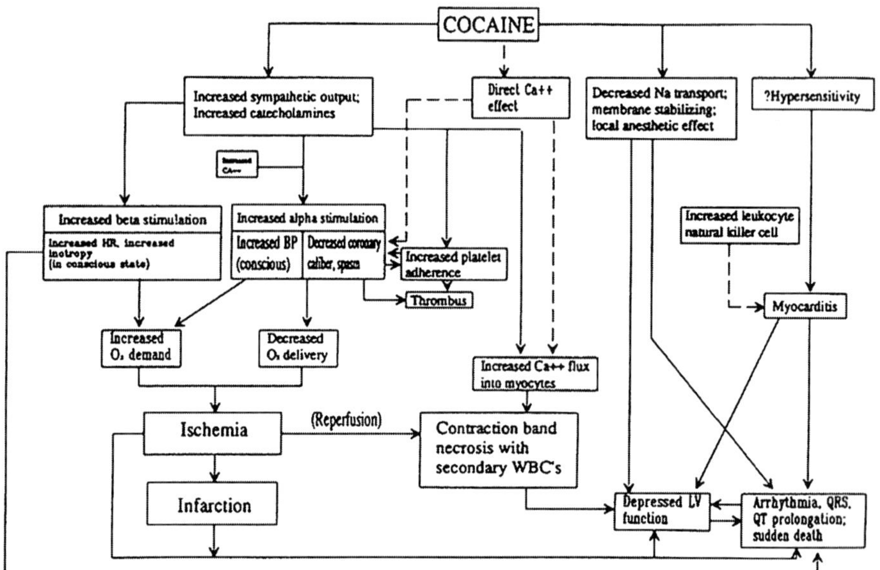

Figure 3.3.   Schematic diagram illustrating the potential mechanisms of cocaine's cardiotoxic effects. From Kloner RA, Hale S, Alker K, Rezkalla S. The effects of acute and chronic cocaine use on the heart. *Circulation* 85:407–419, 1992. Reprinted with permission from author and publisher.

In both the central and peripheral nervous systems, cocaine blocks the presynaptic reuptake of catecholamines, including norepinephrine and dopamine, and increases the release of catecholamines. Excess catacholamines at the postsynaptic level result in sympathetic stimulation of alpha- and beta-receptors, producing increases in heart rate, cardiac automaticity, contractility, and vasoconstriction. Adrenergic stimulation increases myocardial oxygen demand by increasing heart rate, contractility, and blood pressure. Some patients with evanescent ST segment elevation, chest pain, and angiographically normal coronary arteries may have coronary artery spasm. Spasm may occur through two mechanisms: alpha-adrenergic stimulation and a calcium-mediated effect on smooth muscle contraction. In vitro, cocaine-induced vasoconstriction may be blocked by pretreatment with a calcium antagonist. Intranasal cocaine, in doses used for rhinolaryngologic surgery, has been shown to produce reductions in coronary artery diameter and coronary sinus blood flow.[2] These effects are reversed by alpha-adrenergic blockade. Circulating catecholamines are elevated following cocaine ingestion. This increased sympathetic tone enhances electrical instability, particularly in the setting of ischemia, and predisposes to arrhythmias. The increased intracellular calcium levels resulting from sympathetic stimulation may promote after depolarizations, which have been implicated in arrhythmogenesis.

Cocaine also has a local anesthetic or membrane-stabilizing effect, with electrophysiologic properties similar to those of class I antiarrhythmics. By blocking myocardial fast sodium channels, cocaine produces a depression of depolarization, a slowing of conduction velocity, and a prolongation of atrial and ventricular refractoriness. Such effects result in a prolongation of the PR, QRS, and QT intervals. Furthermore, impaired impulse conduction produced by sodium channel blockade provides a substrate for reentry.

In vitro, cocaine induces platelets to release their alpha-granule contents and bind fibrinogen to their surfaces, produces increased platelet aggregability, and potentiates platelet thromboxane production.[3] Platelet aggregation and coronary thrombosis may occur in the presence or absence of underlying atherosclerotic disease, but while patients with cocaine-induced myocardial ischemia and infarction may have angiographically normal coronary arteries, several autopsy reports have identified an association between cocaine use and the prevalence of atherosclerosis.

Cocaine may also cause marked depression in myocardial function. In a dog model, acute administration of cocaine resulted in a rise in left ventricular end-diastolic pressure and a significant reduction in left ventricular ejection fraction.[4] These effects are magnified by concomitant administration of ethanol—a combination often seen clinically. Cardiomyopathy and heart failure have been reported in patients who used cocaine chronically and in whom no other cause could be found. Histologic evaluation has shown the presence of contraction band necrosis and evidence of myocarditis. Left ventricular dysfunction may resolve with abstinence. The mechanisms by which cocaine results in a depression of ventricular function are not fully understood but include (1) direct toxic effects of cocaine, (2) repeated microvascular injury from vasospasm and ischemia, (3) deleterious effects of prolonged sympathetic stimulation such as that seen in pheochromocytoma, (4) hypersensitivity myocarditis secondary to cocaine or associated contaminants (e.g., heavy metals), and (5) noncocaine causes related to patients' lifestyles (e.g., alcohol abuse and nutritional deficiencies).

Intravenous drug use in general is a risk factor for endocarditis, but intravenous use of cocaine in particular appears to pose an additional risk.[5] The reasons for this are not fully known but have been suggested to be due to the following. Cocaine is not heated prior to injection, as some other drugs are (e.g., heroin), and this may allow the injection of more pathogens. Stress predisposes to endocarditis, and cocaine use can produce intense physiologic stress. Prolonged use of cocaine may result in interstitial and endothelial damage, providing a site for bacterial attachment and subsequent endocarditis.

NATURAL HISTORY OF THE DISEASE

Although it lacks the lengthy historical tradition that ethanol enjoys in Western societies, cocaine use can be traced back to several hundred years B.C. in South American natives, who chewed or sucked the leaves of the *Erythroxylon coca* plant. In those societies, its use was often restricted to religious ceremonies and some other circumstances; more casual use was taboo. In more recent times, however, the use of products prepared from those leaves (ben zoylecgonine or cocaine, the crystalline, water-soluble alkaloid, and crack, the nonsalt form prepared from cocaine hydrochloride by organic extraction with ether) has become a major social and medical problem.[6] The natural history of long-term cocaine use is unknown, though as mentioned, chronic use may result in cardiomyopathy. The difficulty in achieving abstinence may result in repeated hospitalizations for myocardial ischemia and arrhythmias.

CURRENT METHODS OF TREATMENT

The treatment of cocaine-induced myocardial ischemia and infarction is directed to blockade of adrenergic stimulation and reversal of intracoronary thrombosis. Selective beta-blockade leads to unopposed alpha-adrenergic stimulation, resulting in a further reduction in coronary sinus blood flow and coronary arterial diameter and an increase in coronary vascular resistance. It should therefore be avoided. Instead, treatment with an alpha-receptor blocker such as phentolamine or with a combined alpha and beta blocker such as labetalol has been advocated. Thrombolytic therapy has been used safely in cocaine-related myocardial infarction, but no significant effect on peak MB fraction of creatine kinase (CK-MB) or clinical complications has been demonstrated.[7] The treatment of cocaine-induced cardiomyopathy includes abstinence and standard therapy of left ventricular dysfunction. Treatment of cocaine-induced arrhythmias should be directed to the underlying cause (e.g., ischemia), but class I antiarrhythmic agents should be avoided. Routine therapy should be employed for cocaine-related endocarditis.

REFERENCES

1. Brody SL, Slovis CM, Wrenn KD: Cocaine-related medical problems: Consecutive series of 233 patients. *Am J Med* 88:325–331, 1990.
2. Lange RA, Cigarroa RG, Yancy CW, et al: Cocaine-induced coronary-artery vasoconstriction. *N Engl J Med* 321:1557–1562, 1989.
3. Kugelmass AD, Atsushi O, Monahan K, et al: Activation of human platelets by cocaine. *Circulation* 88:876–883, 1993.
4. Uszenski RT, Gillis RA, Schaer GL, et al: Additive myocardial depressant effects of cocaine and ethanol. *Am Heart J* 124:1276–1283, 1992.
5. Chambers JF, Morris DL, Tauber MG, et al: Cocaine use and the risk for endocarditis in intravenous drug users. *Ann Intern Med* 106:833–836, 1987.
6. Mouhaffel AH, Madu EC, Satmary WA, et al: Cardiovascular complications of cocaine. *Chest* 107:1426–1434, 1995.
7. Hollander JE, Burstein JL, Hoffman RS, et al: Cocaine-associated myocardial infarction. Clinical safety of thrombolytic therapy. *Chest* 107:1237–1241, 1995.

Miscellaneous Drugs/ Prescription Medications

Thomas D. Conley, M.D.
J. David Talley, M.D.

PRESENTING MANIFESTATIONS

History

A history of drug use associated with symptoms of chest discomfort, myocardial infarction without coexisting classic risk factors, cardiac arrest, or shortness of breath suggesting congestive heart failure are clues to the use of illicit or excessive use of drugs.

Physical Examination

Patients who ingest the stimulant phenylpropanolamine may have episodic systemic arterial hypertension and cardiac arrest. Hypertensive urgencies have been associated with the use of phencyclidine.

Laboratory Evaluation

Cardiac arrest may follow ingestion of the newer, long-acting H-1 antihistamines (e.g., terfenadine and astemizole). Patients may present with syncope. The electrocardiogram may show prolongation of the QT interval and malignant ventricular arrhythmias including torsades de pointes. These complications typically occur after an overdose, in the presence of liver disease, or with concomitant administration of a medication that interferes with hepatic cytochrome P-450 enzymatic metabolism (e.g., macrolide antibiotics). In vitro studies suggest that this proarrhythmic effect is due to potassium channel blockade leading to delayed repolarization, QT-interval prolongation, and enhanced susceptibillity to the development of premature ventricular depolarization.[1]

DIAGNOSTIC CRITERIA

No diagnostic criteria exist solely for illicit drug use and the development of cardiovascular diseases. Illicit drug use should be suspected in the presence of severe cardiovascular diseases, especially in the young or when symptoms are intermittent. The presence of the compound in either serum or urine is associated with ingestion.

DIFFERENTIAL DIAGNOSIS

There is no distinct differential diagnosis associated with illicit drug use.

PATHOPHYSIOLOGY

Amphetamines possess stimulant properties similar to those of cocaine and their use may result in similar cardiac complications, including myocardial injury and cardiomyopathy. Autopsy series have shown right ventricular hypertrophy and evidence of pulmonary hypertension, common findings in patients chronically using illicit substances that cause scarring and inflammation of the pulmonary arteries.

Caffeine is a common constituent of many foods and beverages and has received much attention concerning its potentially detrimental cardiac effects. Conflicting reports on the effect of caffeine intake and coffee drinking on cardiovascular morbidity and mortality led to a prospective study to evaluate the relationship between coffee consumption and the risk of myocardial infarction, the need for coronary artery bypass grafting or angioplasty, and the risk of a stroke. No evidence that caffeine or coffee consumption increases the risk of coronary heart disease or stroke was found.[2]

Many substances have been abused through sniffing (e.g., glue, gasoline, aerosolized household cleaners), and sudden cardiac death associated with their use has been reported. The emetic ipecac has been abused by patients an attempt to achieve weight loss. Associated electrolyte abnormalities may lead to arrhythmias, but cardiomyopathy has been seen and attributed to the accumulation of the cardiotoxic substance emetine.[3]

Anabolic steroids have been used by athletes to enhance performance, and have been associated with aggressive, accelerated atherosclerosis related to their ability to reduce HDL cholesterol markedly.

The list of prescription drugs that can produce cardiovascular side effects including arrhythmias, sudden cardiac death, and cardiomyopathy is long. A partial list of some common agents is presented in Table 3.1.

TABLE 3.1. Some Drugs with Cardiovascular Side Effects

Amphotericin B	Ergot alkaloids	Interleukin-2
Astemizole	Erythromycin	Lithium
Beta-adrenergic antagonists	5-Fluorouracil	Oral contraceptives
Carbamazepine	Fluoxetine	Pentamidine
Cyclophosphamide	Haloperidol	Steroid hormones
Dexamethasone	Ifosfamide	Paclitaxel (Taxol)
Doxorubicin	Ipecac	Tricyclic antidepressents

NATURAL HISTORY OF THE DISEASE

Continued ingestion of cardiotoxic drugs leads to progressive symptoms and signs of cardiac decompensation.

CURRENT METHODS OF TREATMENT

While it is generally advisable to stop illicit drug use, it is not known that the detrimental effects are reversible.

REFERENCES

1. Berul CI, Morad M: Regulation of potassium channels by nonsedating antihistamines. *Circulation* 91:2220–2225, 1995.
2. Grobbee DE, Rimm EB, Giovannucci E, et al: Coffee, caffeine, and cardiovascular disease in men. *N Engl J Med* 323:1026–1032, 1990.
3. Adler AG, Walinsky P, Krall RA, et al: Death resulting from ipecac syrup poisoning. *JAMA* 243:1927–1928, 1980.

— IV —
Cardiovascular Involvement with Infectious Diseases

Robert W. Bradsher M.D.
Section Editor

Cardiac Manifestations of Human Immunodeficiency Virus

Rebecca E. Martin, M.D.
Richard W. McDonnell, M.D.
Robert W. Bradsher, M.D.

DEFINITION AND PRESENTING MANIFESTATIONS

The acquired immunodeficiency syndrome (AIDS) was first recognized in 1981 and is the result of infection with a virus first isolated in 1983; the name *human immunodeficiency virus (HIV)* was given to this virus in 1986.[1,2] HIV is an RNA virus belonging to the lentivirus family.[2] Two major forms have been described, HIV-1 and HIV-2. HIV-2 is found primarily in West Africa, while HIV-1 is worldwide in distribution. Since 1981, 1 to 2 million persons in the United States have been infected with HIV, with approximately 45,000 cases of AIDS diagnosed each year.[3] It is estimated that 4.5 million cases of AIDS had been diagnosed worldwide by 1994.

Transmission of HIV occurs through sexual contact, parenteral exposure to infected blood or blood products, and perinatally. Early in the epidemic the primary populations infected in the United States were homosexual and bisexual men, intravenous drug users (IVDU), and hemophiliacs.[4] Worldwide, however, heterosexual transmission is the most common means of acquisition,[5] and in the United States this is the most rapidly growing epidemiologic category.[3,5]

HIV can infect many types of human cells but has a particular tropism for the CD4 lymphocyte. Depletion of this cell line results in profound immunosuppression over time and eventual development of opportunistic infections and certain neoplasms. Approximately 50% of seropositive persons will develop AIDS within 11 years of initial HIV infection.[5,6]

A paraphrase of a quote attributed to Osler is "Know syphilis and all of medicine is given to you." In the current era, *syphilis* could be replaced by *HIV*. Significant cardiac disease occurs in approximately 6–7% of HIV-infected persons and is the attributable cause of death in 1–6%.[7] As prophylaxis and treatment for opportunistic infections extend the life expectancy of AIDS patients, morbidity and mortality from cardiac involvement will likely increase. The cardiac manifestations associated with HIV infection will now be described.

Pericardial Disease

PRESENTATION AND NATURAL HISTORY

Pericardial disease is the most common cardiac abnormality seen in AIDS patients, with a spectrum ranging from asymptomatic pericarditis to tamponade.[8] Signs and symptoms of pericardial disease in HIV patients are variable. When present, chest pain may be atypical and intermittent. For example, in a patient with *Listeria monocytogenes* pericarditis, chest pain occurred only with hiccups.[9] Dyspnea, peripheral edema, cardiac rub, and the usual signs of tamponade may be present, as well as an enlarged or globular heart on chest radiography. HIV-infected patients with tamponade are often febrile, 62% in one study.[10] As previously mentioned, the patient may also be asymptomatic. Left ventricular function is usually normal, arguing against cardiomyopathy as the pathogenesis of pericardial effusions. The fluid usually is a serosanguinous exudate with nonspecific characteristics. HIV infection should be considered when a patient presents with fever, pulmonary infiltrates, and tamponade.[10]

Echocardiography performed on HIV-infected patients without cardiac complaints has shown pericardial effusions to be present in 10–40% in six studies summarized by Kaul et al.[8] Autopsy studies have documented pericardial effusions in 18–32%; effusions are more likely to occur in persons with advanced HIV disease, a low CD4 count, and a decreased body surface area.[11] Effusions in these patients often resolve spontaneously. In one report, 9 of 33 patients followed sequentially demonstrated resolution without therapeutic intervention.[11] Large effusions complicated by tamponade are also common. In a series of U.S. and European HIV patients with cardiac disease, 20 of 67 patients with pericardial effusions had tamponade. Death from tamponade occurred in four of these patients.[7]

DIAGNOSIS AND DIFFERENTIAL ETIOLOGY

Although many different infectious agents and neoplasms can cause pericarditis in HIV-infected persons, usually no etiology is identified despite thorough evaluation. Reynolds et al. reviewed 14 patients who had undergone paracentesis and found that a definitive cause was established in only 3.[12] Another series analyzed 13 patients presenting with tamponade; 2 were shown to have *Mycobacterium tuberculosis,* 2 had bacterial processes, and the remainder had no identified etiology.[10] Except for *M. tuberculosis,* there is usually no correlation between the microorganisms causing simultaneous infection in other organ systems and those causing pericarditis.[11]

M. tuberculosis is particularly common in HIV-infected persons, either with primary disease or with reactivation as the CD4 lymphocyte count falls. Compared to the estimated 5-fold risk of tuberculosis reactivation with steroid use, HIV infection is estimated to increase the risk of tuberculosis reactivation by an incredible 150-fold. Therefore, it is not surprising that *M. tuberculosis* is particularly common in HIV-infected persons, either with primary disease or with reactivation as the CD4 lymphocyte count falls.[7] Tuberculous pericarditis usually occurs in conjunction with another active focus of tuberculosis distant from the heart.[13] When a person has symptomatic pericarditis and active tuberculosis at another site, tuberculous pericarditis should be presumed and antituberculous therapy begun. If there is no appropriate clinical response to antituberculous therapy, then pericardiocentesis and further diagnostic studies should be performed. *Mycobacterium avium-intracellulare* (MAI) is likewise common, especially in end-stage HIV infection, and it too has been reported to cause pericarditis.[14] MAI is a ubiquitous, atypical mycobacterium which is usually pathogenic only in HIV patients when the CD4 count is less than $50/mm^3$. Other bacterial causes of pericarditis are rare in AIDS but have been reported. As in non-HIV-infected patients with purulent pericarditis, *Staphylococcus aureus* pericarditis has been described several times in HIV-infected persons.[15] HIV-infected persons have a high rate of staphylococcal nasal colonization. Furthermore, they are prone to frequent skin diseases and often require intravenous therapy, thereby increasing the risk of staphylococcal infection. Pneumococcal pericarditis has been reported in HIV patients and is more likely to occur after pneumonia. Other bacterial causes of pericarditis in HIV patients described in the literature include *Listeria monocytogenes,*[9] *Proteus mirabilis,*[12] *Nocardia asteroides,* and *Salmonella typhimurium.*[7]

Cytomegalovirus (CMV) is a common cause of morbidity in very advanced HIV disease, usually causing colitis or retinitis. The intranuclear inclusions typically formed by CMV have been demonstrated at autopsy in the pericardium of an AIDS patient who presented with tamponade, even with an unremarkable antemortem pericardial examination. Herpes simplex pericarditis has been diagnosed by pericardial fluid culture, so viral culture should be done on fluid from HIV-infected patients. *Cryptococcus neoformans* and *Toxoplasma gondii* have also been reported to cause pericardial disease in HIV-infected persons.[7]

B-cell lymphomas and Kaposi's sarcoma (KS) are the most common neoplastic causes of pericardial effusions in HIV patients. KS of the pericardium is often silent clinically.[16] B-cell lymphoma in HIV disease is particularly aggressive, and is more likely to cause symptoms and tamponade if metastatic to the pericardium.[16]

DIAGNOSIS AND TREATMENT

Diagnostic evaluation and treatment for HIV-associated pericarditis should proceed in the same manner as for the HIV-negative patient. A discussion of the specific treatment for each pathogen or condition is beyond the scope of this chapter, but we must note that in AIDS patients the potential for relapse is high after therapy has been discontinued. However, since more than one pathogen may occur concurrently, repeated diagnostic evaluations may be required.

Myocardial Disease

PRESENTATION

Myocarditis is a common finding in autopsy reports of HIV-infected patients. In a tabulation of postmortem results taken from six studies, Kaul et al. found that of 402 patients evaluated, 184 (46%) had evidence of myocarditis.[8] In more than 80% of these patients, however, no specific cause was identified. Classic myocarditis requires that both inflammatory cells and myocyte necrosis be present. Although some studies have demonstrated both lymphocytic infiltrates and myocyte necrosis in HIV-infected patients,[17] a nonspecific inflammatory infiltrate without myocyte damage is the usual histologic finding.[8]

DIFFERENTIAL ETIOLOGY

Infectious agents—viral, bacterial, fungal, and protozoan—have been demonstrated in the myocardium of 15–20% of HIV patients with myocarditis.[8] *T. gondii* is commonly found in myocardial autopsy specimens in patients from France, where the prevalence of toxoplasmosis is particularly high. Myocardial toxoplasmosis is usually associated with central nervous system toxoplasmosis, although occasionally *T. gondii* is found only in the myocardium. Cardiac involvement was considered prior to death in only 4 of 21 patients with proven myocardial toxoplasmosis at autopsy.[18] When diagnosed early enough, treatment with appropriate antimicrobials such as sulfadiazine or clindamycin and pyrimethamine has been successful.[19] Other organisms that have been identified as potential causes of myocarditis in AIDS patients are *M. tuberculosis, MAI, C. neoformans, Aspergillus fumigatus, Coccidioides immitis, Candida albicans, Histoplasma capsulatum, Trypanosoma cruzi,* CMV, coxsackie B virus, and herpes simplex virus.[8,20,21] HIV has been identified in cardiac tissue by various techniques, including Southern blot, in situ hybridization, and culture,[17,22] and is therefore a possible primary cause of myocarditis as well. However, no definitive link between histologic findings in the myocardium and actual clinical disease has been established.[8] An "innocent bystander" theory has been proposed whereby, instead of directly damaging myocardium, HIV replication might cause a release of cellular enzymes or lymphokines that are toxic to nearby myocytes.

Cardiomyopathy

PRESENTATION

Among U.S. and European HIV-infected patients, dilated cardiomyopathy accounts for 31% of all cardiac-related deaths.[7] The first cases of congestive, dilated cardiomyopathy were described by Cohen et al. in 1986.[23] These three patients had rapid cardiac decompensation following several months of recurrent opportunistic infections. Postmortem examination revealed four-chamber dilatation, myofibrillar loss, and focal myocarditis. In all three patients, the histologic processes were myopathic and generalized.[23]

Estimates of the frequency of dilated cardiomyopathy in HIV disease are variable. Herskowitz et al.[24] prospectively studied a group of asymptomatic, ambulatory HIV-infected patients with two-dimensional echocardiography and calculated the prevalence of global hypokinesis to be 14.5%. However, over the ensuing 18 months, only 5.8% of these patients developed symptomatic congestive heart failure,[24] and those with clinically apparent left ventricular dysfunction were more likely to have CD4 counts $<100/mm^3$. In another serial echocardiographic study, an 11% prevalence of left ventricular dysfunction was found in a group of 80 ambulatory HIV patients without symptoms of heart disease.[25] Three of these patients had normal left ventricular function when repeat echocardiography was performed. Persistence of left ventricular abnormality was associated with a poor prognosis.[25] Other prevalence estimates of left ventricular dilatation range from 0% to 41%. On the whole, it is apparent that dilated cardiomyopathy encompasses a wide clinical spectrum. It is often present but unsuspected clinically and is frequently reversible. When persistent, however, it is a poor prognostic sign.

ETIOLOGY

The etiology of dilated cardiomyopathy in HIV-infected patients is unknown, but it is likely multifactorial. HIV has been demonstrated to infect human fetal myocyte cells via the Fc receptor, and HIV has been cultured from a subendocardial biopsy specimen of the right ventricular septal wall in a patient with congestive cardiomyopathy and no other pathology.[22] Even though there is no direct proof that myocyte infection by HIV causes the injury resulting in cardiomyopathy, this remains a possible mechanism. Alternatively, HIV has been proposed to cause cardiomyopathy indirectly through immunologic mechanisms.[26] Many autoimmune phenomena, such as hypergammaglobulinemia, circulating immune complexes, and idiopathic thrombocytopenic purpura, have been associated with HIV-infected patients. Herskowitz et al. have found evidence of cardiac-specific autoimmunity in HIV patients with symptomatic cardiac dysfunction.[27] A role for cytokines in the development of cardiomyopathy has also been proposed. Tumor necrosis factor a (TNFa) and interleukin-6 (IL-6) have been shown to inhibit directly cardiac contractility of isolated papillary muscles.[28] Herskowitz et al. have also shown that IL-6 is significantly elevated in HIV patients with biopsy-proven myocarditis compared to levels in patients without myocarditis.[29] There appears to be an association between left ventricular dysfunction and lymphocytic myocarditis as well. Biopsies have shown foci of inflammation containing increased numbers of CD8 and mature T cells (CD2+ and CD3+).[29] Accelerated atherosclerotic lesions have been demonstrated in postmorten specimens of young HIV-positive patients with no other cardiac risk factors.[30] Fibrosis of the large and small arteries was also seen, which suggests that ischemic disease may also be a factor in the development of cardiomyopathy.[30]

In addition to the infectious agents discussed above as causes of myocardial disease, several drugs have been associated with cardiomyopathy. Zidovudine, the most common antiretroviral drug used in the treatment of HIV disease, has been reported to cause a reversible cardiomyopathy. Herskowitz et al. described four patients who developed symptomatic cardiomyopathy while taking zidovudine.[31] Myocardial biopsy in two of these patients showed active myocarditis with a predominance of CD8+ cells. Two of the patients had active skeletal myositis as well. Symptoms resolved when the zidovudine was discontinued but recurred when the patients were challenged again with the drug.[31] Both dideoxyinosine (ddI) and dideoxycytidine (ddC) caused depressed cardiac function in some of these patients as well.[31] Reversible cardiomyopathy has also been described in patients receiving alpha-interferon therapy for KS and foscarnet for CMV esophagitis. Patients with advanced HIV disease often have significant weight loss and, consequently, are often malnourished. Selenium deficiency has been demonstrated in AIDS patients and has also been proposed as a cause of cardiomyopathy.

Nondilated cardiomyopathy may be seen in patients with infiltrative neoplastic disease resulting in restrictive disease or a low cardiac output syndrome. Thirty-one percent of cardiac deaths in HIV patients have been attributed to nondilated heart failure.[7]

Right ventricular abnormalities are common in HIV patients. Blanchard and colleagues found right-sided cardiac enlargement in 24% of HIV patients screened with echocardiograms[25]; many of these abnormalities resolved spontaneously.[25] Many etiologies have been proposed for right ventricular cardiomyopathy: generalized myopathy, primary pulmonary hypertension, pulmonary emboli, recurrent chest infections, and tricuspid incompetence secondary to endocarditis.

CURRENT METHODS OF TREATMENT

The treatment of HIV congestive cardiomyopathy should follow the same course as the treatment of non-HIV cardiomyopathy, using diuretics, digoxin, and preload- and afterload-reducing agents. Since the cause is often multifactorial, a careful search for possible reversible causes such as drug toxicity or infection should be undertaken. Physicians treating HIV-infected patients should remember that HIV cardiomyopathy often regresses spontaneously, so therapy should be reviewed periodically and appropriate adjustments made.

Endocarditis

PRESENTATION

The most common endocardial lesion found in AIDS patients is nonbacterial thrombotic endocarditis.[8] Marantic endocarditis in this population is usually right-sided or multivalvular. It has previously been associated with cancer and chronic wasting diseases, both of which are common in HIV disease.[7] Most cases are asymptomatic and are discovered only at autopsy. An antemortem presentation is likely to include systemic embolization.

Endocarditis should be considered in any AIDS patient with a puzzling and unexplained fever. Because of the high-level bacteremia that often occurs in AIDS, extracardiac manifestations are often seen. Encapsulated organisms such as *Staphylococcus aureus, Streptococcus pneumoniae,* and *Hemophilus influenzae* are the most common causes of bacterial endocarditis in HIV-infected patients,[32] and with appropriate therapy, the prognosis is typically as good as it is in the drug using population. A number of more unusual organisms have been reported to cause endocarditis in AIDS patients. *Bartonella quintana,* an organism similar to the one causing bacillary angiomatosis and peliosis hepatis in AIDS patients, was isolated from the blood of an AIDS patient with endocarditis. Both the bacteremia and the endocardial lesion resolved with erythromycin therapy.[33] *Salmonella* endocarditis has been reported and successfully treated in an AIDS patient. Fungal endocarditis has been increasingly recognized in HIV-infected patients. Endocardial infections with *C. neoformans,* *Aspergillus* species, and *Pseudallescheria boydii* have been reported. Fungal vegetations are large and especially prone to embolization.

CURRENT METHODS OF TREATMENT

Treatment of endocarditis in the HIV-infected person should include appropriate antibiotics and valve replacement when necessary. Cardiac surgery has been shown to be well tolerated and does not seem to depress immune function further in an HIV-infected individual.

Arrhythmias

Pentamidine isethionate and trimethoprim-sulfamethoxazole are drugs commonly used in HIV-infected patients to treat *Pneumocystis carinii* infection. Both have been associated with cardiac arrhythmias. There are reports of torsade de pointes induced by intravenous or even inhaled pentamidine,[34] a compound similar in structure to procainamide. In one study, 14 subjects were given usual doses of intravenous pentamidine and monitored daily with 12-lead echocardiograms (ECGs) and weekly 250-beat, signal-averaged ECGs and 24-hr ambulatory ECGs.[35] Five of these patients developed a prolonged rate-corrected QT interval of greater than 0.48 sec (maximum QT interval mean, 0.55 sec) by the fourth day of therapy. Three of these five patients developed torsades de pointes.[35] Thus, patients receiving intravenous pentamidine should be closely monitored during the first week of therapy, and a different antibiotic for prophylaxis for *Pneumocystis* should be chosen if the QT interval becomes prolonged. Ganciclovir, an antiviral agent used primarily in the treatment of CMV, has also been reported to cause ventricular tachycardia.

Cardiac Malignancies

The incidence of neoplasia is higher in HIV-infected persons than in the general population. KS and non-Hodgkin's lymphoma are the most common cardiac malignancies affecting HIV-infected patients.[36] In one autopsy series, when KS was found anywhere in the body, there was a 19% incidence of cardiac involvement as well.[37] KS of the heart, which is often clinically silent, has been found in the pericardium, epicardium, and myocardium. Primary cardiac lymphoma was distinctly unusual prior to the AIDS epidemic; however, as the life span of AIDS patients has increased, more cases of cardiac lymphoma have been reported.[38] Most of these tumors are of the diffuse large-cell or small noncleaved cell types. Clinical manifestations of cardiac lymphoma include arrhythmias, congestive heart failure, pericardial effusion, and tamponade; however, some of these lesions are silent.[38] Diagnosis is usually made at autopsy. The prognosis is poor, and survival is usually very short even when the diagnosis is made antemortem, but complete responses have been achieved in patients with large-cell cardiac lymphoma. It is important, therefore, to consider the possibility of cardiac malignancy in HIV-infected persons with arrhythmias or congestive heart failure and to proceed with appropriate diagnostic studies and treatment.

REFERENCES

1. Barre-Sinoussi F, Nugeyre M, Dauguet C, et al: Isolation of a T-lymphotropic retrovirus from a patient at risk for acquired immune deficiency syndrome. *Science* 220:868–871, 1983.
2. Coffin J, Haase A, Levy J, et al: Human immunodeficiency viruses. *Science* 232:697, 1986.

3. Centers for Disease Control. *HIV/AIDS Surveillance Report* 7:1–34, 1995.

4. Curran J, Morgan W, Hardy A, et al: The epidemiology of AIDS: Current status and future prospects. *Science* 229:1352–1357, 1985.

5. Quinn TC: The epidemiology of AIDS in the 1990's. *Emerg Clin North Am* 13:1–25, 1995.

6. Rutherford G, Lifson A, Hessol N, et al: Course of HIV infection in a cohort of homosexual and bisexual men: An 11 year follow-up study. *Br Med J* 301:1183–1187, 1990.

7. Anderson D, Virmani R: Emerging patterns of heart disease in human immunodeficiency virus infection. *Hum Pathol* 21:253–259, 1990.

8. Kaul S, Fishbein M, Siegel R: Cardiac manifestations of acquired immune deficiency syndrome: A 1991 update. *Am Heart J* 122:535–544, 1991.

9. Ferguson R, Yee S, Finide H, et al: *Listeria*-associated pericarditis in an AIDS patient. *J Natl Med Assoc* 85:225–228, 1993.

10. Kwan T, Karve M, Emerole O: Cardiac tamponade in patients infected with HIV. *Chest* 104:1059–1062, 1993.

11. Hsia J, Ross A: Pericardial effusion and pericardiocentesis in human immunodeficiency virus infection. *Am J Cardiol* 74:94–96, 1994.

12. Reynolds M, Hecht S, Berger M, et al: Large pericardial effusions in the acquired immunodeficiency syndrome. *Chest* 102:1746–1747, 1992.

13. Pedro-Botet L, Auguet T, Coll J, et al: Tuberculous pericarditis as the first manifestation of AIDS. *Infection* 21:334–335, 1993.

14. Woods G, Goldsmith J: Fatal pericarditis due to *Mycobacterium avium-intracellulare* in acquired immunodeficiency syndrome. *Chest* 95:1355–1357, 1989.

15. Decker C, Tuazon C: *Staphylococcus aureus* pericarditis in HIV-infected patients. *Chest* 105:615–616, 1994.

16. Anderson D, Virmani R: Cardiac pathology of HIV disease. In: Joshi VV (ed): *Pathology of AIDS and Other Manifestations of HIV Infection*. New York, NY, Igaku-Shoin, 1990, p 165–186.

17. Beschorner W, Baughman K, Turnicky R, et al: HIV-associated myocarditis. *Am J Pathol* 137:1365–1371, 1990.

18. Hofman P, Drici M, Gibelin P: Prevalence of toxoplasma myocarditis in patients with the acquired immunodeficiency syndrome. *Br Heart J* 70:376–381, 1993.

19. Grange F, Kinney E, Monsuez J, et al. Successful therapy for *Toxoplasma gondii* myocarditis in acquired immunodeficiency syndrome. *Am Heart J* 120:443–444, 1990.

20. Rocha A, de Meneses A, da Silva A, et al: Pathology of patients with Chagas' disease and acquired immunodeficiency syndrome. *Am J Trop Med Hyg* 50:261–268, 1994.

21. Altieri P, Climent C, Lazala G, et al: Opportunistic invasion of the heart in Hispanic patients with acquired immunodeficiency syndrome. *Am J Trop Med Hyg* 51:56–59, 1994.

22. Calabrese L, Proffitt M, Yen-Leiberman B, et al: Congestive cardiomyopathy and illness related to the acquired immunodeficiency syndrome (AIDS) associated with isolation of retrovirus from myocardium. *Ann Intern Med* 107:691–692, 1987.

23. Cohen I, Anderson D, Virmani R, et al: Congestive cardiomyopathy in association with the acquired immunodeficiency syndrome. *N Engl J Med* 315:628–630, 1986.

24. Herskowitz A, Vlahov D, Willoughby S, et al: Prevalence and incidence of left ventricular dysfunction in patients with human immunodeficiency virus infection. *Am J Cardiol* 71:955–958, 1993.

25. Blanchard D, Hagenhoff C, Chow L, et al: Reversibility of cardiac abnormalities in human immunodeficiency virus (HIV)-infected individuals: A serial echocardiographic study. *J Am Coll Cardiol* 17:1270–1276, 1991.

26. Ho D, Pomerantz R, Kaplan J: Pathogenesis of infection with human immunodeficiency virus. *N Engl J Med* 317:278–286, 1987.

27. Herskowitz A, Ansari A, Neumann D, et al: Cardiomyopathy in acquired immunodeficiency syndrome: Evidence for autoimmunity (abstract). *Circulation* Suppl II:322, 1989.

28. Finkel M, Oddis C, Jacob T, et al: Negative inotropic effects of cytokines on the heart mediated by nitric oxide. *Science* 257:387–389, 1992.

29. Herskowitz A, Willoughby S, Wu T, et al: Immunopathogenesis of HIV-1-associated cardiomyopathy. *Clin Immunol Immunopathol* 68:234–241, 1993.

30. Paton P, Tabib A, Loire R, et al: Coronary artery lesions and human immunodeficiency virus infection. *Res Virol* 144:225–231, 1993.

31. Herskowitz A, Willoughby S, Baughman K, et al: Cardiomyopathy associated with antiretroviral therapy in patients with HIV infection: A report of six cases. *Ann Intern Med* 116:311–313, 1992.

32. Brown J, King A, Francis C: Cardiovascular effects of alcohol, cocaine, and acquired immune deficiency. *Cardiovasc Clin* 21:341–376, 1991.

33. Spach D, Callis K, Paauw D, et al: Endocarditis caused by *Rochalimaea quintana* in a patient infected with human immunodeficiency virus. *J Clin Micro* 31:692–694, 1993.

34. Stein K, Haronian H, Mensah G, et al: Ventricular tachycardia and torsades de pointes complicating pentamidine therapy of *Pneumocystis carinii* pneumonia in the acquired immunodeficiency syndrome. *Am J Cardiol* 66:888–889, 1990.

35. Eisenhauer M, Eliasson A, Taylor A, et al: Incidence of cardiac arrhythmias during intravenous pentamidine therapy in HIV-infected patients. *Chest* 105:389–395, 1994.

36. Currie P, Boon N: Cardiac involvement in human immunodeficiency virus infection. *Q J Med* 86:751–753, 1993.

37. Cammarosano C, Lewis W: Cardiac lesions in acquired immune deficiency syndrome (AIDS). *J Am Coll Cardiol* 5:703–706. 1985.

38. Holladay A, Siegel R, Schwartz D: Cardiac malignant lymphoma in acquired immune deficiency syndrome. *Cancer* 70:2203–2207, 1992.

Spirochetal Disease

Rebecca E. Martin, M.D.
Richard W. McDonnell, M.D.
Robert W. Bradsher, M.D.

One old (*Treponema pallidum;* syphilis) and one relatively new (*Borrelia burgdorferi;* Lyme disease) spirochetal infectious disease can have major manifestations in the cardiovascular system. The rate of syphilis in the United States had been decreasing over the past 50 years until recently, when increased numbers of cases were observed, particularly in the southern states.[1,2] This infection has been known as the "great imitator" because of its protean presentations. Lyme disease could also claim that title since it too can mimic many other diseases. The illness, first described with the aid of a grandmother who noted an epidemic of juvenile rheumatoid arthritis in Old Lyme, Connecticut,[3] is the most common tick-borne disease in the United States and has been reported from 46 of the 48 contiguous states.[4] Both syphilis and Lyme disease produce local infection (primary), disseminated infection (secondary), and chronic (tertiary) disease. The manifestations related to the heart will be highlighted below.

PRESENTING MANIFESTATIONS

History and Physical Examination

Patients with acquired syphilis have a history of sexual exposure and usually a history of a primary lesion or chancre. Classically, the lesion is a painless ulcer with sharp borders and a clean base, but superinfection with bacteria may cause both pain and an exudate. Because of the lack of pain, the ulcer may be unnoticed. Either with or without therapy, the chancre resolves within 2–4 weeks. Regional lymphadenopathy accompanying the lesion may take longer to resolve. Secondary, or disseminated, syphilis is caused by bloodstream distribution of the spirochete to various locations and may cause a number of signs or symptoms. Most have a skin rash, which may be at any site but classically is described on the palms and soles. *Condyloma lata* are verrucous lesions found in most skinfold areas (perineum, scrotum, vulva, etc). Generalized adenopathy at this stage is common. Denuded, painless mucosal lesions are found in 15–20% of patients and are known as *mucous patches.* Constitutional symptoms of fever, malaise, or weight loss are common. Neurologic involvement in secondary syphilis is not usually symptomatic, but meningismus may be found. Other uncommon presentations at this stage include glomerulonephritis, hepatitis, or arthritis. This secondary stage of syphilis also resolves with or without therapy. *Latent syphilis* is the asymptomatic phase following secondary syphilis. The *early latent period* is a time with potential for relapse into secondary syphilis manifestations. By contrast, in the *late latent period,* syphilis does not relapse into secondary disease. Late syphilis is classified as either late latent (asymptomatic), neurosyphilis, gummatous syphilis, or cardiovascular syphilis.

Lyme disease begins with inoculation of *B. burgdoferi* from a tick bite, usually a tick from the *Ixodes* complex of ticks. As with syphilis, the primary stage is local infection, known as *erythema chronicum migrans,* which begins as a red papule on the skin, with expansion of the red border but clearing of the erythema centrally. This lesion is very common, if not universal, in cases of confirmed Lyme disease. Without a history of such a lesion, diagnosis of later manifestations as Lyme disease is difficult. Again, as with syphilis, the lesion fades, with or without therapy, over approximately 1 month. Other symptoms and signs of early Lyme disease are nonspecific and include adenopathy, myalgias, backache, arthralgias, and fatigue. Days to weeks after the skin lesion appears, hematogenous dissemination may deliver spirochetes to virtually any organ, but particularly the heart, joints, and nervous system. Stage 3 or chronic manifestations of Lyme disease occur months to years after the tick bite and involve mainly the joints, but the skin or central nervous system may also be affected.

LABORATORY EVALUATION AND DIAGNOSTIC CRITERIA

Syphilis and Lyme disease are usually diagnosed by serologic tests since *B. burgdorferi* is very difficult to cultivate in the lab and since *T. pallidum* can be grown only by inoculation of animals. Fortunately, patients with either spirochetal illness are highly likely to have the specific antibody test to be positive; unfortunately, many people without infection may have a positive screening serologic study for either infection. Confirmatory tests following a screening test exclude a false-positive screening study result and give a clear diagnosis.

For syphilis, the initial study is either the Veneral disease research laboratory (VDRL) or rapid plasma reagin (RPR), the modern descendants of the Wassermann test. These tests, also called *reaginic,* are nonspecific and are therefore called *nontreponemal antibody studies.* Their major value is their ability to quantitate and, therefore, to assess the adequacy of therapy. The specific treponemal tests are used qualitatively and usually, but not always, persist for the life of the patient. These are the fluorescent treponemal antibody, absorbed (FTA-ABS), and the microhemagglutination *T. pallidum* (MHA-TP) studies. By the stage of secondary syphilis virtually all patients have a positive treponemal test, which remains positive throughout life in the vast majority of patients even with effective therapy.

To diagnose cardiovascular syphilis, a nontreponemal test is performed, with determination of the highest titer with a positive result. If the test is positive and the titer is >1:4 or 1:8, confirmation is obtained with either the MHA-TP or FTA-ABS test. Following therapy, the titer of the VDRL test is reevaluated in 3–6 months to make sure that at least a fourfold decline in titer has occurred; if not, retreatment may be required.

Lyme disease serology has been somewhat controversial. Early in the course of infection, antibodies may be absent and early therapy may abort the titer rise usually observed. Cross-reactions of false-positive results may be found with other infections (syphilis, bacterial endocarditis, mononucleosis) or with rheumatic disorders (juvenile rheumatoid arthritis, systemic lupus erythematosus). These cross-reactions are seen with immunofluorescent antibody or enzyme-linked immunosorbent assays and are typically reported as borderline or low-level positive. Western blot analysis to detect antibodies for specific *Borrelia* antigens can confirm the presence of infection. Standardization among laboratories has been improving, but further work is needed.

For clinical diagnosis of cardiac complications of Lyme disease, sera should be sent for testing for immunoglobulins M and G for *B. burgdorferi*. A second serum specimen test may be repeated over a period of time for titer changes. The confirming Western blot analysis may also be performed. However, antibiotic therapy would likely be started based on a history of tick bite or exposure, plus a complication such as heart block, plus a positive screening assay for antibody.

PATHOPHYSIOLOGY AND NATURAL HISTORY OF THE DISEASE

Syphilitic involvement of the heart causes dilation of the ascending aorta and results in complications of aortic insufficiency, aneurysm, or coronary ostial stenosis. Prior to effective therapy for syphilis, Boeck performed a prospective study of Europeans with syphilis.[5] Cardiovascular syphilis was clinically diagnosed in 13.6% of males and 7.6% of females.[6] In another study started in Tuskeegee, Alabama, in 1932, men with syphilis were followed without therapy. This unethical study found that cardiovascular syphilis was clinically diagnosed in 50% of men infected for more than 10 years.[7] Other studies suggest that aortitis may be found in up to 50–70% of untreated patients with syphilis.[8–10]

The pathology of syphilis is one of inflammatory changes in the vasa vasora secondary to the presence of organisms, leading to endarteritis and aortic wall scarring with medial necrosis. The intima of the aorta develops "tree barking" from diffuse atherosclerosis; calcification may occur. The scarring can lead to coronary ostial stenosis, and the weakening of the aortic wall may lead to aneurysm formation. Aortic insufficiency results from the aortic root dilatation manifested by the classical cardiac findings of valvular damage. The prognosis is poor, with estimates of 10-year survival of 30%.[11] Angina is the manifestation of coronary ostial stenosis, but myocardial infarction is said to be relatively rare.[12] Aneurysms are usually saccular, involving the aortic arch, and are clinically silent. Symptoms usually occur only with compression of surrounding anatomic structures, with pain, hoarseness, dysphagia, or dyspnea. Because the aneurysm may be very large, symptoms of superior vena cava syndrome may be the first clue to the condition.[11] Once symptoms occur, the prognosis is poor, with a life expectancy of less than a year.

The cardiac manifestations of Lyme disease occur because *B. burgdorferi* can cause infection in either the conduction system or the myocardium.[13] Conduction abnormalities are more common but still occur only in a small minority of patients with Lyme disease.[14] Lyme carditis in the secondary or early disseminated phase occurs most commonly with a heart block of first or second degree, although complete, irreversible heart block has also been described.[15–17] Electrophysiologic studies have found the block to be located most commonly above the bundle of His, although multiple sites may be affected.[14] Diagnosis begins with consideration of the infection and/or other manifestations of Lyme disease. The serologic studies are usually positive if Lyme disease involves the heart. The prognosis at this stage of Lyme disease is usually good with antimicrobial therapy, although deaths due to Lyme carditis are reported.[14]

The myocardial involvement with *B. burgdorferi* is thought to be associated with late-stage Lyme disease and manifests as cardiomyopathy. This spirochete has been isolated from the myocardium of patients with long-standing cardiomyopathy.[18] Interstitial inflammation with lymphocytes and plasma cells, with associated cardiac cell necrosis or edema, leads to the dilated cardiomyopathy seen clinically. Antibiotic therapy was reported to improve the ejection fraction in a small series of patients with this diagnosis.[19]

In an endemic area in the United States for Lyme disease, Sonnesyn and colleagues conducted a prospective study of seroprevalence of this disease in patients with severe heart failure.[20] Although 33% of patients reported tick bites, only 4.6% were seropositive on screening serology tests. Patients with severe heart failure were a bit more likely to be seropositive (8%) than a control group (3%), but false-positive results were fairly frequent in both groups.

CURRENT METHODS OF TREATMENT

Syphilis remains sensitive to penicillin. For early-stage disease (primary, secondary, and early latent), a single injection with benzathine penicillin is effective. For late-stage infection, including cardiovascular syphilis, three weekly injections of benzathine penicillin are recommended. Many authorities use intravenous high-dose penicillin for 10 days for neurosyphilis, and some would argue for the same regimen for cardiovascular syphilis. Obviously, anatomic changes are not reversed by antibiotics, but further progression is aborted. For penicillin-allergic patients, doxycycline for a month is the recommended therapy.

Lyme disease therapy is likewise dependent on the stage of the infection. In early infection, oral amoxicillin or oral doxycycline is effective, but in Lyme carditis, intravenous therapy with ceftriaxone in a dose of 2 g/day for 4 weeks is recommended. Oral therapy has been suggested by some authorities for first-degree atrioventricular block.

REFERENCES

1. Tramont EC. Syphilis in adults: From Christopher Columbus to Sir Alexander Fleming to AIDS. *Clin Infect Dis* 21:1361–1371, 1995.
2. Division of STD/HIV prevention. Syphilis. Sexually transmitted disease surveillance, 1993. Center for Disease Control and Prevention. Atlanta GA. 1994, p 17–23.
3. Steere AC, Malawista SE, Snydman DR, et al. Lyme arthritis: An epidemic of oligoarticular arthritis in children and adults in three Connecticut communities. *Arthritis Rheum* 20:7–17, 1977.
4. CDC. Lyme disease—United States, 1993. *MMWR* 43:564–572, 1993.
5. Gjestland T: The Oslo study of untreated syphilis. An epidemiologic investigation of the natural course of untreated syphilis based on a restudy of the Boeck–Bruusgaard material. *Acta Derm Venereol* 35(Suppl 34):1–368, 1955.
6. Clark EG, Danbolt N: The Oslo study of the natural course of untreated syphilis. *Med Clin North Am* 48:613–623, 1964.
7. Peters JJ: Untreated syphilis in the male Negro: Pathologic findings in syphilitic and nonsyphilitic patients. *J Chronic Dis* 1:127–148, 1955.
8. Cole HN, Usilton LJ, Moore JE, et al: Cooperative clinical studies in the treatment of syphilis. *JAMA* 108:1861–1866, 1937.
9. Warthin AS. The lesions of latent syphilis. *South Med J* 24:273–278, 1931.
10. MacFarlane WV, Swan WGA, Irvine RE. Cardiovascular disease in syphilis: A review of 1330 patients. *Br Med J* 1:827–832, 1956.
11. Jackman JD, Radolf JD: Cardiovascular syphilis. *Am J Med* 87:425–433, 1989.
12. Burch GE, Winsor T: Syphilitic coronary stenosis with myocardial infarction. *Am Heart J* 24:740–751, 1942.
13. Cooke WD, Dattwyler RJ: Complications of Lyme borreliosis. *Annu Rev Med* 43:93–103, 1992.
14. Sigal LH: Early disseminated Lyme disease: Cardiac manifestations. *Am J Med* 98:4A-25S–29S, 1995.
15. McAlister HF, Klementowicz PT, Andrews C, et al: Lyme carditis: An important cause of reversible heart block. *Ann Intern Med* 110:339–345, 1989.

16. Mayer W, Kleber FX, Wilske B, et al: Persistent atrioventricular block in Lyme borreliosis. *Klin Wochenschr* 1990;68:431–435, 1990.
17. Artigao R, Tores G, Guerrero A, et al: Irreversible complete heart block in Lyme disease. *Am J Med* 90:531–533, 1991.
18. Stanek G, Klein J, Bittner R, et al: Isolation of *Borrelia burgdorferi* from the myocardium of a patient with longstanding cardiomyopathy. *N Engl J Med* 322:249–252, 1990.
19. Gasser R, Dusleag J, Reisinger E, et al: Reversal of ceftriaxone of dilated cardiomyopathy *Borrelia burgdorferi* infection (letter). *Lancet* 339:1174–1175, 1992.
20. Sonnesyn SW, Diehl SC, Johnson RC, et al: A prospective study of the seroprevalence of *Borrelia burgdorferi* infection in patients with severe heart failure. *Am J Cardiol* 76:97–100, 1995.

Sepsis

Rebecca E. Martin, M.D.
Richard W. McDonnell, M.D.
Robert W. Bradsher, M.D.

The frequency of sepsis and sepsis-related death has increased significantly in recent decades to 400,000–500,000 cases annually in the United States, with sepsis now the 13th leading cause of death in the United States.[1] Cardiac manifestations play a major role in the mortality secondary to sepsis.[2] Changes in demographics and medical care have resulted in a growing population of seriously ill and immunocompromised patients, which, combined with the increasing use of invasive procedures and devices, has resulted in an increasing risk of sepsis in an enlarging group of high-risk patients.

Septic shock is associated with a mortality in excess of 40%.[3] Despite the development of numerous effective antibiotics and advances in the intensive care support of these patients, no significant improvement in the mortality rates for sepsis has occurred over the last 30 years, although it can be argued that the severity of illness has increased for these patients over the same time period.

Increasing knowledge of the host response to infection has led to the understanding of the critical role played by inflammatory mediators released in response to infection or other stimuli. Seemingly excessive activation of host responses correlates with the development of shock and increased mortality. Advances in biotechnology have resulted in the increasing consideration of potential therapeutic agents designed to modify the cascade of physiologic events which leads to the occurrence of shock and organ dysfunction. However, several experimental therapies have failed to show benefit in clinical trials of sepsis therapy. Other potential useful agents are being developed, and several are undergoing clinical trial.

The optimal management of patients with severe sepsis and shock in the intensive care unit remains a vexing problem, with continued high morbidity and mortality. Defining optimal fluid and pharmacologic support remains an area of significant investigation.

DEFINITIONS

Infections can lead to physiologic changes that are commonly referred to as *signs of sepsis*. There are noninfectious disorders such as pancreatitis, burns, trauma, and tissue ischemia that can result in clinical syndromes indistinguishable from those caused by infection. The term *systemic inflammatory response syndrome (SIRS)* has been proposed to encompass all such inflammatory conditions.[4] SIRS is defined as the presence of two or more of the following: (1) abnormal thermoregulation, (2) tachycardia, (3) tachypnea, and (4) abnormal white blood cell count.

Sepsis is therefore SIRS caused by infection. Severe SIRS or sepsis exists when organ dysfunction, hypoperfusion, or hypotension is present. Shock due to sepsis or SIRS exists when persistent hypotension or hypoperfusion occurs.

Multiorgan dysfunction syndrome (MODS) is a common occurrence in critically ill patients, often those who have an infection. Data from the Acute Physiology and Chronic Health Evaluation (APACHE) studies have documented the substantial mortality associated with organ dysfunction in critical care patients, with no change in occurrence rates and outcome in recent years.[5] MODS can develop in the absence of shock and correlates with mortality in patients with sepsis or SIRS.

Patients with possibly infectious processes are extremely heterogeneous in terms of clinical presentation, underlying etiology, and prognosis. It is recognized that the definition of SIRS includes patients with relatively mild disease. Increasing morbidity and mortality occur in patients with severe sepsis and septic shock. Risk stratification is important to predict the clinical outcome, and there is a need to define subsets of patients who may benefit from specific therapy.

A recent study prospectively followed patients meeting the definition of SIRS at a tertiary health care center.[6] Of these patients with SIRS, 26% developed sepsis, 18% developed severe sepsis, and 4% developed septic shock. Mortality from SIRS, sepsis, severe sepsis, and septic shock was 7%, 16%, 20% and 46%, respectively.[6] Patients with similar clinical pictures but negative cultures occurred in equal numbers, and virtually all received antibiotics. Most had been placed on empiric antibiotics, and their morbidity and mortality rates were similar to those of patients with positive cultures. Patients who met three or four of the SIRS criteria instead of two were more likely to develop sepsis and organ dysfunction and had higher mortality rates. The concept of a continuum of increasingly inflammatory responses in SIRS and related disorders appears to be valid in approaching patients with possible sepsis.

CLINICAL PRESENTATION

Common signs and symptoms at the onset of sepsis include fever, chills, hyperventilation, and changes in mental status. Elderly and debilitated patients may not manifest fever and other clinical signs in an obvious manner. Hypothermia can occur as well and is associated with a poor prognosis. Monitoring data from intensive care patients who become septic has demonstrated that hyperventilation and apprehension are the earliest clinical signs of sepsis, frequently preceding the onset of chills and fever. Unexplained respiratory alkalosis can therefore herald the onset of sepsis. Lethargy, obtundation, or other mental status changes are common.

Patients can progress, sometimes quite rapidly, to manifest hypotension, organ dysfunction, and bleeding complications. Leukopenia can be seen early, and usually converts within hours to leukocytosis in patients with normal hematologic status. Thrombocytopenia is common, and should prompt consideration of serious infection if not already suspected. Bleeding is relatively uncommon, occurring in 3% of patients with gram-negative sepsis.[7]

Oliguria is a frequent early sign of sepsis and shock. Liver dysfunction can also be an early clue that serious infection is present. Any initial respiratory alkalosis is usually replaced by metabolic acidosis. Hypoxia may indicate that the patient is developing the adult respiratory distress syndrome (ARDS) or noncardiogenic pulmonary edema.

Tachycardia is nearly always present with sepsis. Transient hypotension is common and frequently responds to fluid administration. The term *septic shock* is reserved for hypotension and hypoperfusion that persist after fluid challenge. The appearance of tachycardia, vasodilatation, and hypotension is associated with increased cardiac output and is referred to as *warm shock*. Hypotension may not be suspected during such a hyperdynamic phase. Vasoconstriction with decreased cardiac output may intervene, with *cold shock* carrying high mortality rates.[8]

DIAGNOSIS AND DIFFERENTIAL ETIOLOGY

A vigorous effort is needed to try to define the source and etiology of suspected sepsis. Pneumonia, urinary tract infection, and meningitis are considerations, as well as surgical conditions such as cholecystitis, perforated viscus, or abscess. Sepsis is commonly a nosocomial event, affecting many patients already under care for other conditions. Urinary tract infections, line sepsis, and pneumonia are common in this setting. Postsurgical patients have the same risks plus problems with wound infections, deep infections, and sometimes ischemic complications. Foreign bodies such as orthopedic prostheses, ventriculoperitoneal catheters, pacemakers, and vascular grafts are all potential sites of infectious complications.

Cutaneous manifestations of infections can occur and can help determine the etiology of the infection. Some streptococcal and staphylococcal strains can cause a diffuse erythroderma related to toxin formation. Focal metastatic infections occur as well. Ecthyma gangrenosum lesions are 1–5 cm in diameter, with a raised rim of induration around a central area that can blister and then form a necrotic ulcer. Such lesions are usually caused by *Pseudomonas aeruginosa* but can be due to other gram-negative organisms as well. Any cutaneous lesions may help in making the diagnosis, and aspiration or biopsy may help define the specific cause of sepsis.

Neutropenic patients may not manifest local infections such as cellulitis, with the usual swelling and erythema, because of a lack of white blood cells at the site, although pain is usually present. Bacteremia is more likely to occur in the absence of a focal source. In postchemotherapy patients with mucositis, bacteremia is believed to originate commonly from the gastrointestinal tract.

In addition to the common bacterial causes of sepsis, it is important to remember that fungal diseases, miliary tuberculosis, and parasitic diseases can present as sepsis, as can a variety of noninfectious illnesses. Diarrhea or an abdominal presentation should include workup for enteric pathogens, including *Clostridium difficile*. These conditions are usually preceded by antibiotic use but can occur after chemotherapy and spontaneously.

PATHOPHYSIOLOGY

Bacteria, fungi, protozoa, and viruses, as well as noninfectious causes, may initiate SIRS. In recent years, there has been increasing understanding that these diverse stimuli produce similar host responses, and that host-derived factors appear to mediate detrimental physiologic responses such as hypotension, coagulopathies, and hypoperfusion of organs.

Gram-negative bacterial infection is the most thoroughly studied initiator of sepsis and shock. Gram-negative bacteria contain endotoxin or lipopolysaccharide (LPS) in their outer membrane, LPS, a heat-stable molecule, has been extensively studied. LPS interacts with LPS-binding proteins found in normal serum and forms complexes that can bind to specific receptors on inflammatory cells, causing release of numerous inflammatory mediators.[9] Cytokines that appear to be central to the inflammatory response include tumor necrosis factor (TNF), interleukin-1 (IL-1), and interferon gamma (IFN-gamma).

TNF appears to play a central role in sepsis and shock.[9] High levels have correlated with a poor outcome in some but not all studies of septic shock. TNF, when administered to animals and humans, mimics most of the clinical and laboratory findings of sepsis and septic shock. It appears to act synergistically in animal models with other cytokines, such as IL-1 and IFN-gamma. LPS is not the only stimulator of TNF release, which occurs in a wide variety of disease states including gram-positive, fungal, and parasitic infections. TNF, along with other cytokines, appears to be a primary mediator of SIRS, sepsis, and septic shock.

Many of the deleterious effects of sepsis are not caused directly by cytokines but result instead from secondary mediators induced by cytokines.[9] Nitric oxide (NO), previously referred to as *endothelium-derived relaxant factor,* controls normal vascular tone. TNF in combination with other cytokines can induce the production of NO synthases, and there is considerable evidence that NO production leads to vascular relaxation and hypotension, which respond poorly to vasoconstrictors. Cytokines also stimulate the release of prostaglandins from endothelial cells, with the potent vasodilator PGI_2 being most prominent.

Endotoxin induces the release of platelet-activating factor (PAF) from macrophages, neutrophils, endothelial cells, and platelets.[10] PAF increases cell adhesion and activates endothelial cells. In conjunction with cytokines and hematologic growth factors, PAF appears to amplify mediator release. It may mediate many of the toxicities of TNF and IL-1.

Tissue injury from hypoperfusion can lead to free radical production with tissue injury and attraction of neutrophils, with resultant further damage from enzymes and superoxide release. Neutrophils appear to be a major cause of organ injury in septic shock.

Disseminated intravascular coagulation can lead to fibrin deposition in small blood vessels, with resultant thrombosis in the microvasculature. Consumption of clotting factors can lead to bleeding as well. TNF appears to play a role in this activation of the coagulation scheme.

Complement activation can be stimulated by a variety of microbial products, and can include both direct and indirect pathways. Complement activation has been associated with shock in patients with gram-negative bacteremia. Complement components such as C5a are involved in the recruitment of neutrophils to the lung in ARDS.

The large number of host factors which may be involved in the cytokine cascade makes full understanding seem remote. Both positive and negative feedback loops exist, and counterregulatory mechanisms are likely to be critical to survival and the return to homeostasis. Too much suppression of the host response may be detrimental, and presumably some patients may need augmented host defense mechanisms.

CARDIAC PHYSIOLOGY OF SEPTIC SHOCK

The usual hemodynamic profile of patients presenting with septic shock is increased cardiac output and decreased systemic vascular resistance.[8] Venous pooling and fluid accumulation in tissues frequently result in low filling pressures at presentation. In many septic patients with initial hypotension, the administration of fluid results in elevation of blood pressure to levels within the normal range. Those who remain hypotensive or who require pressors to maintain blood pressure are in septic shock. Survival of septic shock correlates strongly with elevation of the cardiac index above the normal range. Mortality is markedly higher in patients with normal or low cardiac output, who are more likely to develop vasoconstriction and progressive declines in cardiac output.

Sepsis and septic shock are hypermetabolic conditions with an increased oxygen demand.[8] The failure to meet this demand results in a tissue energy deficit and marked lactic acidosis. This occurs in the hyperdynamic state and is consistent with circulatory maldistribution. Impaired tissue oxygen utilization and shifts in the oxygen dissociation curve have been postulated as well. Hyperdynamic shock is usually associated with increased oxygen delivery and oxygen consumption inadequate for the demand, frequently with an elevated mixed venous oxygen content.

While the primary pathophysiology of septic shock occurs peripherally, alterations of cardiac function have also been documented.[11] A reversible decrease in left and right ventricular ejection fractions by radionuclide ventriculography has been seen in several studies.

End-diastolic volumes are increased. These abnormalities return toward normal in survivors 7 to 10 days after the onset of shock.

Survivors of septic shock tend to have higher levels of oxygen delivery and consumption than nonsurvivors. The concept of supranormal targets of the cardiac index and oxygen metabolism has been tested in the management of critically ill surgical patients, and increased survival has been seen.[12] Applying the concept to patients with septic shock may improve survival. Target levels for the cardiac index in these studies have ranged from 4.5 to 6.0 L/min/m^2. Other targets such as lactic acid clearance might be valid.

With the increased demands on the heart in sepsis, it is not surprising that the underlying cardiac dysfunction is associated with a poor outcome. In gram-negative sepsis there is more likelihood of developing shock and less likelihood of recovery in patients with underlying cardiovascular disease.

TREATMENT

The workup and care of potentially septic patients must be done in a timely manner. The clinical status may demand initiation of vigorous resuscitative efforts at presentation, but this does not obviate the need for a complete history and physical examination. There may be symptoms or signs which suggest specific problems such as pneumonia, meningitis, a urinary tract focus, or an intra-abdominal process. Antecedent events such as surgery, trauma, or instrumentation should be looked for. Underlying conditions or diseases such as transplantation, malignancy, diabetes mellitus, or collagen vascular disease can predispose to infection. Treatment of underlying disorders should be analyzed. It is important to determine if the patient has a history of significant corticosteroid use, as adrenal suppression may be present. If the patient is on corticosteroids or has been on chronic corticosteroids within months of presentation, it is prudent to administer stress-level doses of corticosteroids intravenously to compensate for the potentially inadequate adrenal reserve. Appropriate dosing is a corticosteroid dose equivalent to 200–300 mg/day of hydrocortisone.

Many patients are already under medical care and may have devices such as central venous catheters or urinary catheters in place. Patients may already be on antibiotics or may have had recent treatment for infection, and prior culture results may be available. Prolonged, complex medical care has commonly been given prior to presentation with sepsis. At the other end of the spectrum are patients in relatively good health presenting with community-acquired diseases. Exposure history, travel history, and recent dietary intake are pertinent.

A complete physical exam should be performed, with special attention to finding any focal process that is serving as a source of sepsis. Immunocompromised or neutropenic patients may manifest fewer signs of local processes. A focal process may suggest specific etiologies for empiric coverage. A major goal is to identify the presence of processes that require surgery, as the prognosis is bleak when necessary surgery is not done.

Appropriate laboratory studies should be obtained based on the history and physical examination. Two or more blood cultures from separate sites should be obtained in all patients with suspected sepsis. Aggressive attempts to obtain potentially infected body fluids and secretions are warranted. A lumbar puncture should be performed. Although scanning may be difficult to accomplish, seriously ill patients should undergo any imaging studies that appear appropriate to aid in making the diagnosis.

Circumstances may allow an orderly progression from a thorough exam to testing and consideration of appropriate therapy. However, when patients need prompt intensive care support, their workup can become disjointed, and there is danger of missing clues to the etiology and of failing to obtain all appropriate specimens. This can lead to empiric therapy that is not optimal and may delay necessary surgery. Every effort should be made to ensure that the workup is complete, including obtaining an additional history from family members and reexamining the patient as needed.

EMPIRIC ANTIMICROBIAL THERAPY IN SEPSIS

Instituting empirical antibiotic coverage is routine in the initial care of septic patients. In some instances, such as suspected endocarditis, therapy can be withheld pending diagnosis if the patient is physiologically stable. Febrile neutropenic patients should always be treated with antibiotics for potential sepsis. In patients with gram-negative bacteremia and shock, survival is roughly twice as likely with appropriate initial antibiotic coverage.[13] This is likely true for patients who harbor other organisms producing shock.

The underlying disease status plays a strong role in survival.[14] Patients with underlying, rapidly fatal illnesses have extremely high mortality with or without appropriate antibiotics. Survival in cancer patients correlates with disease remission and bone marrow recovery. Bone marrow transplant recipients who need intensive care or ventilatory support rarely survive, regardless of what underlying processes are present.[15]

It is useful to consider the likely flora of the patient at the onset of illness. Healthier patients with no recent medical care or antibiotic therapy are not likely to be colonized with bacteria highly resistant to antibiotics. Those patients already or recently hospitalized may have had prior antibiotics, which puts them at substantial risk of disease caused by highly resistant hospital bacterial flora, which tend to be particular to each institution.

If a clear source of sepsis is present, such as pneumonia, pyelonephritis, or intra-abdominal abscess, then therapy can be tailored to the likely pathogens. Many patients lack a clear source of infection and must be covered for all likely possibilities. Infection by gram-negative bacteria is present in roughly half of the patients with severe sepsis and shock. Empiric coverage should include agents active against gram-negative organisms, and it is common to use two agents initially. Synergistic killing of bacteria such as *Pseudomonas* may be beneficial, but it is probably more important that the spectrum of activity be very broad to avoid missing adequate coverage for the infecting organism(s). Third-generation cephalosporins, extended-spectrum penicillins, and imipenim-cilastatin are commonly used, often with the addition of an aminoglycoside. Local antibiotic resistance patterns should be taken into consideration.

Gram-positive coverage is particularly important if intravenous catheter infection is possible. In that setting, the possibility of methicillin-resistant staphylococci makes vancomycin use appropriate until culture and antimicrobial sensitivity data are available. Outpatient-acquired infections are less likely to require vancomycin coverage. Patients with a polymicrobic source, such as intra-abdominal abscess, should be given anaerobic coverage.

Sepsis and shock can be associated with rapid changes in renal and hepatic metabolism. Many antibiotics need dosage adjustment secondary to altered clearances with organ dysfunction. Aminoglycosides can be safely used, but diligence is required to maintain appropriate levels. There is potential neurotoxicity with imipenim-cilastatin, usually in the setting of high dosage regimens or renal dysfunction. All drugs should be reviewed for potential dosage adjustment.

SUPPORTIVE THERAPY

Fluid management is a critical element in the care of septic patients. Many patients have initially low cardiac filling pressures and improve with fluid administration. When hypotension persists, it can be difficult to predict the hemodynamic status accurately and to respond promptly to changes in status based on the clinical appearance alone. Catheters that allow monitoring of left and right heart filling pressures can aid management and allow a more aggressive approach to volume management. Authorities differ regarding the relative merits of colloid and crystalloid solution in fluid management, but the central role of fluid and electrolyte management in the care of septic shock is not in dispute.

The benefits and relative merits of various sympathomimetic amines in the therapy of septic shock have never been adequately investigated.[16] Dopamine, dobutamine, and isoproterenol are commonly used when fluid management alone fails to correct blood pressure and tissue perfusion. These agents can have a positive inotropic effect on the heart coupled with selective peripheral perfusion improvements. Dopamine causes an increased heart rate and blood pressure while increasing renal perfusion. Dobutamine has less chronotropic activity but is otherwise similar.[17] Because norepinephrine causes intense peripheral vasoconstriction and may compromise organ perfusion, it is usually used only when other agents have failed.

It is important that adequate fluid replacement occur prior to the use of pressor agents, as beta-adrenergic stimulation can cause vasodilatation and can adversely affect cardiac output and tissue perfusion. Many experts recommend fluid challenge until the pulmonary wedge pressure is at the upper limit of normal prior to considering the use of sympathomimetic amines.[18]

For many years, there was controversy regarding the possible benefit of corticosteroids in the setting of septic shock. In animal models of sepsis, pretreatment with corticosteroids can have beneficial effects. However, benefit is hard to demonstrate when treatment is given after infectious challenge has occurred. The results of large multicenter clinical trials failed to show any benefit of glucocorticoid therapy,[19,20] and their use cannot be recommended in the therapy of septic shock. Stress-level replacement of corticosteroids in suspected adrenal insufficiency is clearly a different situation and is to be recommended.

EXPERIMENTAL THERAPIES IN SEPSIS AND SEPTIC SHOCK

With the increasing knowledge of the cytokine cascade and the role that host responses appear to play in the adverse events of sepsis, it is widely believed that much of the morbidity and mortality seen in sepsis is related to excessive activation of host defense mechanisms. Alteration of host responses has become a major focus of sepsis research. Utilizing modern biotechnology, a variety of potentially useful agents have been developed that are designed to either augment desirable host responses or inhibit undesirable responses.

Decreasing the host response to LPS in gram-negative infections has been an early approach. It has the disadvantage of targeting only patients with gram-negative infections, which cause fewer than half of all cases of clinical sepsis.[21] Therapies that modulate host defenses through TNF-a, IL-1, and other agents are potentially beneficial in sepsis, regardless of the etiology. A variety of experimental agents are being developed and tested.[21]

A number of these agents have undergone clinical trials, with disappointing results. Antiendotoxin monoclonal antibodies, anti-TNF monoclonal antibodies, TNF receptor, and IL-1 receptor-blocking protein and others have failed to show a clear benefit in clinical trials. Several of these agents are no longer undergoing development.

While more potential therapies are being tested, many experts feel that no one agent is likely to show clear-cut improvement in mortality from sepsis and shock. Some experts suggest that multiple agents working at different stages of sepsis may be required to produce measurable benefit.

Sepsis is a leading cause of morbidity and mortality, and there is increasing understanding of the risk factors and prognosis of this highly lethal condition. However, despite great increases in our knowledge of the pathophysiology of sepsis and septic shock, very little improvement in outcome has occurred. Continued study of intensive care management is likely to clarify treatment goals that achieve optimal survival. While studies of the alteration of the host response have been disappointing so far, it is premature to conclude that an improved outcome with this approach will not occur. There is marked heterogeneity among patients with sepsis, and there is a need to define subsets of patients that may benefit from specific therapies that do not help others. Some episodes of sepsis are preventable, and avoidance of this complication is clearly the best approach of all.

REFERENCES

1. Centers for Disease Control: Increase in national hospital discharge survey cases for septicemia. *MMWR* 39:31–34, 1990.
2. Carleton SC: The cardiovascular effects of sepsis. *Cardiol Clin* 13:249–256, 1995.
3. Lowrey SF: Sepsis and its complications: Clinical definitions and therapeutic prospects. *Crit Care Med* 22:1–2, 1994.
4. Bone RC, Balk RA, Cerra FB, et al: Definition for sepsis and organ failure and guidelines for the use of innovative therapies in sepsis: The American College of Chest Physicians/Society of Critical Care Medicine Consensus Conference Committee. *Chest* 101:1644–1655, 1992.
5. Sun X, Wagner DP, Knaus WA: Evaluation of prognosis from MSOF: Data from APACHE III study. Supplement. *Proceedings of the 6th European Congress on Intensive Care Medicine,* 1992.
6. Rangel-Frausto MS, Pittet D, Constigan M, et al: The natural history of the systemic inflammatory response syndrome (SIRS). *JAMA* 273:117–123, 1995.
7. Kreger BE, Craven DE, McCabe WR: Gram-negative bacteremia IV. Re-evaluation of clinical features and treatment in 612 patients. *Am J Med* 68:344–355, 1980.
8. Nishijima H, Weil MH, Shubin H, et al: Hemodynamic and metabolic studies on shock associated with gram negative bacteremia. *Medicine* 52:287–294, 1973.
9. Natanson C, Hoffman WD, Suffredini AF, et al: Selected treatment strategies for septic shock based on proposed mechanisms of pathogenesis. *Ann Intern Med* 120:771–780, 1994.
10. Touvay C, Vilain B, Carre C, et al: Role of a platelet-activating factor (PAF) in the bronchopulmonary alterations and beta adrenoceptor function induced by endotoxin. *Biochem Biophys Res Commun* 152:527–533, 1988.
11. Parker MM, Ognibene FP, Parrillo JE: Peak systolic pressure/end-systolic volume ratio, a load-independent measure of ventricular function, is reversibly decreased in human septic shock. *Crit Care Med* 22:1955–1959, 1994.
12. Shoemaker WC, Appel P, Kram H, et al: Prospective trial of supranormal values of survivors as therapeutic goals in high risk surgical patients. *Chest* 94:1176–1186, 1988.
13. Weil MH, Shubin H, Biddle M: Shock caused by gram-negative microorganisms: Analysis of 169 cases. *Ann Intern Med* 60:384–400, 1964.
14. Kreger B, Craven DE, Carling PC, et al: Gram-negative bacteremia III. Reassessment of etiology, epidemiology and ecology in 612 patients. *Am J Med* 68:332–343, 1980.
15. Afessa B, Tefferi A, Hoagland HC, et al: Outcome of recipients of bone marrow transplants who require intensive-care unit support. *Mayo Clin Proc* 67:117–122, 1992.
16. DiBona GF: Hemodynamic support: Volume management and pharmacological cardiovascular support. *Semin Nephrol* 14:33–40, 1994.
17. Shoemaker WC, Appel PL, Kram HB: Oxygen transport measurements to evaluate tissue perfusion and titrate therapy: Dobutamine and dopamine effects. *Crit Care Med* 19:672–688, 1991.
18. Tuchschmidt J, Fried J, Astiz M, et al: Elevation of cardiac output and oxygen delivery improves outcome in septic shock. *Chest* 102:216–220, 1992.
19. Veterans Administration Systemic Sepsis Cooperative Study Group: Effect of high dose glucocorticoid therapy on mortality in patients with clinical signs of systemic sepsis. *N Engl J Med* 317:659–665, 1987.
20. Bone RC, Fisher CJ, Clemmer TP, et al: A controlled clinical trial of high-dose methylprednisolone in the treatment of severe sepsis and septic shock. *N Engl J Med* 317:653–658, 1987
21. Ziegler EJ, Fisher CJ, Sprung CL, et al: Treatment of gram-negative bacteremia and septic shock with HA-1A human monoclonal antibody against endotoxin. The HA-1A Sepsis Study Group. *N Engl J Med* 324:429–436, 1991.

— V —

Cardiovascular Involvement with Renal Disease

Sameh R. Abul-Ezz, M.D.
Section Editor

Left Ventricular Dysfunction

Sameh R. Abul-Ezz, M.D.

The relationship between pathophysiologic alterations in renal failure and cardiovascular disorders are detailed in Table 5.1. Diminished cardiac output is commonly encountered in acute renal failure. Although a common underlying disease could be responsible for both cardiac and renal failure, several lines of evidence implicate uremia as an important etiologic factor in left ventricular dysfunction. Echocardiographic studies in chronic renal failure reported a prevalence of 74% of left ventricular hypertrophy. One-third of these patients had left ventricular dilatation, and 15% had systolic dysfunction which was independently associated with mortality.[1]

PRESENTING MANIFESTATIONS

History

Congestive heart failure is the most common presentation of left ventricular dysfunction. General symptoms of weakness and easy tiredness are commonly found in patients with heart failure but are nonspecific, especially in patients with renal failure. Respiratory symptoms are more helpful but may not be obvious in the sedentary patient. Dyspnea on exertion is an important symptom, especially when it represents a change from a previous level with a given degree of exertion. Orthopnea may be described by the patient as shortness of breath on recumbency, necessitating the use of more pillows, or as a cough when lying down. Description of paroxysmal nocturnal dyspnea helps differentiate it from orthopnea, since patients usually describe a sudden onset of shortness of breath during sleep, which is usually relieved after sitting up for 20 to 30 min. Wheezing may be noticeable, but the rapid improvement obtained by sitting up helps differentiate left ventricular dysfunction from bronchial asthma.

Physical Examination

Attention should be paid to the general manifestation of cardiac insufficiency, which may not be evident until cardiac decompensation takes place. Dyspnea at rest is not uncommon in patients with renal failure, as volume overload may not be tolerated by an otherwise compensated left ventricle. Cardiac cachexia, usually found in the late stages of classic heart failure, may manifest with generalized loss of muscle mass and bitemporal wasting. These late stages are usually associated with right ventricular failure, as well as with hepatic congestion

88

TABLE 5.1. Metabolic and Hemodynamic Disorders in Renal Failure and Their Effect on the Heart

Disorder Resulting from Renal Failure	Mechanism	Cardiac Effect
Sodium and fluid retension	Increased blood return	Increased preload
A-V fistula		
Increased renin secretion	Hypertension	Increased preload
Sodium and fluid retention		
Possible renovascular disease		
Anemia	Increased cardiac output	Cardiac overwork
Malnutrition		
High carbohydrate diet		
Increased insulin peripheral resistance	Hyperlipidemia	Coronary artery disease
Glucose administration with dialysis		
Impaired lipid metabolism		
Metastatic calcification	Mitral and aortic valve damage	Valvular heart disease
Increased incidence of endocarditis		
Hypertension	Myocardial hypertrophy and pulmonary hypertension	Left and right ventricular dysfunction
Uremic toxins		
Hyperparathyroidism		
Electrolytes and mineral imbalance	Electrophysiologic disturbances	Arrhythmias
Hyperadrenergic state		
Dialysis shifts in electrolytes		

which could result in the icteric tinge found on skin examination. Examination of the jugular veins commonly reveals elevated jugular venous pressure and hepatojugular reflux, but these signs are nonspecific. Cardiac examination could reveal signs of cardiac enlargement, with lateral and downward displacement of the apical impulse, and palpation may demonstrate right ventricular lift. On auscultation, the first and second heart sounds may be normal, but gallop sounds are common. An atrial gallop (S_4) is common but nonspecific. A left ventricular S_3 gallop, heard best over the apical area, or a right ventricular gallop, heard best over the subxiphoid area, are more specific signs of decreased ventricular compliance. Mitral and tricuspid regurgitation murmurs could be secondary to ventricular dilatation with incomplete closure of the valve leaflets. Extracardiac manifestations such as bibasilar crackles on lung examination, enlarged liver with or without ascites, and peripheral edema are important signs.

Laboratory Evaluation

Hematologic or blood chemistry evaluations are not helpful in diagnosing or ruling out left ventricular dysfunction. They are useful in investigating complicating and precipitating factors such as anemia, infection, thyroid function abnormality, calcium and phosphorus abnormalities leading to secondary hyperparathyroidism, inadequate dialysis, and congestive hepatic dysfunction.

On chest x-ray, an increased cardiothoracic ratio and left ventricular volume, pulmonary venous congestion with cephalization of flow, linear densities in interlobular regions, and pleural effusions are specific signs of left ventricular dysfunction, but they are not very sensitive. Electrocardiographic (ECG) findings of left ventricular hypertrophy are nonspecific. Old infarct patterns may suggest the etiology of ischemic heart disease.

DIAGNOSTIC CRITERIA

Echocardiography is extremely valuable in evaluating the structure and function of the left ventricle. Measurement of left ventricular mass, cavity volume, and fractional shortening can not only establish the diagnosis but also differentiate between left ventricular hypertrophy, dilatation, systolic dysfunction, and diastolic dysfunction.[2]

DIFFERENTIAL DIAGNOSIS

Noncardiac causes of dyspnea and peripheral edema should be differentiated from congestive heart failure. Volume overload in dialysis patients could produce a clinical picture which is difficult to distinguish from that of left ventricular failure. Primary liver disease with cirrhosis, ascites, and edema may resemble light ventricular failure. Also, primary lung disease with asthma, chronic obstructive pulmonary disease, recent pulmonary embolism, and infections can occasionally be misdiagnosed as heart failure.

PATHOPHYSIOLOGY

Many of the risk factors for the development of cardiac failure are often present in patients with renal failure. These include hypertension, coronary artery disease, and salt and fluid retention, in addition to a high output state precipitated by arteriovenous fistula, anemia, a hypercatabolic state, and nutritional deficiencies.[3]

Evidence from animal studies in uremia demonstrates increased interstitial collagen deposition in the myocardium, which ultimately results in decreased left ventricular compliance.[4] Other studies have shown a depressant effect of uremia on N-K ATPase and depression of sacrolemmal calcium transport.[5] Human studies have demonstrated that in the absence of all other risk factors, uremia is associated with a decreased left ventricular ejection fraction and increased end-diastolic volume and pressure. Autopsy findings have demonstrated interstitial edema and patchy myocardial necrosis.[6]

On the other hand, it is possible that uremic cardiomyopathy is a result of deficiencies in uremic sera rather than added toxic effects. Evidence for the association between selenium and carnitine deficiencies and echocardiographic abnormalities have been reported, with measurable improvement in these indices when supplementation was provided.[7]

NATURAL HISTORY OF THE DISEASE

Serious clinical consequences with increased morbidity and mortality could be attributed to the progressive cardiomyopathy associated with uremia. Increased hypotensive episodes on dialysis could interfere with the delivery of needed dialysis treatment. Arrhythmia is a complication of left ventricular hypertrophy and could result in sudden death on dialysis. Also, an increased oxygen demand could contribute to worsening ischemic heart disease in a patient with renal failure.[8]

CURRENT METHODS OF TREATMENT

Prevention of cardiac failure through careful evaluation and management of known risk factors is of the utmost importance. In a patient with renal failure, control of hypertension, hyperlipidemia, hyperparathyroidism, acidosis, and volume overload should be optimized. Anemia should be treated with erythropoietin to keep the hematocrit above 30%. Hypotension on dialysis should be prevented, as it could lead to significant morbidity.[9] Use of a cooler dialysis solution composed of bicarbonate rather than acetate, with adequate sodium and calcium contents, should help decrease the incidence of hypotension on dialysis.[10]

Avoiding overzealous ultrafiltration and vasodilators is important in patients with left ventricular hypertrophy. This emphasizes the need for a baseline echocardiogram upon starting dialysis. ACE inhibitors and nondihydropyridine calcium channel blockers are preferred for hypertension management.

REFERENCES

1. Foley RN, Parfrey PS, Harnett JD, et al: Clinical and echocardiographic disease in patients starting end-stage renal disease therapy. *Kidney Int* 47:186–192, 1995.
2. Huwez FU, Pringle SD, Macfarlane PW: A new classification of left ventricular geometry in patients with cardiac disease based on M-mode echocardiography. *Am J Cardiol* 70:681–688, 1992.
3. Collins AJ, Hanson G, Umen A, et al: Changing risk factor demographics in end-stage renal disease patients entering hemodialysis and the impact on long-term mortality. *Am J Kid Dis* 15:422–432, 1990.
4. Harnett JD, Parfrey PS: Cardiac disease in uremia. *Semin Nephrol* 14:245–252, 1994.
5. Smolens P, Stein JH: Pathophysiology of acute renal failure. *Am J Med* 70.479–482, 1981.
6. Drueke T, Le Pailleu C, Meilhac B, et al: Congestive cardiomyopathy in uraemic patients on long term haemodialysis. *Br Med J* 1:350–353, 1977.
7. Pierpont ME, Judd D, Goldenberg IF, et al: Myocardial carnitine in end-stage congestive heart failure. *Am J Cardiol* 64:56–60, 1989.
8. Parfrey PS, Griffiths SM, Harnett JD, et al: Outcome of congestive heart failure, dilated cardiomyopathy, hypertrophic hyperkinetic disease, and ischemic heart disease in dialysis patients. *Am J Nephrol* 10:213–221, 1990.
9. Daugirdas JT: Preventing and managing hypotension. *Semin Dialysis* 7:276–283, 1994.
10. Levy FL, Grayburn PA, Foulks CJ, et al: Improved left ventricular contractility with cool temperature hemodialysis. *Kidney Int* 41:961–965, 1992.

Ischemic Heart Disease

Sameh R. Abul-Ezz, M.D.

Advances in dialysis and transplantation over the last decade have improved the survival of patients with end-stage renal disease. Despite this steady improvement, however, myocardial infarction and other cardiac causes contributed to approximately 40% of the deaths in this patient population in 1991. Mortality from coronary artery disease in the dialysis and transplant populations far exceeds the rates observed in the general population.[1]

PRESENTING MANIFESTATIONS

History

Typically, patients with coronary artery disease complain of chest discomfort. The most common description is that of indigestion. Less common is a feeling of heaviness, squeezing, burning or sharp pain. The symptoms are usually felt in a sternal or retrosternal location or to the left of the sternum. Radiation is commonly felt in the left upper extremity, but sometimes it extends to the back, the neck, the jaw, or the left shoulder. Dyspnea, weakness, dizziness, diaphoresis, nausea, and belching are the usual associated symptoms. In stable angina, pain usually follows physical or mental stress and is relieved with rest and sublingual nitroglycerin. In unstable angina and myocardial infarction, chest pain is more intense, may not be related to exertion, and lasts significantly longer. A history of angina is less reliable when sought in patients with chronic renal failure. A large proportion of patients on dialysis are diabetics. The typical retrosternal or left precordial chest pain may not be present. Twenty-eight percent of asymptomatic diabetic patients with end-stage renal disease have angiographic evidence of 75% or higher-grade stenosis in one or more coronary arteries.[2] Furthermore, chest pain from the imbalance between oxygen supply and demand during hemodialysis without fixed coronary artery lesions or from pericarditis may add to the difficulty of the diagnosis.

Physical Examination

The physical examination of patients during an episode of angina or myocardial infarction usually reveals anxiety and restlessness. Tachycardia with hypotension, normal blood pressure, or hypertension may be present. The skin may be pale and clammy. Jugular venous pressure is usually elevated when significant left ventricular failure or right ventricular infarction is present. Chest examination may reveal wheezing and basilar inspiratory crackles, and the cardiac examination commonly is significant for the presence of an S_4 gallop, but occasionally an S_3 gallop and the systolic murmur of mitral regurgitation are auscultated. Other signs of right ventricular failure may be manifested with hepatomegaly and hepatojugular reflux. Following myocardial infarction, signs of fluid retention with peripheral edema and occasionally ascites may be observed. In the patient with renal failure these signs are difficult to interpret, since most of them are usually attributed to volume overload, hyperdynamic state, anemia, and left ventricular dysfunction.

Laboratory Evaluation

Because myocardial ischemia is reversible during angina, no hematologic or chemical investigation would help diagnose a patient with ischemic heart disease. Only in myocardial infarction will serum creatine phosphokinase rise within 6–8 hr and peak within 24 hr, then return to the normal range within 3 days. The MB fraction of that enzyme is specific for myocardial cell origin. Similarly, lactic dehydrogenase (LDH) is helpful in diagnosing myocardial cell injury. Reversal of the normal LDH1/LDH2 pattern is a specific marker for a recent myocardial infarction, as it rises 1–2 days after injury and lasts for 8–14 days after peaking at 3–6 days. The pattern of serum glutamic-oxaloacetic transaminase (SGOT) rise and fall is between that of the previous two enzymes and consequently is utilized less often as a marker of myocardial infarction. Renal failure does not affect the reliability of these chemical tests in diagnosing myocardial infarction.

The frequently encountered nonspecific ST-T changes on ECGs performed on patients with renal failure makes interpretation of ischemic changes more challenging. Nonetheless, horizontal or down-sloping ST segments during episodes of chest pain are helpful, especially when they represent change from the baseline ECG. Development of Q waves and loss of R waves in certain leads is of value in diagnosing transmural myocardial infarction and pointing to its location.

DIAGNOSTIC CRITERIA

The diagnostic value of noninvasive exercise stress screening in end-stage renal disease is limited. The high prevalence of nonspecific ST-T segment changes and poor exercise tolerance in these patients seriously limit the diagnostic yield of these tests. This not uncommon effort limitation encountered in the dialysis population similarly restricts the utility of exercise thallium and exercise echocardiographic studies. Compared to quantitative angiography, the positive and negative predictive values of dipyridamole thallium were 82% and 83%, respectively.[3] Since more than half of the patients in that study had coronary occlusive lesions of at least 70%, decreased reliability of the test should be expected when coronary artery lesions are less prevalent. A positive predictive value of 29% and a negative predictive value of 68% have been reported with the single photon emission computed tomography (SPECT) thallium test in end-stage renal disease patients. Preliminary results of the dobutamine echocardiographic test appear more promising. A positive predictive value of 62% and a negative predictive value of 100% were reported when the prevalence of 70% occlusive coronary artery disease was 28%.[4]

Therefore, if the purpose of noninvasive testing is to rule out the presence of significant coronary artery occlusive disease, thallium exercise testing should be used when the exercise capacity of the renal patient is not impaired. In patients with severe arthritis, lower extremity amputations, and poor exercise tolerance, dobutamine echocardiography seems to offer the highest negative predictive value.

Evaluation of the perioperative cardiac risk in asymptomatic patients with renal failure is even more difficult. This question is usually raised when the dialysis patients are evaluated for kidney transplantation. Eighty-seven percent of type I diabetic patients 45 years or older referred for kidney transplant evaluation had significant coronary occlusive disease.[5] Since coronary angiography cannot be done on all transplant candidates, strategies for risk stratification in this population should be attempted. Clinical factors such as age, diabetes mellitus, angina, congestive heart failure, and an abnormal ECG have been found to identify a subgroup of patients at high risk of postoperative cardiac death. When exercise thallium testing in this subgroup has demonstrated reversible ischemia, the risk of perioperative cardiac death was the highest.[6]

Coronary arteriography is the gold standard for diagnosing coronary artery disease in renal failure. An algorithm that utilizes clinical data for risk stratification and the limited utility of some noninvasive cardiac tests to guide the most cost-effective use of coronary angiography is shown in Figure 5.1.

DIFFERENTIAL DIAGNOSIS

Because of the higher incidence of pericarditis in the dialysis population, the possibility of a pericardial origin of the chest pain should always be considered. The relationship of the pain to position and breathing, as well as specific changes in the ECG, would help to differentiate the two. Upper gastrointestinal disorders are common in patients with renal failure and may produce chest pain that might be difficult to differentiate from angina. These disorders include

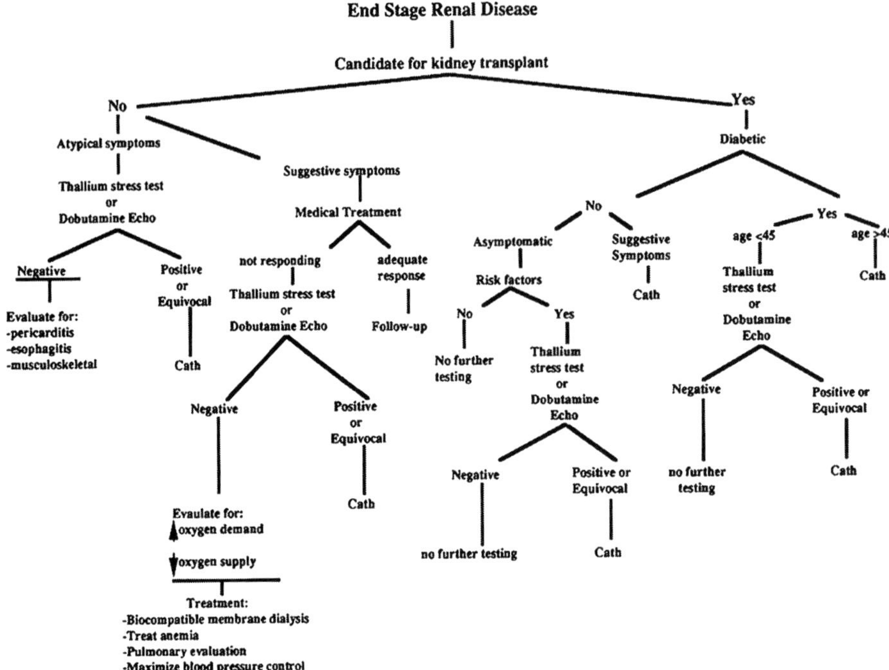

Figure 5.1. Algorithm for evaluation of coronary artery disease in end-stage renal disease.

esophagitis, esophageal spasm, gastroesophageal reflux, hiatal hernia, gastritis, and duodenal peptic ulcer disease as well as symptomatic cholelithiasis and gallbladder disease. Suggestive symptoms include the relation to meals and relief with antacids. These symptoms are helpful but inconclusive, as patients with angina and myocardial infarction occasionally describe heartburn and belching. The possibility of a cardiac etiology of these symptoms should be examined before subjecting patients to stressful gastrointestinal investigations. A musculoskeletal etiology of chest pain from cervical osteoarthritis or osteochondritis of the chest wall is usually reproducible by pressure or by movement of the involved joints.

PATHOPHYSIOLOGY

Structural changes in the coronary arteries are known to occur early in renal insufficiency and to increase progressively while on dialysis and after transplantation. Increased calcium X phosphate product and secondary hyperparathyroidism are known to result in metastatic calcification which could involve the coronary arteries. Increased thrombotic tendencies have been described in chronic renal failure and may contribute to the high incidence of atherosclerosis. Platelet dysfunction, decreased thrombolytic activity, and increased procoagulants such as the von Willibrand factor and factor VIII have been reported. This could contribute to endothelial changes and plaque formation.

Concomitant with these factors are the dyslipidemias associated with chronic renal failure. The most prevalent lipid disorder in this patient population is a pattern similar to that of patients with type IV hyperlipidemia. Cholesterol levels may not be increased, but very low density lipoprotein (VLDL) and triglyceride levels are invariably elevated. Other patterns with increased intermediate density lipoprotein (IDL) and low high density lipoprotein (HDL) levels have been reported. These dyslipidemias have been attributed to impaired glucose tolerance, increased insulin resistance, diminished lipoprotein lipase activity, carnitine deficiency, and the use of glucose and acetate in dialysis solutions.[7] Immunosuppressive agents administered after transplantation are known to affect lipid metabolism adversely. Cyclosporine is associated with hypercholesterolemia, mainly through increased LDL levels. Increased insulin resistance and hypercholesterolemia are other important side effects of corticosteroid treatment in this population.

Other hormonal and hemodynamic factors can contribute to a further decrease in coronary blood flow in addition to the decrease produced by fixed atherosclerotic lesions. The hyperadrenergic state frequently observed in the dialysis population can result in decreased coronary blood flow through two mechanisms: increased coronary vascular reactivity and tachycardia with decreased diastolic time. Impaired coronary flow can also result from diastolic dysfunction. A further decrease in the oxygen supply could result from anemia and dialysis-induced hypoxemia. Together with the decreased oxygen-carrying capacity due to the decreased hemoglobin content, hypoxemia has been reported in hemodialysis as a result of complement activation and decreased alveolar ventilation.[8] Also, the normal state of myocardial oxygen demand is significantly altered. The creation of an arteriovenous fistula results in increased preload. Changes in volume homeostasis with fluid and sodium retention could increase both pre- and afterload. Myocardial hypertrophy as a result of hypertension, hyperparathyroidism, valvular heart disease, and possibly uremic toxins can significantly increase the oxygen demand. Concomitant with these changes is the tachycardia associated with anemia, a hyperadrenergic state, and thiamine deficiency. Understanding these pathophysiologic changes is necessary to evaluate ischemic heart disease properly in patients with renal failure and to select the best management techniques.

NATURAL HISTORY OF THE DISEASE

When the diagnosis of ischemic heart disease is missed and the patient is not treated, myocardial infarction and sudden death from arrhythmia are the likely consequences. Diabetic patients with renal failure are at especially high risk because their ischemic heart disease is often asymptomatic.

CURRENT METHODS OF TREATMENT

As in nonrenal patients, all identifiable risk factors for coronary artery disease should be addressed. Patients should be counseled against smoking and unhealthy dietary habits. At the same time, every effort should be made to achieve maximum blood pressure and volume control. Hyperlipidemia should be treated aggressively with dietary modification and medication if necessary, and anemia should be treated with erythropoietin.

Patients with significant coronary artery disease should be considered for percutaneous transluminal balloon angioplasty. However, although this procedure has been reported to be effective in end-stage renal disease patients, high rates of restenosis have been reported.[9] Patients who have more than 75% stenosis and meet the criteria for revascularization prior to transplantation have significantly better survival than those treated medically.[10] Higher morbidity and mortality rates in the perioperative period have been reported in end-stage renal disease patients undergoing bypass surgery. These were mostly due to an increased bleeding tendency and greater susceptibility to infection.

Medical treatment should be tried initially to control symptoms and to treat patients who are not candidates for revascularization. Attention should be paid to the possible drawbacks of standard antianginal therapy in chronic renal failure. For example, patients with renal failure exhibiting diastolic dysfunction could be dependent on a relatively increased preload for compensation. Reduction with excessive doses of nitrates might further compromise ventricular function in these patients. Beta-blocking agents administered before hemodialysis could interfere with the sympathetic response of these patients to excessive ultrafiltration and hypotension. Similarly, calcium channel blockers with negative inotropic effects could further compromise the cardiac output in hemodialysis patients with marginally compensated heart failure. When the above precautions are kept in mind, these therapeutic approaches can be extremely valuable in treating renal failure patients with ischemic heart disease.

REFERENCES

1. Rostand SG, Gretes JC, Kirk KA, et al: Ischemic heart disease in patients with uremia undergoing maintenance hemodialysis. *Kidney Int* 16:600–611, 1979.
2. Manske CL, Wilson RF, Wang Y, et al: Prevalence of and risk factors for angiographically determined coronary artery disease in type I diabetes patients with nephropathy. *Arch Intern Med* 152:2450–2455, 1992.
3. Boudreau RJ, Strony JT, duCret RP, et al: Perfusion thallium imaging of type I diabetes patients with end-stage renal disease: Comparison of oral and intravenous dipyridamole administration. *Radiology* 175:103–105, 1990.
4. Marwick TH, Steinmuller DR, Underwood DA, et al: Ineffectiveness of dipyridamole spect thallium imaging as a screening technique for coronary artery disease in patients with end-stage renal failure. *Transplantation* 49:100–103, 1990.
5. Manske CL, Thomas W, Wang Y, et al: Screening diabetic transplant candidates for coronary artery disease: Identification of a low risk subgroup. *Kidney Int* 44:617–621, 1993.
6. Le A, Wilson R, Douek K, et al: Prospective risk stratification in renal transplant candidates for cardiac death. *Am J Kidney Dis* 24:65–71, 1994.
7. Lindner A, Charra B, Sherrard DJ, et al: Accelerated atherosclerosis in prolonged maintenance hemodialysis. *N Engl J Med* 290:697–701, 1974.
8. Francos GC, Besarab A, Burk JF Jr, et al: Dialysis-induced hypoxemia: Membrane-dependent and membrane-independent cause. *Am J Kidney Dis* 5:191–198, 1985.
9. Kahn JK, Rutherford BD, McConahay DR, et al: Short- and long-term outcome of percutaneous transluminal coronary angioplasty in chronic dialysis patients. *Am Heart J* 119:484–489, 1990.
10. Manske CL, Wang Y, Rector T, et al: Coronary revascularisation in insulin-dependent diabetic patients with chronic renal failure. *Lancet* 340:998–1002, 1992.

Pericarditis

Sameh R. Abul-Ezz, M.D.

Pericardial disease may occur during the course of acute renal failure, in chronic renal insufficiency before the institution of dialysis, or in end-stage renal disease patients already receiving maintenance dialysis. The incidence of pericarditis in renal failure patients has been reported to vary between 0.5% and 44%. Uremic pericarditis encountered before the start of dialysis appears to be part of the generalized serositis associated with the uremic syndrome. Before the improvement of dialysis techniques, it was regarded as a preterminal sign in the natural history of renal failure.[1] By contrast, pericarditis developing in patients already on dialysis may represent a distinct form of pericardial disease. Although the question of dialysis adequacy in these patients is always raised, correlation with the parameters of inadequate dialysis is not consistently demonstrated. Less than 50% of these patients demonstrate improvement when their dialysis prescription is increased. Because of the immunosuppressed state of the dialysis population, the possibility of infectious pericarditis, either viral or bacterial, should always be sought. Also, the possibility that autoimmune disease is responsible for the original renal disease and the later development of pericarditis should be entertained.[2]

PRESENTING MANIFESTATIONS

History

The most common complaint of approximately two-thirds of patients with pericarditis and renal failure is chest pain. The most common description is that of squeezing pain, sharp pain, or heaviness located retrosternally. Radiation to the neck close to the trapezius ridge or to the back is most commonly described. Less commonly, the pain is described as severe crushing pain retrosternally or sharp pain of pleuritic quality away from the midchest. It is usually aggravated by deep inspiration, cough, or lying flat and is partially relieved by sitting up and leaning forward.

In the dialysis population, the presentation of pericarditis can differ. Chest pain may be mild or nonexistent, while dyspnea becomes more manifest. Malaise, weakness, and low-grade fever are commonly associated symptoms. When pericardial tamponade is present, patients usually complain of worsening dyspnea, weakness, dizziness, and diaphoresis.[3]

Physical Examination

The signs of pericarditis with or without effusion are easily detectable in the nonrenal patient. These signs are often modified by the underlying heart disease in end-stage renal disease. Early diagnosis requires recognition of subtle changes in the cardiac and hemodynamic examination. The presence of pluses paradoxes and more than a 10 mm Hg drop in blood pressure during inspiration are late, ominous signs of cardiac tamponade. Hypotension on dialysis, especially when it represents a change from the usual course of dialysis in a specific patient, should alert the physician to include the possibility of tamponade in the differential diagnosis. A large proportion of end-stage renal disease patients have volume overload and cardiac dysfunction. Accordingly, increased venous pressure is not uncommon. Further increases in jugular venous pressure and change in the venous pulse waveform, with a more pronounced x descent, should alert the astute physician. If constrictive pericarditis develops, a further increase in venous pressure may be noticed with inspiration, and the y descent becomes most noticeable. The pericardial friction rub is the classical physical sign of pericarditis. From 80% to 90% of the dialysis population with pericarditis demonstrates a pericardial rub on auscultation. This is usually present even after the accumulation of a large pericardial effusion. The grating quality of the pericardial rub should help differentiate it from the functional and organic murmurs commonly encountered in the dialysis population. Although the classical rub is of triphasic components, commonly it is biphasic.[4]

Laboratory Evaluation

Patients with renal failure who develop pericarditis should undergo a complete laboratory evaluation, as for pericarditis in the nonrenal patient. This should include white blood cell count for leukocytosis, platelet count, and prothrombin and partial thromboplastin times for hemorrhagic complications. Cardiac enzymes and isoenzymes (CPK, LDH, and SGOT) should be evaluated to rule out myocardial infarction. One should also include the erythrocyte sedimentation rate as a measure of inflammation and antinuclear antibody for the possibility of collagen vascular disease. An infectious etiology of pericarditis should be evaluated with bacterial cultures, a tuberculin skin test, streptozyme, antimycoplasma, or cold agglutinin titers. The most common viral etiology of pericarditis can be evaluated by examining antibody titers against coxsackie virus B_5 and B_6 subtypes, Epstein-Barr virus, and cytomegalovirus. Thyroid-stimulating hormone is most valuable in ruling out the possibility of hypothyroidism.

In the patient already on chronic dialysis, urea clearance measurements should be employed to rule out inadequate dialysis.

A chest roentgenogram is helpful in the nonrenal patient when a global increase in the cardiac silhouette is demonstrated. This is more difficult to evaluate in the renal patient because of the common finding of cardiomegaly and failure. Also, accumulation of pericardial fluid without pericardial disease could be a manifestation of fluid retention, with transudative pleural and pericardial effusions.

DIAGNOSTIC CRITERIA

Pathognomonic electrocardiographic changes with ST elevation and PR depression are often encountered. Underlying nonspecific ST-T segment changes associated with left ventricular hypertrophy and electrolyte imbalance may modify these changes. The upward concavity of the elevated ST segment and its presence in all limb leads and most chest leads would help differentiate these changes from the injury pattern of ischemic heart disease. In pericarditis, reciprocal changes are encountered only in leads AVR and V1. Premature atrial depolarizations, atrial fibrillation, and flutter are the most frequently encountered arrhythmias.

Small amounts of effusion could be missed by echocardiography. Also, as part of the generalized fluid retention, moderate amounts of effusion could be present in renal failure patients without pericardial disease. This could further decrease the positive predictive value of this technique. Nonetheless, echocardiography is important in early detection of pericardial tamponade and in treatment evaluation. Right atrial or ventricular collapse in diastole is considered specific evidence of tamponade.[5] When tamponade is suspected, placement of a Swan-Ganz catheter can confirm the diagnosis. As pericardial pressure increases with accumulation of effusion, pressures in the right and left atria will increase in order to maintain cardiac output. A finding of equilibration of the pulmonary wedge pressure, pulmonary diastolic pressure, right ventricle pressure and right atrial diastolic pressure is diagnostic. Monitoring of the venous pulse wave and the finding of a deep x descent could help differentiate cardiac tamponade from constrictive pericarditis. Further increase in venous pressure during inspiration and a prominent y descent are considered hallmarks for the diagnosis of constrictive pericarditis.[6]

DIFFERENTIAL DIAGNOSIS

Pericarditis-related chest pain should be differentiated from chest pain caused by myocardial infarction, aortic dissection, pulmonary embolism or infarction, and pleurisy of infectious or inflammatory etiology. Because of the high prevalence of coronary artery disease in the dialysis population, emphasis should be placed on ruling out myocardial infarction with serial ECGs and cardiac isoenzyme tests. Right ventricular infarction could present with a clinical picture similar to that of constrictive pericarditis. Transesophageal echocardiography is extremely valuable when thoracic aortic dissection is suspected. A transudative pericardial fluid collection without pericardial disease can be ruled out only with pericardiocentesis.

PATHOPHYSIOLOGY

The histopathologic changes in uremic pericarditis are not dissimilar to those observed in acute pericarditis in patients without renal failure. The classic bread-and-butter histologic changes, with thickening of both the visceral and parietal pericardium, have been described. Fibrinous deposits with hemorrhagic and vascular involvement are variable, and correlate with the amount and type of effusion present. No clear explanation for the high incidence of pericarditis in renal failure is available. The higher incidence of pericarditis in hemodialysis patients compared to peritoneal dialysis patients is not well explained either. Theoretically, better clearance of the so-called middle molecules and a reduced requirement for systemic heparinization could be important etiologic factors, but these remain unproved.

NATURAL HISTORY OF THE DISEASE

The natural history of uremic pericarditis is well documented. If left untreated, pericardial tamponade with hemodynamic compromise is life-threatening. Before the advent of dialysis, pericarditis was rightfully regarded as a sign of imminent death. Renal failure patients with uremic pericarditis require meticulous attention to detail to avoid lethal consequences. Excessive ultrafiltration may further compromise venous return, leading to serious hemodynamic instability. Whether liberal heparinization during dialysis adversely affects the prognosis remains controversial. Chronic constrictive pericarditis may subsequently develop in 12% of patients who experienced acute uremic pericarditis with or without hemopericardium.[7] Typically, these patients appear chronically ill, with progressive weight gain secondary to fluid retention. Pleural effusions, hepatic congestion, ascites, and increasing peripheral edema become evident. Increasing jugular venous pressure during inspiration (Kussmaul's respiration) and prominent y descent are diagnostic. Hemodynamic instability with frequent hypotensive episodes on dialysis are signs of tamponade.

CURRENT METHODS OF TREATMENT

When uremic pericarditis develops in the course of acute or chronic renal failure approaching end-stage renal disease, dialysis is indicated. These patients usually respond to approximately 10 days of intensive daily dialysis. Use of heparin should be restricted to the minimum necessary to prevent clotting in the extracorporeal circuit. When the patient is hemodynamically unstable, acute peritoneal dialysis is preferred to avoid sudden fluid shifts. Close monitoring of the hemodynamic and volume status in an intensive care setting is advisable. Echocardiography should be repeated to evaluate the change in the size of the effusion in response to dialysis.

When acute pericarditis develops in patients already on dialysis, a meticulous search for a variety of underlying disorders should be undertaken. Since underdialysis is always suspected, intensified dialysis should be administered to all patients, even though indicators of underdialysis may not be present. Approximately 59% of these patients will respond to a daily dialysis regimen for 1–2 weeks. Precautions concerning volume shifts and heparinization, as in the previous group, should be followed. Signs of unresponsiveness to intensive hemodialysis, hemodynamic instability, or echocardiographic evidence of tamponade are indications for drainage.[8]

Treatment with nonsteroidal anti-inflammatory drugs, though effective in nonuremic pericarditis, is less successful in patients with renal failure.[9] In addition, the dialysis population is more prone to the side effects of these agents, especially gastric ulceration and bleeding. Although in some cases of uremic pericarditis circulating immune complexes have been demonstrated, the response to systemic corticosteroids has been disappointing.

Subxiphoid pericardiocentesis, with catheter drainage and instillation of nonabsorbable steroids, should be attempted in urgent situations with evidence of hemodynamic instability.[10] Patients with large effusions and those unresponsive to conservative treatment modalities should be recommended for subxiphoid pericardiotomy. A pericardial biopsy should be done at the time of surgery. This limited procedure is usually well tolerated and appears to be successful in over 90% of patients. Reaccumulation of effusion or later development of constrictive pericarditis is an indication for pericardiectomy.

REFERENCES

1. Beaudry C, Nakamoto S, Kolff WJ: Uremic pericarditis and cardiac tamponade in chronic renal failure. *Ann Intern Med* 64:990–995, 1966.
2. Kumar S, Lesch M: Pericarditis in renal disease. *Prog Cardiovasc Dis* 22:357–369, 1980.
3. Luft FC, Gilman JK, Weyman AE: Pericarditis in the patient with uremia: Clinical and echocardiographic evaluation. *Nephron* 25:160–166, 1980.
4. Spodick DH: Pericardial rub. Prospective, multiple observer investigation of pericardial friction in 100 patients. *Am J Cardiol* 35:357–362, 1975.
5. Di Segni E, Beker B, Arbel Y, et al: Left ventricular pseudohypertrophy in pericardial effusion as a sign of cardiac tamponade. *Am J Cardiol* 66:508–511, 1990.
6. Guberman BA, Fowler NO, Engel PJ, et al: Cardiac tamponade in medical patients. *Circulation* 64:633–640, 1981.
7. Lindsay J Jr, Crawley IS, Callaway GM Jr; Chronic constrictive pericarditis following uremic hemopericardium. *Am Heart J* 79:390–395, 1970.
8. De Pace NL, Nestico PF, Schwartz AB, et al: Predicting success of intensive dialysis in the treatment of uremic pericarditis. *Am J Med* 76:38–46, 1984.
9. Suki WN: Pericarditis. *Kidney Int* 33(Suppl 24):S10–S12, 1988.
10. Leehey DJ, Daugirdas JT, Popli S, et al: Predicting need for surgical drainage of pericardial effusion in patients with end stage renal disease. *Int J Artif Org* 12:618–625, 1989.

Disorders of Potassium Balance

Sameh R. Abul-Ezz, M.D.

Intracellular potassium represents up to 98% of the total body stores. The gradient between the serum potassium concentration (3.5–5.0 mEq/L) and the intracellular concentration (150 mEq/L) is responsible for the transmembrane potential, which is essential for conductivity in the heart and the neuromuscular system. The effect of dietery or exogenous potassium administration is significant only when renal potassium handling is impaired. This is because the kidney is responsible for the excretion of over 90% of dietary intake, with gastrointestinal excretion accounting for the remaining 10%. The kidneys can adjust to changes in serum potassium by decreasing or increasing distal tubular secretion from less than 10 meq/day to 10 mEq/kg/day. This high degree of flexibility in potassium handling is usually preserved until the glomerular filtration rate (GFR) declines below 20 mL/min.[1]

HYPERKALEMIA

A gradual decline in GFR by itself seldom results in severe hyperkalemia because of a compensatory increase in renal potassium secretion and gastrointestinal secretion from 10% to more than 30% of dietary potassium intake. Hyperkalemia should be suspected in acute renal failure in the setting of a rapid decrease in urine output; in chronic renal failure when noncompliance with dietary restrictions or dialysis is suspected; when large amounts of endogenous potassium are released, as in rhabdomyolysis, hemolysis, and resorption of large hematomas; and in states of acidosis, aldosterone deficiency, and insulin deficiency.

PRESENTING MANIFESTATIONS

History

Symptoms of generalized muscle weakness, paresthesias, and tingling usually indicate severe hyperkalemia.

Physical Examination

Muscle fasciculations and hyporeflexia can be detected. Flaccid paralysis is a late manifestation since it is always preceded by severe cardiac toxicity.[2]

Laboratory Evaluation

Because of the wide availability of electrolyte testing in outpatient and emergency settings, hyperkalemia is usually diagnosed by a serum potassium determination prior to the presentation of significant clinical symptoms or signs.

DIAGNOSTIC CRITERIA

Laboratory diagnosis of hyperkalemia may be misleading since artifactual elevation of serum potassium can be encountered.[3] These errors can be prevented by avoiding hemolysis in sample collection and by determining plasma potassium levels in cases of malignant erythrocytosis, leukocytosis, or thrombocytosis. ECG changes in hyperkalemia are pathognomonic, although not consistently correlated with the severity of the hyperkalemia. As shown in Figure 5.2, the earliest change is reflected in peaking of the T waves. A further increase in serum potassium leads to flattening of the P waves, prolongation of the PR interval, and widening of the QRS complex. Ultimately, the blending of a wide QRS complex into the T wave will result in the sine wave.

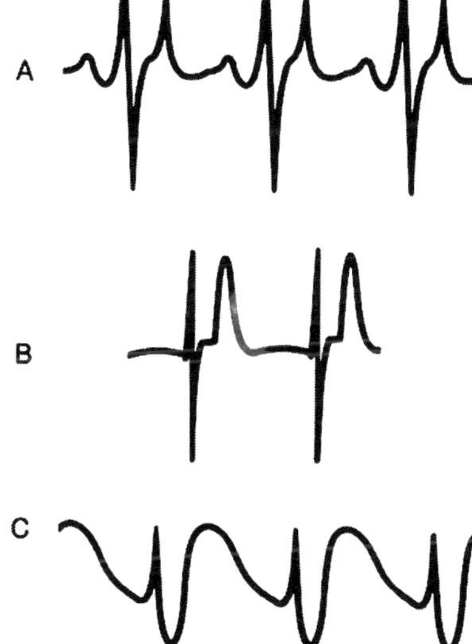

Figure 5.2. ECG findings in hyperkalemia. The initial variation from the normal complex is tall, peaked T waves (A). This is followed by a decrease in amplitude of the P waves and widening of the QRS complex. The P waves disappear as the PR interval widens (B). The final change is a blending of the QRS complex into the T waves, forming the classic sine wave pattern (C). Adapted from Andreoli, et al, in *Cecil Essentials of Medicine,* Philadelphia, PA, W.B. Saunders Company. Reprinted with permission of author and publisher.

DIFFERENTIAL DIAGNOSIS

Once artifactual hyperkalemia is ruled out, urinary potassium secretion and renal function should be determined. In patients with chronic renal failure (GFR <20 mL/min), the sudden development of hyperkalemia should alert the physician to the possibility of overwhelming the residual renal function with excessive dietary intake, especially the use of salt substitute containing potassium salts, or the release of large amount of intracellular potassium, as in hemolysis, rhabdomyolysis, or resorption of a large hematoma.

In cases of adequate renal reserve (GFR >20 mL/min), causes of the transcellular shift in potassium should be investigated. The effect of such shifts between intracellular and extracellular potassium are usually transient since the normal kidney can adapt quickly to maintain potassium homeostasis. Acidosis, beta-adrenergic blockade, hyperosmolar disorders, and periodic paralysis should be sought. When urinary potassium excretion is diminished in the presence of hyperkalemia, drugs that interfere with potassium secretion, hypoaldosteronism, and diseases associated with type IV renal tubular acidosis should be investigated.[4] Figure 5.3 summarizes these disorders.

The most common cause of hyperkalemia in patients with chronic renal insufficiency is hyporeninemic hypoaldosteronism. The majority of these patients are diabetics with a distal tubular disorder characterized by hyperkalemia, hyperchloremic acidosis, and low plasma and urinary aldosterone levels. A low renin level in these patients is thought to be secondary to chronic volume expansion or to an abnormality in the conversion of prorenin to renin. There is also evidence of primary renal aldosterone secretion defect in these patients.

PATHOPHYSIOLOGY

The clinical presentation of hyperkalemia is a manifestation of the disturbed transmembrane potential in the cardiac and neuromuscular systems. The earliest ECG changes with peaked T waves reflect an increased rate of repolarization. This is induced by the altered transmembrane resting potential (TRP), with a decreased intracellular:extracellular potassium ratio. Normally, the transmembrane resting potential is highly negative and is dependent on the gradient between intracellular and extracellular potassium. Any further increase in extracellular potassium would result in conduction delay. Since sensitivity to hyperkalemia is not uniform, different patterns of conduction delays are manifest in the ECG. Initially, conduction above the bundle of His is affected, leading to a prolonged PR interval. A further increase in hyperkalemia affects conduction in the Purkinje system below the bundle of His, with widening of the QRS complex. Because of its depressant effect on conductivity, the arrhythmia associated with hyperkalemia is thought to be due to the reentrant mechanism. Junctional and ventricular ectopic arrhythmias could rapidly deteriorate into ventricular fibrillation, with grave consequences.[5] Furthermore, hyperkalemia can interfere with pacemaker-induced depolarization, resulting in failure of atrial capture.[6]

In the clinical setting, cardiac toxicity secondary to hyperkalemia is unpredictable. This is because the rate of increase in extracellular potassium is more important as a determinant of cardiac toxicity than in terms of its absolute value. This is true especially in patients with chronic renal failure who present with few or no ECG changes despite serum potassium levels that are sometimes above 6 mEq/L. On the other hand, associated hyponatremia, hypocalcemia, hypermagnesemia, and acidosis can potentiate hyperkalemia-induced cardiac toxicity.

NATURAL HISTORY OF THE DISEASE

Untreated hyperkalemia is life-threatening because of its effect on cardiac conduction. Widening of the QRS complex on the ECG is indicative of impending ventricular fibrillation and cardiac arrest.[7]

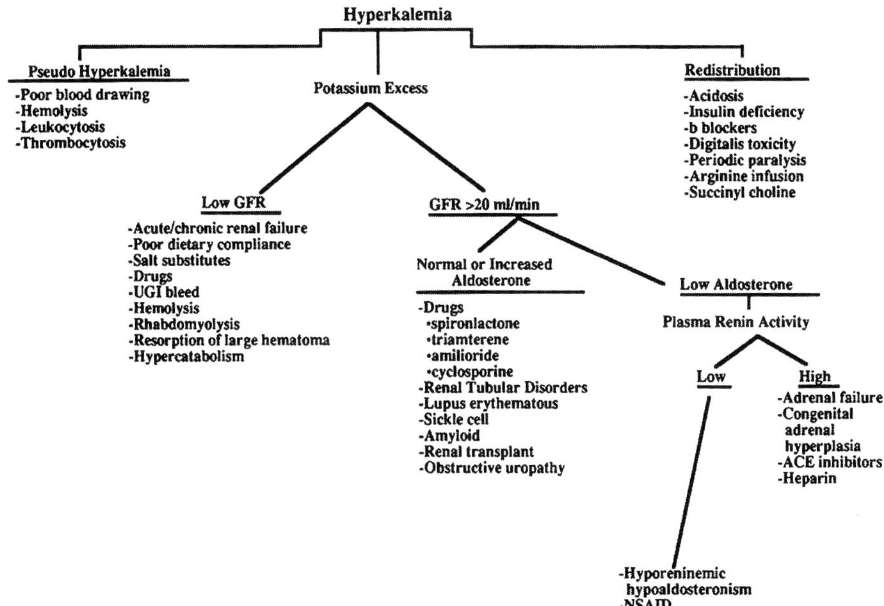

Figure 5.3. Differential diagnosis of hyperkalemia. Adapted from Tannen RL in *Schrier RW (ed) Manual* of Nephrology Diagnosis and Therapy, second edition, Boston, MA, Little, Brown. p. 44. Reprinted with permission of author and publisher.

CURRENT METHODS OF TREATMENT

Hyperkalemia with serum potassium levels above 6.5 mEq/L is considered a medical emergency. Early ECG changes such as peaking of the T wave are an indication for calcium administration in order to stabilize the cell membrane. Calcium gluconate, 10–30 mL of a 10% solution should be administered intravenously.[5] Caution should be exercised in patients who are on digitalis in order to avoid hypercalcemia-induced digitalis toxicity. Acute measures to facilitate an intracellular potassium shift should be started since removal of excess total body potassium might take hours to accomplish. The most effective method is to administer regular insulin, 5 μm/kg/min intravenously, with 20% glucose at a rate of 5 mu/kg/min in order to avoid hypoglycemia. Diabetics with hyperglycemia should receive boluses of regular insulin, which will promote an intracellular potassium shift and control their hyperosmolality. The role of sodium bicarbonate infusion is controversial. In renal failure patients with acidosis and hyperkalemia, sodium bicarbonate in doses ranging from 44 to 132 mEq/L could be given. Compared to insulin, its effect is short lived and may lead to volume overload.[8] Administration of beta agonists such as epinephrine at a rate of 0.05 μg/kg/min intravenously or salbutamol by aerosol can cause a significant intracellular potassium shift. Unfortunately, these agents are not as effective in renal failure patients.[9] The dose of albuterol is 10–20 mg by aerosol inhaler over 10 min. Intravenous saline or sodium bicarbonate and diuretics will help increase sodium and fluid delivery to the distal tubules and increase potassium diuresis except in cases of oliguria. Removal of excess body potassium by cation exchange resin through the gastrointestinal tract is effective but requires 1–2 hr before the onset of action. Sodium polysterene sulfonate (Kayexalate) can be given orally up to 40 g. Higher doses are not well tolerated. Greater potassium removal and a more rapid onset of action could be achieved with 50–100 g of Kayexalate in 200 mL of 20% sorbitol as an enema. This should be retained for 30 min and preceded by a cleansing enema. In patients with acute or chronic renal failure and severe hyperkalemia, hemodialysis or peritoneal dialysis should be initiated as soon as possible. Measures to stabilize the cell membrane and to achieve an intracellular shift in potassium should be started, as waiting for the dialysis setup might expose the patient to undue risks.

Chronic hyperkalemia in renal tubular acidosis, hypoaldosteronism, and hyporeninemic hypoaldosteronism require patient education and dietary counseling on potassium restriction in the diet.[10] Avoidance of potassium-sparing diuretics and nonsteroidal anti-inflammatory drugs should be emphasized. In hypoaldosteronism, fludrocortisone, 0.1 mg orally daily, and a high salt intake should be used. In hyporeninemic hypoaldosterone states, fludrocortisone is less effective, and may further complicate hypertension and fluid retention.

HYPOKALEMIA

As in hyperkalemia, alterations in the intracellular:extracellular potassium ratio can lead to serious neuromuscular and cardiac sequelae.[11]

PRESENTING MANIFESTATIONS

History

Although most patients with serum potassium levels between 3.0 and 3.5 mEq/L are asymptomatic, some patients may complain of malaise, easy fatigability, generalized muscle aches, and cramping. As the potassium level decreases below 3.0 mEq/L, symptoms of skeletal muscle dysfunction become more pronounced. Symptoms related to smooth muscle dysfunction are usually manifested in gastrointestinal symptoms. Constipation is common at mild levels of hypokalemia and could deteriorate to paralysis of the gastrointestinal tract with the development of ileus.[12]

Physical Examination

Physical examination of the neuromuscular system may reveal restless leg, tetany, and even paralysis with severe hypokalemia.

Laboratory Evaluation

Typical ECG changes include T-wave flattening, depression of ST segments, and prominent U waves. The prominent U waves may be mistaken for the T waves and may lead to overestimation of the QT interval.[13] Serum potassium levels below 3.0 mEq/L are usually associated with peaked P waves. Prolongation of the PR and QRS intervals is uncommon. In hypokalemia, the heart is predisposed to a wide range of arrhythmias. Atrial, junctional, and ventricular premature beats are common.

DIAGNOSTIC CRITERIA

The diagnosis of hypokalemia rests on determination of the serum potassium level.

DIFFERENTIAL DIAGNOSIS

Transcellular shift of potassium can result in moderate to severe hypokalemia. Alkalemia, insulin administration and hereditary hypokalemic periodic paralysis are associated with acute

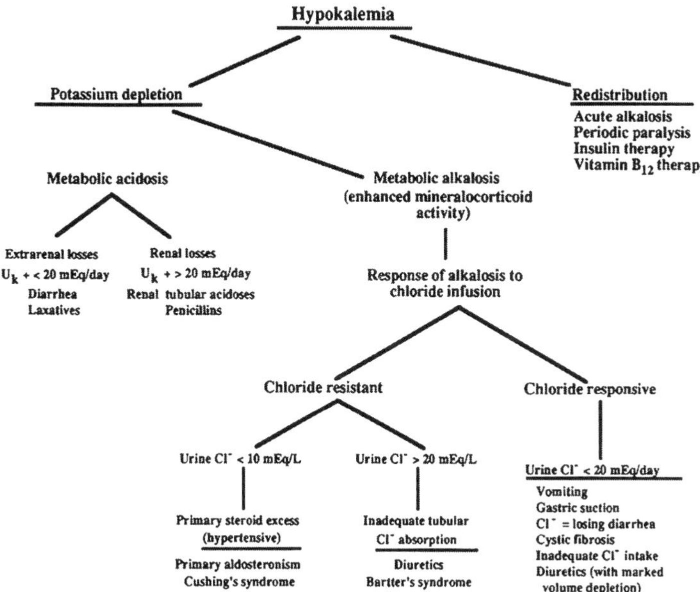

Figure 5.4. Differential diagnosis of hypokalemia. Adapted from Andreoli, et al, in *Cecil Essentials of Medicine* third edition, Philadelphia, PA, W.B. Saunders Company. Reprinted with permission of author and publisher.

intracellular shifts of potassium. Common medications such as beta-adrenergic agonists used in the treatment of asthma and chronic obstructive pulmonary disease can cause intracellular potassium shifts even with inhalation aerosols. Addition of theophylline could have a synergistic effect in these patients. Intoxication with toluene and barium produces a similar effect. In order to differentiate between renal and gastrointestinal potassium losses, determination of urinary potassium and its fractional excretion, together with the acid-base, volume, and blood pressure statuses, will help reach the specific diagnosis.[14] Figure 5.4 shows a diagnosis tree based on these determinations. Renal potassium conservation with a urinary potassium concentration <20 mEq/day and fractional excretion <6% points to an extrarenal etiology such as diarrhea, laxative abuse, or excessive perspiration. Renal potassium losses >20 mEq/day in the presence of hypokalemia with decreased volume status should suggest the possibility of vomiting and the use or abuse of diuretics. The presence of hypertension should raise the possibility of primary or secondary hyperaldosteronism or implicate the administration of exogenous steroids and compounds with steroid-like action. Renal potassium losses with non–anion gap acidosis should point to type I or type II renal tubular acidosis. Renal potassium losses in the presence of a variable acid-base status are seen in patients receiving nonresorbable anions like penicillin and carbenicillin, as well as in patients with hypomagnesemia and Barter's syndrome.[14]

PATHOPHYSIOLOGY

Cardiac toxicity secondary to hypokalemia can be attributed to hyperpolarization. Delay in atrioventricular conduction can be attributed to the alteration in transmembrane resting potential with an increased threshold to provoke an action potential as a result of the increased intracellular:extracellular potassium ratio. This altered ratio may also affect termination of the action potential, resulting in reduction of the takeoff potential before complete repolarization.[15]

NATURAL HISTORY OF THE DISEASE

In the setting of underlying cardiac disease, especially in acute myocardial infarction, hypokalemia has been shown to be arrhythmogenic, with increased susceptibility to the development of ventricular tachycardia and fibrillation.[16] The potentiation of digitalis toxicity with the development of a wide range of arrhythmias is well recognized. Even in the presence of mild hypokalemia, the spectrum of arrhythmia attributed to digitalis toxicity may include supraventricular tachycardia, heart block, ventricular premature beats, and ventricular tachyarrhythmia.[17]

CURRENT METHODS OF TREATMENT

When left untreated, hypokalemia may have serious cardiac and systemic effects. Mild hypokalemia in patients with underlying heart disease, especially in acute myocardial infarction, and in patients on digitalis should be treated promptly. Digitalis toxicity could occur with normal digitalis levels in the presence of hypokalemia. Hypokalemia could also result in increased ammoniagenesis, which could precipitate hepatic encephalopathy in patients with marginal hepatic reserve. Symptoms attributed to hypokalemia, especially muscle weakness, dictate emergency treatment before progression to paralysis.[18] The underlying cause of hypokalemia should be identified and its treatment initiated. In nonemergency situations without symptoms or arrhythmia, oral potassium supplementation with potassium chloride is well tolerated and ensures safe replenishment of the potassium deficit. When symptoms are evident or cardiac manifestations are demonstrated on the ECG, intravenous potassium chloride should be administered. Estimation of the potassium deficit for replacement is not accurate since an intracellular shift could accompany true potassium losses.[19] Serial determinations of serum potassium levels during treatment are necessary. Intravenous potassium administration is rarely needed unless oral intake is restricted. The peripheral venous route should be used with potassium concentrations ≤ 40 mEq/L to avoid phlebitis. Sodium chloride solutions are preferred to dextrose solutions to avoid glucose loading with increased insulin secretion, with a further intracellular potassium shift. In high-risk patients who need long-term diuretic treatment, as in congestive heart failure, especially patients on digitalis, therapy with potassium-sparing diuretics should be considered.[20]

REFERENCES

1. Tannen RL: Potassium metabolism. In Gonick HC (ed): *Current Nephrology,* Vol. 12. St. Louis, MO, Year Book, 1989, pp 87–134.
2. Pollen RH, Williams RH: Hyperkalemic neuromusculopathy in Addison's disease. *N Engl J Med* 263:273–277, 1963.
3. Sterns RH, Spital A: Disorders of internal potassium balance. *Semin Nephrol* 7:206–221, 1987.
4. West M: Disorders of serum potassium. *Med North Am* 28:5208–5222, 1988.
5. Rardon DP, Fisc C. Electrolytes and the heart. In Hurst JW (ed): *The Heart.* New York, NY, McGraw-Hill, 1994, pp 759–774.
6. Barold SS, Kalkoff MD, Ong LS, et al: Hyperkalemia-induced failure of atrial capture during dual-chamber cardiac pacing. *J Am Coll Cardiol* 10:467–469, 1987.
7. Ewy GA, Karliner J, Bedynek JL Jr: Electrocardiographic QRS axis shift as a manifestation of hyperkalemia. *JAMA* 215:429–432, 1971.
8. Blumberg A, Weidmann P, Shaw S, et al: Effect of various therapeutic approaches on plasma potassium and major regulating factors in terminal renal failure. *Am J Med* 85:507–512, 1988.
9. Du Plooy WJ, Hay L, Kahler CP, et al: The dose-related hyper- and hypo-kalaemic effects of salbutamol and its arrhythmogenic potential. *Br J Pharmacol* 111:73–76, 1994.

10. Williams ME, Rose RM: Hyperkalemia: Disorders of internal and external potassium balance. *J Intens Care Med* 3:52–64, 1988.

11. Welt LG, Holander W Jr, Blythe WB: The consequences of potassium depletion. *J Chronic Dis* 2:213–254, 1960.

12. Tannen RL: Potassium disorders. In Kokko JP, Tannen RL (eds): *Fluid and Electrolytes,* ed 2. Philadelphia, PA, WB Saunders, 1990, pp 195–300.

13. Surawicz B, Lepeschkin E: Electrocardiographic pattern of hypopotassemia with and without hypocalcemia. *Circulation* 8:801–828, 1953.

14. Wright RS: Renal potassium handling. *Semin Nephrol* 7:174–184, 1987.

15. Rardon DP, Fisc C: Electrolytes and the heart. In Hurst JW (ed): *The Heart,* ed 8. New York, NY, McGraw-Hill, 1994, pp 759–774.

16. Coronel R: Heterogeneity in extracellular potassium concentration during early myocardial ischemia and reperfusion: Implications for arrhythmogenesis. *Cardiovasc Res* 28:770–777, 1994.

17. Aronson JK: Digitalis intoxication. *Clin Sci* 64:253–258, 1983.

18. Tannen RL: Hypo-hyperkalemia. In Cameron S, Davison AM, Grunfeld J-P, et al (eds): *Textbook of Clinical Nephrology.* Oxford, Oxford University Press, 1992, pp 895–917.

19. West M: Disorders of serum potassium. *Med North Am* 28:5208–5222, 1988.

20. Hoes AW, Grobbee DE, Peet TM, et al: Do non-potassium-sparing diuretics increase the risk of sudden cardiac death in hypertensive patients? Recent evidence. *Drugs* 47:711–733, 1994.

Disorders of Calcium Homeostasis

Sameh R. Abul-Ezz, M.D.

The normal total body content of calcium is 1000 to 1500 g in a 70-kg adult. Most of it occurs in the skeleton, and 1% is found in the extracellular fluid. This small percentage of total body calcium is kept within a narrow range, as it critically affects the neuromuscular activity. The total plasma calcium concentrate is divided into 40% protein bound, 13% complexed, and 47% ionized. Ionized calcium is kept between 4 and 5 mg/dL by several homeostatic mechanisms, including the parathyroid hormone, vitamin D, the gastrointestinal tract, and the kidneys. Although the kidney plays only a secondary role in calcium balance, acute and chronic renal failure are commonly associated with disorders of calcium metabolism. Directly related to calcium homeostasis is the secondary hyperparathyroidism commonly encountered in patients with chronic renal failure on maintenance dialysis.[1]

HYPERCALCEMIA

The many causes of hypercalcemia and the differential diagnosis in the general population are extensively covered in several excellent reviews. In this section, the causes and differential diagnosis of hypercalcemia in the renal patient will be emphasized.

Hypercalcemia is commonly seen in the setting of acute renal failure, in end-stage renal disease patients on dialysis, and shortly after kidney transplantation. It is uncommon in patients with chronic renal insufficiency who have not developed end-stage disease. In some forms of acute renal failure such as rhabdomyolysis, hypercalcemia is one of the manifestations of the disease resulting from resorption of calcified, necrotic muscle tissue. In other cases, resolution of acute renal failure is followed by hypercalcemia due to a persistent state of secondary hyperparathyroidism even after the recovery of renal function. This same phenomenon is observed soon after kidney transplantation.

Chronic dialysis patients exhibit hypercalcemia as a result of several factors: an autonomous parathyroid gland, increased use of calcium compounds as phosphate binders, hydroxylated vitamin D supplementation with increased intestinal absorption, and increased calcium concentration in the dialysate with a net calcium gain from the dialysate.

Hypercalemia may be nonrenal in etiology and may lead to acute renal failure. With normal renal function, hypercalcemia always raises the suspicion of malignancy or primary hyperparathyroidism. Commonly used thiazide diuretics are frequent causes of hypercalcemia, manifested through increased calcium tubular reabsorption and volume contraction.[2] Increased absorption of calcium, through either vitamin D intoxication or vitamin D hydroxylation in sarcoid tissues, is a less common cause of hypercalcemia.

PRESENTING MANIFESTATIONS

History

Symptoms that can be attributed to elevated serum calcium include skin itching and mental status change with mental dulling, lethargy, and confusion.[3] The gastrointestinal tract is commonly involved, with symptoms ranging from anorexia, nausea, vomiting and constipation to severe symptoms attributed to peptic ulceration and acute pancreatitis. Patients without renal insufficiency commonly manifest nephrogenic diabetes insipidus with polyuria and polydipsia. Nephrolithiasis secondary to hypercalcemia is common in primary hyperparathyroidism.[4]

Physical Examination

Hypertension is often demonstrated. The mental status examination may reveal emotional lability, disorientation, and occasionally psychosis. The neurologic examination usually reveals generalized muscle weakness and decreased deep tendon reflexes.

Laboratory Evaluation

The predominant ECG change in hypercalcemia is shortening of the ST segment. Extreme elevation in serum calcium could lead to complete disappearance of the ST segment, with the T wave directly joining the end of the QRS complex.[5] Correlation between the degree of hypercalcemia and the QT interval is poor. By contrast, the interval from the beginning of the Q to the apex of the T wave offers a strong inverse correlation with the serum calcium level.[6] Arrhythmias are rarely encountered in hypercalcemia, especially when no other electrolyte disorder is present. Only extreme elevations in serum calcium have been associated with conduction delay. Prolongation of the PR interval and widening of the QRS complex are demonstrated in some cases and in experimental calcium infusion.

DIAGNOSTIC CRITERIA

The demonstration of increased serum calcium level is diagnostic.

DIFFERENTIAL DIAGNOSIS

The diagnosis of the specific etiology of hypercalcemia is usually obvious from the underlying disease presentation. In end-stage renal disease patients on dialysis with hypercalcemia, the etiology is likely iatrogenic. Review of the dialysis calcium concentration and the dosage of hydroxylated vitamin D is necessary. Aluminum bone disease is common in the dialysis population and often results in hypercalcemia secondary to decreased bone turnover. When renal

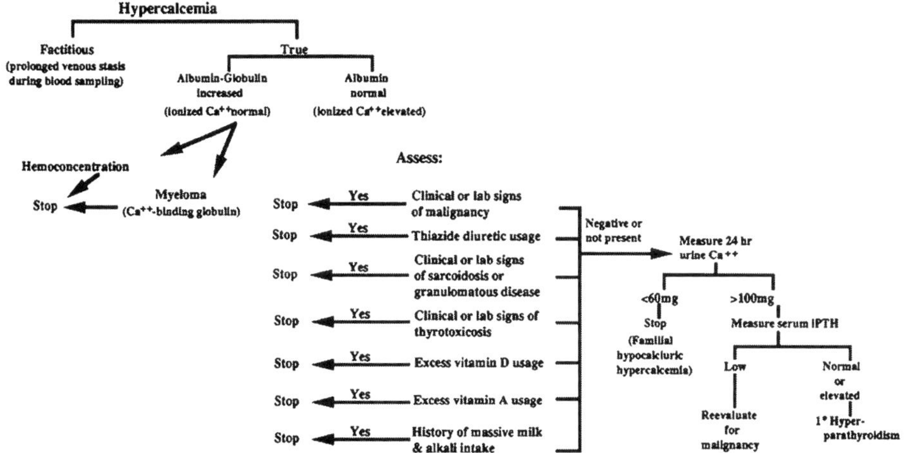

Figure 5.5. Algorithm for the differential diagnosis of hypercalcemia. Adapted from Garrick R, Goldfarb S, *Am J Kid Dis* 13:161; 1989. Reprinted with permission of author and publisher.

function is normal, determination of 24-hr urinary calcium excretion and intact parathyroid hormone will help in the differential diagnosis of hypercalcemia, as shown in Figure 5.5.

PATHOPHYSIOLOGY

Increased serum calcium affects phase 2 of the transmembrane action potential. This is manifested in decreased duration and reduced amplitude of the plateau. These effects are responsible for the shortening of the ST segment. Hypercalcemia decreases the velocity of the propagated action potential, resulting in conduction delays, most consistent with first degree atrioventricular block. Despite the increase in diastolic depolarization seen with hypercalcemia, arrhythmias are not commonly seen. This is thought to be due to a simultaneous increase in the threshold potential.[7]

Neuropsychiatric manifestations of hypercalcemia have been correlated with the increase in cerebrospinal fluid calcium ion concentration, which is thought to decrease conduction in the nerve terminals. The conduction delay associated with an increased calcium concentration inside the nerve cells has been proposed as the mechanism for neuromuscular manifestations associated with hypercalcemia.

NATURAL HISTORY OF THE DISEASE

Untreated hypercalcemia results in metastatic calcification and pancreatitis. Serum calcium levels above 15 mg/dL may cause hypercalcemia crisis, resulting in stupor and coma.

CURRENT METHODS OF TREATMENT

Acute treatment of hypercalcemia is based on saline diuresis.[8] Increased urinary sodium results in decreased tubular reabsorption of calcium and increased urinary calcium excretion. Before starting to use diuretics, patients should achieve normal intravascular volume, as hypovolemia increases tubular calcium reabsorption. Once normal intravascular volume is achieved, high rates of saline infusion (200–250 mL/hr) should be accompanied by an intravenous loop diuretic to maintain high urinary calcium excretion and avoid volume overload.

Loop diuretics also interfere with calcium reabsorption, while thiazide diuretics promote it and should be avoided.[9] Serum potassium and magnesium levels should be monitored closely and supplements added to intravenous fluids, especially in patients already on digitalis.[10]

Chronic management of hypercalcemia is best achieved by treating the underlying disease. Parathyroidectomy is curative in primary hyperparathyroidism. It is rarely needed in the dialysis population since early, aggressive management of hyperphosphatemia, the wide use of hydroxylated vitamin D, and adjustment of the dialysate calcium level have reduced the incidence and severity of secondary hyperparathyroidism. Patients with malignancy awaiting definitive surgical or chemotherapeutic therapy should be treated with agents which suppress the osteoclastic activity. Calcitonin has often been used, with effective reduction in hypercalcemia, but the frequent complaints of nausea and flushing reduce its long-term use. Also, tachyphylaxis is frequently encountered. The diphosphonates are quite effective in reducing serum calcium through inhibition of bone resorption. Several compounds are available for clinical use, of which etidronate, clodrinate, and pamidronate are the most commonly used.

HYPOCALCEMIA

PRESENTING MANIFESTATIONS

History

Clinical manifestations of hypocalcemia are directly related to the critical influence of extracellular ionized calcium on the integrity of the neuromuscular system. Patients with chronic renal insufficiency commonly have hypocalcemia manifested in two distinct clinical pictures. The first presentation occurs when serum calcium levels decrease precipitously. This presentation is commonly seen in chronic renal failure patients with hyperparathyroidism undergoing parathyroidectomy. Clinically, these patients may present with dramatic and sometimes life-threatening symptoms of neuromuscular irritability. Initially, symptoms of mental confusion, irritability, and occasionally psychosis are associated with circumoral and acral paresthesia. Symptoms of muscle stiffness, cramping, and carpopedal spasm may deteriorate rapidly into tetany and convulsions.[11]

The second presentation of hypocalcemia is seen in chronic renal failure patients in whom the serum calcium level decreases slowly over a long period of time, usually in association with secondary hyperparathyroidism and hyperphosphatemia. These patients seldom present with symptoms of neuromuscular irritability. Instead, their symptoms are related to secondary hyperparathyroidism. They also develop metastatic calcifications in spite of having borderline low serum calcium levels. Cardiovascular and pulmonary calcifications in these patients ultimately produce symptoms of heart failure with progressive dyspnea and fluid retention.[12] Coronary artery calcification contributes to the development of ischemic heart disease in these patients.

Physical Examination

Patients with acute hypocalcemia may be hypotensive. Mental obtundation may be apparent. The neurologic examination may elicit signs of latent neuromuscular irritability such as facial twitching upon tapping over the facial nerve (Chvostek's sign). Also, raising the pressure in a blood pressure manometer over the patient's systolic blood pressure for 3 min may produce carpopedal spasm (Trousseau's sign). Both of these signs are nonspecific.

In patients with chronic renal failure, signs of hyperparathyroidism with metastatic calcification should be looked for in the eye, with the development of premature cataract, and in the musculoskeletal system in the form of tendon and ligament calcification and calcium pyrophosphate crystal-induced arthritis (pseudogout).

Valvular calcifications commonly affect the mitral valve. In one study the prevalence of mitral annular calcification in end-stage renal disease was 40%.[13] Signs of heart failure are commonly seen in the dialysis population, but the etiology is most likely multifactorial rather than metastatic calcification alone.[14]

Laboratory Evaluation

ECG changes consistent with hypocalcemia typically reveal prolongation of the QT interval.[15] Severe hypocalcemia may interfere with ventricular conduction and result in ventricular fibrillation. ECG demonstration of left and right ventricular hypertrophy, mitral annular calcification, and, less commonly, aortic valve calcification are predominant findings in patients on dialysis. Indirect evidence of pulmonary calcification is obtained with increased Technetium-99 uptake by the lungs and decreased carbon monoxide defusing capacity.

DIAGNOSTIC CRITERIA

The diagnosis of hypocalcemia relies on plasma determination of ionized calcium. If the ionized calcium measurement is not available, total serum calcium should be corrected for protein binding to rule out artifactual hypocalcemia. In cases of hypoalbuminemia, each 1 g/L drop in serum albumin is approximately corrected by adding 0.8 mg/dL to the total serum calcium. If this correction still does not result in a normal serum calcium level, true hypocalcemia is present.

DIFFERENTIAL DIAGNOSIS

The differential diagnosis of hypocalcemia requires the determination of renal function, magnesium level, phosphorus level, and intact parathormone level.[16] With these determinations, the etiology of hypocalcemia can be determined by following the approach presented in Table 5.2.

TABLE 5.2. Causes of Hypocalcemia

Normal or increased parathyroid hormone
    Renal failure
    Renal tubular acidosis
    Vitamin D disorder
        Decreased intake
        Malabsorption
        Liver or renal disease
        Medications; phenobarbitol phenytoin
    Osteoblastic metastases
    States of excess phosphate
        Rhabdomyolysis
        Hyperalimentation
        Tumor lysis syndrome
    Pseudohypoparathyroidism
    Hypomagnesemia

Decreased parathyroid hormone
    Hypoparathyroidism
        Idiopathic
        Postsurgical
        Hypomagnesemia
        Infiltrative
        Irradiation

PATHOPHYSIOLOGY

Hypocalcemia produces prolongation and decreased amplitude of the plateau of phase 2 of the transmembrane action potential.[17] This is translated into prolongation of the ST segment and the QT interval on the ECG. Since calcium is known to provide a critical link for excitation-contraction coupling, it is believed to play an important role in the contraction of cardiac muscle. Long-standing hypocalcemia has been shown to affect the left ventricular stroke volume and cardiac index.[18] When accompanied by secondary hyperparathyroidism, myocardial calcification can compound these effects with depression of myocardial contractility. Congestive heart failure resistant to medical treatment has been described in these patients.

NATURAL HISTORY OF THE DISEASE

If left untreated, acute hypocalcemia can be life-threatening. Patients with renal failure and hyperparathyroidism suffer from hungry bone syndrome after parathyroidectomy. Convulsions and multiple fractures may occur.[19] Ventricular arrhythmias are the ultimate result of untreated, rapidly progressing hypocalcemia.

CURRENT METHODS OF TREATMENT

If a precipitous drop is observed or if the patient develops symptoms of neuromuscular irritability, up to 6.0 g of intravenous calcium gluconate in a 10% solution can be administered, either as continuous infusion or by repeated boluses.[20] Chronic hypocalcemia in the dialysis population should be treated with phosphate binders, dialysate containing higher concentration of calcium, and hydroxylated vitamin D. These measures should achieve adequate suppression of the parathyroid gland.

In hypocalcemia with a nonrenal etiology, correction of hypomagnesemia and vitamin D deficiency, when present, is crucial to the successful repletion of calcium. Diagnosing and treating the underlying disease is the most important step in achieving calcium homeostasis.

REFERENCES

1. Akmal M, Brandt RR, Ansari AN, et al: Excess PTH in CRF induces pulmonary calcification, pulmonary hypertension and right ventricular hypertrophy. *Kidney Int* 47:158–163, 1995.
2. Dent DM, Miller JL, Kloff L, et al: The incidence and causes of hypercalcemia. *Postgrad Med J* 63:745–750, 1987.
3. Cogan MG, Covey M, Arieff AI, et al: Central nervous system manifestations of hyperparathyroidism. *Am J Med* 65:963–970, 1978.
4. Heath DA: Primary hyperparathyroidism. Clinical presentation and factors influencing clinical management. *Endocrinol Metabol Clin North Am* 18:631–646, 1989.
5. Harnett JD, Kent GM, Barre PE, et al: Risk factors for the development of left ventricular hypertrophy in a prospectively followed cohort of dialysis patients. *J Am Soc Nephrol* 4:486–490, 1994.
6. Surawicz B, McDonald MG, Kaliot V, et al: Treatment of cardiac arrhythmias with salts of ethylenediamine tetraacetic acid (EDTA). *Am Heart J* 58:493–503, 1959.
7. Nierenberg DW, Ransil BJ: Q-a Tc interval as a clinical indicator of hypercalcemia. *Am J Cardiol* 44:243–248, 1979.
8. Rardon DP, Fisc C: Electrolytes and the heart. In Hurst JW (ed): *The Heart*. New York, McGraw-Hill, 1994, pp 759–774.
9. Harinck HI, Biojvoet OL, Plantingh AS, et al: Role of bone and kidney in tumour-induced hypercalcemia and its treatment with biphosphonate and sodium chloride. *Am J Med* 81:1133–1142, 1987.

10. Kanis JA: Clodronate—a new perspective in the treatment of neoplastic bone disease. *Bone* 8(Suppl 1):1–86, 1987.

11. Vincent RG, Moore GE, Watne AL: Abnormal behavior following parathyroidectomy. *JAMA* 180:372–375, 1962.

12. El-Belbesi S, Brantbar N, Anderson K, et al: Effect of chronic renal failure on heart: Role of secondary hyperparathyroidism. *Am J Nephrol* 6:369–395, 1986.

13. Rostand SG, Sanders C, Kirk KA, et al: Myocardial calcification and cardiac dysfunction in chronic renal failure. *Am J Med* 85:651–657, 1988.

14. Byrg RJ, Gordon PR, Migdal SD: Doppler detected tricuspid, mitral or aortic regurgitation in end stage renal disease. *Am J Cardiol* 63:750–752, 1989.

15. Surawicz B, Lepeschkin E: Electrocardiographic pattern of hypopotassemia with and without hypocalcemia. *Circulation* 8:801–828, 1953.

16. Bourke E, Delaney V: Assessment of hypocalcemia and hypercalcemia. *Clin Lab Med* 13:157–181, 1993.

17. Rardon DP, Fisc C: Electrolytes and the heart. In Hurst JW (ed): *The Heart.* New York, McGraw-Hill, 1994, pp 759–774.

18. Wong CK, Pan KK, Cheng CH, et al: Hypocalcemic heart failure in end stage renal disease. *Am J Nephrol* 10:167–170, 1990.

19. Tohme JF, Bilezikian JP: Hypocalcemic emergencies. *Endocrinol Metab Clin North Am* 22:363–375, 1993.

20. Savazzi GM, Alerg L: The hungry bone syndrome clinical problems and therapeutic approach following parathyroidectomy. *Eur J Med* 2:363–368, 1993.

Disorders of Magnesium Homeostasis

Sameh R. Abul-Ezz, M.D.

HYPOMAGNESEMIA

Magnesium is predominantly an intracellular cation, of which 50% is in bone. Other organs with a high magnesium concentration are the liver, muscle, and red blood cells. Intracellularly, magnesium participates in several membrane and enzymatic functions which are essential for cell survival. A small percentage of total body magnesium is present in the extracellular compartment, with normal serum concentrations between 0.7 and 2.4 mg/dL. Serum magnesium is a poor indicator of total body magnesium. Accordingly, patients with a moderate magnesium deficiency may present with a serum magnesium level that is low normal or slightly below normal. Patients with chronic magnesium depletion, such as alcoholics, usually have their serum magnesium level maintained within the normal limit at the expense of bone and other tissue magnesium depletion. Better indicators of total body magnesium have been sought, but serum magnesium remains the only practical indicator of hypomagnesemia.[1]

The prevalence of hypomagnesemia varies according to the study population. Random serum determinations in hospital in patients reveal a prevalence of 6–11%. In intensive care units, hypomagnesemia is found in as many as 20% of patients.[2] Approximately 19% of patients receiving digitalis were found to be hypomagnesemic when serum magnesium levels were measured. Hypomagnesemia is common in patients with hypokalemia and hypocalcemia. Over 30% of patients on digitalis with hypokalemia or hypocalcemia were found to be magnesium deficient.[3]

PRESENTING MANIFESTATIONS

History

Because of the close association between hypomagnesemia, hypokalemia, and hypocalcemia, there is great deal of overlap between the symptoms and signs of these three ion disorders. Some authors doubted the existence of a separate set of symptoms that are specific to hypomagnesemia.[4] Some patients with overt hypomagnesemia are asymptomatic, and magnesium deficiency in the experimental setting failed to reproduce consistently the same clinical picture of hypomagnesemia. When present, symptoms of magnesium deficiency reflect hyperexcitability in the neuromuscular and cardiovascular systems. The earliest symptoms attributable to magnesium deficiency are neuromuscular and psychiatric. Apathy, confusion, depression, and personality change have all been described. Muscle weakness and paresthesias are common, but convulsions are rare and usually indicate the concurrent presence of other electrolyte imbalances.

Physical Examination

Mental status change and signs of anxiety, agitation, and delirium may be evident. The neurologic examination may reveal coarse tremors, muscle fasciculations, generalized muscle weakness, and positive Chvostek's and Trousseau's signs. When tetany is present, concomitant hypocalcemia is usually present.[5] Evidence of the causal relationship between these manifestations of neuromuscular irritability and hypomagnesemia is based on reversibility of these symptoms and signs with magnesium repletion.

Laboratory Evaluation

Serum magnesium may be normal in the presence of magnesium deficiency. ECG changes with hypomagnesemia are unreliable. Even in severe cases of hypomagnesemia, the ECG may be normal or may reveal nonspecific ST-T segment changes. However, specific ECG changes with peaked T waves and ST segment depression have been described and reproduced in the experimental setting. Widening of the QRS complex in extreme cases of hypomagnesemia has also been described.[6]

Arrhythmias including supraventricular arrhythmias, atrial premature beats and paroxysmal tachycardia, atrial fibrillation, ventricular premature beats, ventricular tachycardia, and ventricular fibrillation may occur in both digitalized and nondigitalized patients with hypomagnesemia.[7] The role of hypomagnesemia in inducing these arrhythmias is debatable, and its effective treatment with magnesium infusion may be secondary to a nonspecific antiarrhythmic effect of magnesium.[8]

DIAGNOSTIC CRITERIA

In order to establish the source of magnesium losses, 24-hr urine magnesium determinations are necessary. When the urinary magnesium level exceeds 36 mg/day in the presence of hypomagnesemia, a renal wasting mechanism is diagnosed. Less than 12 mg/day of urinary magnesium indicates a nonrenal etiology.

In order to establish the diagnosis of magnesium depletion in the presence of a normal serum magnesium level, retention of an intravenous magnesium infusion can be tested. A 24-hr urine collection for baseline magnesium excretion is compared with a second 24-hr urine magnesium determination, starting with the infusion of 7.5 g magnesium sulfate in 500 mL D5W over 8 to 12 hr. Excretion of less than 50% of the infused dose indicates intracellular magnesium depletion.[9]

TABLE 5.3. Causes of Hypomagnesemia

Gastrointestinal disorders
  Malabsorption syndromes
  Chronic diarrhea
  Laxative abuse
  Nasogastric suction
  Intestinal and biliary fistulas
  Pancreatitis
Renal disorders
  Diuretic phase of acute renal failure
  Renal tubular acidosis
  Congenital magnesium wasting
  Diuretic therapy (except potassium-sparing diuretics)
  Drugs
    Cisplatin
    Aminoglycosides
    Alcohol
  After renal transplantation
  Hypercalcemia
Redistribution
  Ketoacidosis
  Hungry bone syndrome
  Hyperalimentation
Endocrine causes
  Diabetes mellitus
  Hyperparathyroidism
  Hyperthyroidism
  Primary hyperaldosteronism
Alcoholism

DIFFERENTIAL DIAGNOSIS

The etiology of magnesium deficiency is probably easy to diagnose. Hospitalized patients with restricted intake, especially those receiving diuretics, will develop hypomagnesemia if a magnesium supplement is not administered. Magnesium redistribution should be suspected in alcoholic withdrawal, diabetic ketoacidosis, hyperalimentation, and acute pancreatitis. When magnesium loss is suspected to be the etiology, gastrointestinal losses are usually evident in chronic malabsorption syndromes, diarrhea, laxative abuse, and short bowel syndrome. Renal magnesium wasting is found in patients with primary or secondary hyperaldosteronism and in renal tubular acidosis, especially when induced by medications and following transplantation. Table 5.3 lists the most common causes of hypomagnesemia.

PATHOPHYSIOLOGY

The close link between magnesium deficiency and other ion depletions explains the overlap between the ECG manifestations of hypomagnesemia and those of potassium and calcium.

Serious ventricular arrhythmias, especially torsade de pointes, have been linked to magnesium deficiency. Several studies have demonstrated successful termination of these arrhythmias with magnesium infusion. The mechanism by which magnesium deficiency predisposes to ventricular arrhythmias is not well understood. Several lines of evidence indicate that magnesium deficiency, through impairment of Na-K ATPase, may induce intracellular hypokalemia and hypercalcemia. These conditions may lead to a further increase in the resting membrane electronegativity and lowering of the threshold potential. This, in turn, could predispose to secondary repolarization before the completion of myocardial cell repolarization and hence ventricular tachycardia. Nonspecificity of magnesium therapy in normal and hypomagnesemic patients remains to be resolved. Nonetheless, several cardiac centers have advocated magnesium treatment in the setting of acute myocardial infarction, digitalis toxicity, and ventricular tachycardia despite a normal serum magnesium level. This is due to the lack of major side effects and the effectiveness of magnesium therapy.[10]

CURRENT METHODS OF TREATMENT

In asymptomatic outpatients, treatment should concentrate on prevention and early diagnosis. High-risk populations should be identified, such as congestive heart failure patients on diuretics, diabetics, alcoholics, and patients with chronic diarrhea. When possible, treatment of the underlying disorder should be the highest priority. Loop diuretics should be substituted for potassium-sparing diuretics when possible. Potassium-sparing diuretics such as amilioride, triamterene, and spironolactone are also magnesium sparing. Oral magnesium supplementation should be tried, using magnesium oxide in doses of 2400–3600 mg/day. Diarrhea is the major side effect of oral magnesium preparations. Critically ill patients receiving hyperalimentation should receive 240 mg of elemental magnesium supplementation daily, unless contraindicated by the presence of renal failure.

In symptomatic hypomagnesemic patients, the deficit should be calculated as 125 mg to 250 mg/kg body weight. Because of 50% obligatory renal wasting, twice the deficit should be administered. In nonemergency situations, 10 g magnesium sulfate is given over 24 hr on the first day, followed by 6 g daily.[10] This could be administered by intramuscular injections, although the pain and sclerosing effect of these injections limits its practicality, especially when large amounts need to be administered.

In cases of tachyarrhythmia, 2 g of 50% magnesium sulfate in a 10 mL solution is injected intravenously over 1 min. This is followed by 2–5 g intravenously over 6 hr. Renal function and serum magnesium levels should be monitored closely.

HYPERMAGNESEMIA

Hypermagnesemia is far less common than hypomagnesemia. This disorder is encountered mainly in patients with renal insufficiency.[11] Patients with oliguric acute renal failure are especially susceptible to the development of hypermagnesemia, as magnesium-containing antacids and laxatives are overlooked when medications are adjusted for renal failure. Patients with end-stage renal disease may develop hypermagnesemia if a high-magnesium dialysate is used or if patients are noncompliant with restrictions on over-the-counter medications containing magnesium.[12] A temporary rise in serum magnesium is frequently seen in obstetric wards, as large doses of magnesium infusion are used in the treatment of eclampsia, preeclampsia, and premature labor.[13] In the absence of significant renal impairment, excess magnesium is rapidly excreted by the kidney.

PRESENTING MANIFESTATIONS

History

A moderate increase in serum magnesium, in the range of 4–6 mEq/L, may be associated with nausea, vomiting, headache, and flushing. Serum magnesium levels above 9 mEq/L may be associated with lethargy, generalized weakness, and burning of the skin.

Physical Examination

Hypotension and bradycardia are common, and arrhythmias arising from conduction delays are common. Neuromuscular symptoms in the form of generalized weakness, decreased tendon reflexes, and even paralysis may occur.[14]

Laboratory Evaluation

ECG changes associated with hypermagnesemia are nonspecific. The most common pattern is that of sinoatrial and atrioventricular blocks with extremely high levels of serum magnesium.[15]

DIAGNOSTIC CRITERIA

Hypermagnesemia can be overlooked in the nonrenal patient if serum levels are not closely monitored.[16] Patients with renal impairment should not receive magnesium infusion without serum magnesium monitoring.

DIFFERENTIAL DIAGNOSIS

It is unusual to find hypermagnesemia in the absence of renal failure. When renal failure is not evident, usually large doses of intravenous magnesium in obstetric wards have been used or large doses of antacids and laxatives containing magnesium have been used in elderly patients, with a significant decrease in the GFR in spite of normal serum creatinine levels.

PATHOPHYSIOLOGY

Neuromuscular symptoms associated with severe hypermagnesemia are secondary to the inhibitory effect on acetylcholine release at the neuromuscular junction.[17] Magnesium levels several times higher than those encountered in clinical practice were found to slow the upstroke velocity of phase 0 of the transmembrane action potential. This is believed to be the mechanism through which sinoatrial and atrioventricular blocks are produced. Further increases in serum magnesium can produce cardiac arrest in asystole.[18]

NATURAL HISTORY OF THE DISEASE

Toxic serum levels of magnesium, if left untreated, could result in respiratory and cardiac dysfunction and ultimately death.

CURRENT METHODS OF TREATMENT

The nonoliguric, asymptomatic patient with hypermagnesemia should be treated with loop diuretics to speed urinary excretion of excess magnesium. In the obstetric patient with severe hypermagnesemia resulting in heart block and arrhythmias, emergency administration of 1 g of calcium gluconate intravenously is indicated. If the patient has concomitant renal failure, dialysis with magnesium-free dialysate will ensure speedy removal of excess body magnesium.[19]

The analysis of several randomized trials on the administration of large intravenous doses of magnesium in the setting of acute myocardial infarction revealed a significantly positive impact on mortality.[20] It is important to emphasize that with total intravenous doses between 8 and 18 g, relatively few side effects were reported. These were manifested mainly in flushing of the skin and hypotension. However, it must be kept in mind that patients with atrioventricular block, bundle branch block, and renal insufficiency were excluded from these trials.

REFERENCES

1. Cohen L, Kitzes R: Magnesium sulfate and digitalis-toxic arrhythmias. *JAMA* 249:2808–2810, 1983.
2. Reinhart RA, Desbiens NA: Hypomagnesemia in patients entering the ICU. *Crit Care Med* 13: 506–507, 1985.
3. Whang R: Magnesium deficiency: Pathogenesis, prevalence and clinical implications. *Am J Med* 82(Suppl 3A):24–29, 1987.
4. Kingston ME, Al-Sibai MB, Skooge WC: Clinical manifestations of hypomagnesemia. *Crit Care Med* 14:950–954, 1986.
5. Shills ME: Experimental human magnesium depletion. *Medicine* 48:61–85, 1969.
6. Seeling MS: Electrocardiographic patterns of magnesium depletion in alcoholic heart disease. *Ann NY Acad Sci* 162:906–917, 1969.
7. Gettes LS: Electrolyte abnormalities underlying lethal and ventricular arrhythmias. *Circulation* 8 (Suppl 1):I70–I76, 1992.
8. Wesley RC Jr, Hanes DE, Lerman BB, et al: Effect of intravenous magnesium sulfate on supraventricular tachycardia. *Am J Cardiol* 63:1129–1131, 1989.
9. Halabe A, Sutton RA: Hypomagnesemia. *Med North Am* 28:5278–5282, 1988.
10. Rasmussen HS, Suenson M, McNair P, et al: Magnesium infusion reduces the incidence of arrhythmias in acute myocardial infarction. A double-blind placebo-controlled study. *Clin Cardiol* 10: 351–356, 1987.
11. Contiguglia SR, Alfrey AC, Miller N, et al: Total body magnesium excess in chronic renal failure. *Lancet* 10:1300–1302, 1972.
12. Abate MA: Magnesium content of antacids. *Am J Hosp Pharm* 38:1662–1664, 1981.
13. James MF, Huddle KR, Owen AD, et al: Use of magnesium sulphate in the anaesthetic management of pheochromocytoma in pregnancy. *Can J Anaes* 35:178–182, 1988.
14. Rizzo MA, Fisher M, Lock JP: Hypermagnesemic pseudocoma. *Arch Intern Med* 153:1130–1132, 1993.
15. Wacker WE, Parisi AF: Magnesium metabolism. *N Engl J Med* 278(12):658–663, 278(13): 712–717, 278(14):772–776, concl. 1968.
16. Clark BA, Brown RS: Unsuspected morbid hypomagnesemia in elderly patients. *Am J Neprhol* 12:336–343, 1992.
17. Mordes JP, Wacker WE: Excess magnesium. *Pharmacol Rev* 29:273–300, 1977.
18. Rardon DP, Fisc C: Electrolytes and the heart. In Hurst JW (ed): *The Heart*. New York, McGraw-Hill, 1994, pp 759–774.
19. Reinhart RA: Magnesium metabolism: A review with special reference to the relationship between intracellular content and serum levels. *Arch Intern Med* 148:2415–2420, 1988.
20. Teo KK, Yusuf S: Role of magnesium in reducing mortality in acute myocardial infarction. A review of the evidence. *Drugs* 46:347–359, 1993.

Cardiovascular Involvement with Diseases Related to Gastrointestinal System/Nutrition

Richard A. Wright, M.D.
Section Editor

Noncardiac Chest Pain

Laszlo J.K. Makk, M.D.
Richard A. Wright, M.D.

The suggestion that the gastrointestinal tract might be the cause of chest pain dates back at least to the nineteenth century, when William Osler described "esophagismus" (eosphageal spasm) in hysterical patients.[1] Since that time, clinicians have pondered the etiology of chest pain in patients with a normal cardiac workup. Potential sources of such noncardiac chest pain include musculoskeletal pain with costochondritis, myositis, myalgia and arthralgia, gastroesophageal reflux disease with or without motility abnormalities, primary esophageal motor disorders, enhanced pain perception, panic attacks, and psychoneuroses.

PRESENTING MANIFESTATIONS

History

Patients with noncardiac chest pain typically complain of a substernal discomfort which is often pressure-like, occasionally burning, and frequently associated with dysphagia, odynophagia, and four-point tenderness in the chest musculature or costochondral junctions. Pain is typically not associated with exertion and often wakens the patient from a sound sleep. If the pain is of esophageal origin, it may be exacerbated by eating, drinking hot or cold liquids, or a supine position. Other associated gastrointestinal symptoms such as nausea, vomiting, and dyspepsia may also be present.

Physical Examination

The physical examination is usually normal. Point tenderness over the costochondral junction, xiphoid process, or chest musculature may suggest a musculoskeletal etiology if it replicates the patient's pain.

Upper gastrointestinal radiography and endoscopy can identify mucosal and anatomic abnormalities such as ulcerations, malignancy, stricture, ring, or web. Esophageal motility studies can be used to diagnose nutcracker esophagus or diffuse esophageal spasm.

Laboratory Evaluation

It goes without saying that the initial workup in the patient with chest pain is performed to exclude clinically significant cardiac disease. It is important for the clinician to note that coronary artery disease, gastroesophageal reflux disease, costochondritis, and panic attacks are common in this population and may coexist in the same patient. It would be a grave mistake to neglect potentially fatal coronary artery disease in the initial pursuit of a noncardiac source. Consequently, the patient should undergo an initial screening by a cardiologist prior to referral to a gastroenterologist, rheumatologist, or psychiatrist.

The extent of the cardiology workup in the patient with chest pain is determined by the primary care physician. A minimal workup might consist of a history and physical examination electrocardiogram (ECG), and treadmill exercise test. If these are negative and the patient has no risk factors, it may be appropriate to consider a noncardiac source of the chest pain. Many cardiologists, however, perform coronary angiography, which gives a definitive diagnosis in most cases and allows a very accurate prognosis from the standpoint of the risk of cardiac death.

The preliminary gastrointestinal workup of noncardiac chest pain consists of evaluating the upper gastrointestinal tract for mucosal or structural disease. The optimal initial evaluation is an esophagogastroduodenoscopy, which will detect mucosal disease not visible on a barium radiograph, and will allow photographic documentation and histology. An ultrasound scan of the gallbladder and the pancreas is desirable in patients with suggestive symptoms. Once a structural or mucosal source of the patient's complaints has been excluded, esophageal manometry with provocative testing should be done. In a large series by Katz et al., a standard esophageal motility study in patients with noncardiac chest pain yielded a positive diagnosis in only 28%.[2] Provocative testing with dilute hydrocholic acid (Bernstein test) increases the yield only minimally.[3] The use of edrophonium increases the yield to approximately 40% and is thus considered to be a suboptimal provocative test.[3,4] Balloon distention has been touted as the provocative study of choice in patients with presumed esophageal chest pain, with yields as high as 100% in some series.[3,4] Unfortunately, this modality has not been evaluated in large, double-blind, controlled trials to ascertain its true value as a diagnostic study.[5]

Ambulatory 24-hr pH and motor monitoring has been advocated by many.[6] This allows the monitoring of gastroesophageal reflux and esophageal motor activity associated with symptoms for a continuous 24-hr period.[7,8] However, while 24-hr pH monitoring criteria have been well standardized, the norms for esophageal motor activity have been based on a series of fewer than 50 individuals.[7,8] Consequently, it is often impossible to ascertain whether truly aberrant motor activity is present. Additionally, in evaluating gastroesophageal reflux, many authors have noted that episodes of reflux do not necessarily coincide with chest pain.[4] Thus a patient may have pathologic gastroesophageal reflux, but it may not be relevant to the patient's chest discomfort.[4]

A psychiatric evaluation commonly yields a variety of diagnoses such as panic attacks, depression, anxiety, and hypochondriasis.[9] In addition to the problem of treating these disorders, the question always arises of whether they are the cause or the result of the chest pain. Combining drug therapy with behavioral modification is often helpful, in addition to providing reassurance after a negative workup.[7]

DIAGNOSTIC CRITERIA

The diagnosis of noncardiac chest pain involves the initial exclusion of a cardiac source, often requiring coronary angiography and/or multigated angiography.

DIFFERENTIAL DIAGNOSIS

The differential diagnosis of noncardiac chest pain includes musculoskeletal sources (costochondritis, myalgia, arthralgia, trauma), esophageal (gastroesophageal reflux disease, esophageal motor disorders), pulmonary (pulmonary embolus, bronchospasm, pneumonia), and idiopathic.

PATHOPHYSIOLOGY

Gastroesophageal Reflux Disease

Gastroesophageal reflux disease (GERD) is a frequent source of noncardiac chest pain. Mellow et al. demonstrated that infusion of dilute hydrochloric acid into the esophagus (Bernstein test) resulted in chest pain identical to angina pectoris in patients with known coronary artery disease.[10] At least one-third of patients with noncardiac chest pain have significant gastroesophageal reflux, as documented by 24-hr pH monitoring.[11] Frequently, these patients have gross and histologic evidence of esophageal mucosal damage as a result of the reflux when upper gastrointestinal endoscopy is performed.[11] Intraesophageal pH monitoring for 24 hr reveals that pain episodes do not commonly coincide with the reflux of gastric acid.[12] This raises the possibility that reflux may occur commonly in patients with noncardiac chest pain, but the acid may have little to do with the chest pain.[7,12] Alternatively, substances other than acid such as bile, pancreatic enzymes, and ingested mucosal toxins (alcohol, nonsteroidal antiinflammatory drugs, etc.) could potentially lead to chest pain. To date, however, studies have shown that gastroesophageal reflux is associated with noncardiac chest pain in the majority of patients studied, but not all patients with GERD have pain as a symptom.

Delayed gastric emptying is present in a significant number of patients with GERD. As a result of the decreased emptying, gastric volume is increased, leading to frequent episodes of lower esophageal sphincter relaxation. While there are good studies correlating the degree of acidity with the presence of Barrett's esophagus and esophageal mucosal damage, there are no studies linking hyperacidity with noncardiac chest pain. Likewise, esophageal clearance of refluxed acid is diminished in patients with erosive esophagitis, but it has not been studied in patients with noncardiac chest pain. Finally, mucosal resistance to reflux-induced injury has not been investigated in patients with noncardiac chest pain. Consequently, GERD is a significant concomitant of noncardiac chest pain, but further study is needed to delineate its pathogenesis.

Esophageal Motor Disorders

After GERD, the next most common esophageal source of noncardiac chest pain is esophageal motor disorder. In a large series of more than 900 patients with noncardiac chest pain by Castell and associates, a standard nonprovocative esophageal motility study was positive in only 28% of those studied.[2] The most common disorder was nutcracker esophagus, which was present in nearly half of those with positive test results.[2] The next largest category was a nonspecific esophageal motor disorder indicating some sort of nonclassifiable esophageal motor disturbance that did not meet the criteria for any other accepted esophageal motor disorders (Figure 6.1). Diffuse esophageal spasm occurred in 10%. Hypertensive lower esophageal sphincter occurred in 4% and achalasia in 2%.[2] Breumelhof et al. noted that fewer than one-quarter of patients with a suspected esophageal source of their noncardiac chest pain had documented motility disturbances by 24-hr motor monitoring.[11] A higher percentage (33%) had gastroesophageal reflux as a potential etiology.[11] Thus,

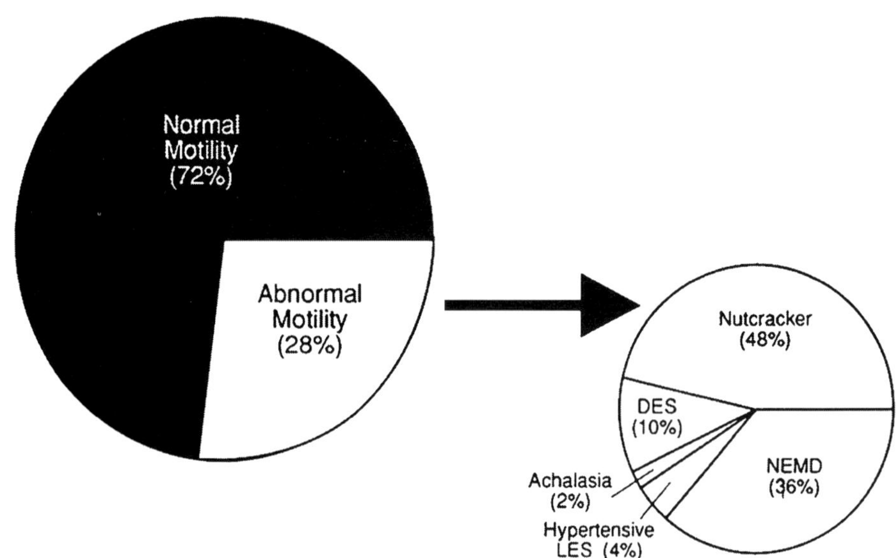

Figure 6.1. Esophageal testing in patients with non cardiac chest discomfort shows that approximately one-fourth of patients will have abnormal motility. Of those patients with abnormal motility, nearly one-half have features characteristic of a nutcracker esophagus. Abbreviations: DES = diffuse esophageal spasm, LES = lower esophageal spasm, NEMD = non-specific esophageal motor disorder. From Katz PO, Dalton CB, Richter JE, et al. Esophageal testing of patients with noncardiac chest pain or dysphagia: Results of three years' experience with 1161 patients. *Ann Intern Med* 106:593–597, 1987. Reprinted with permission of author and publisher.

although esophageal motor disorders are often considered to be the major source of esophageal chest pain, they can be documented in only a small minority of carefully selected patients.

In view of the poor correlation between esophageal motor activity and chest pain, other potential etiologies of esophageal chest pain have been explored. Richter et al. described abnormal sensory perception in patients with presumed esophageal chest pain.[9] Patients were more sensitive to balloon distention of the esophagus at smaller volumes than were matching controls. An abnormally low visceral nociceptive threshold has been described in individuals with noncardiac chest pain, perhaps analogous to the findings of previous lower gastrointestinal tract studies done in patients with irritable bowel syndrome. Additionally, Gignoux et al. described the failure of upper esophageal sphincter relaxation with the belch reflex in a group of patients with noncardiac chest pain.[6,13] The presumed defect is in the mechanoreceptors mediated by the autonomic (sympathetic and vagal) nervous systems.[14] Thus, the "irritable esophagus" appears to be a major category in patients with noncardiac chest pain.

Several published studies have described an increased rate of psychiatric diagnoses in patients with noncardiac chest pain.[15] Among the most common diagnoses are panic attack, depression, agoraphobia, and substance abuse. While the true frequency of psychiatric disorders in patients with noncardiac chest pain varies widely across the literature, it is estimated that nearly one-half of the patients with the diagnosis of noncardiac chest pain have some underlying psychiatric disorder.

Another proposed etiology of noncardiac chest pain is a primary smooth muscle abnormality.[15] The concordance of microvascular angina, Syndrome X, and noncardiac chest pain suggests a potential common pathway: an intrinsic disorder in the smooth muscle that might elicit coronary artery spasm as well as esophageal spasm.[15] This avenue of research holds the best chance of yielding an answer to the riddle of noncardiac chest pain.

Esophagocardiac Reflexes

It has long been presumed that esophageal stimulation can induce chest pain. Kramer and Hollander described ST depression on the ECG after distending the esophagus with a balloon.[16] Roesler described acute myocardial infarction in three individuals with esophageal food impaction and in one individual after consuming cold liquids.[17] This findings led to the expression "cafe coronary."[17] Gayheart et al. found that balloon distention of the canine esophagus led to a significant decrease in mean circumflex blood flow.[18] This was not antagonized by parasympathetic muscarinic blockade (with atropine) or by sympathetic beta-adrenergic blockade (with propranolol). However, sympathetic alpha-adrenergic blockade with phentolamine did abolish the decrease in coronary artery blood flow (Figures 6.2 and 6.3). This observation indicates that stimulation of the esophagus could potentially cause ischemic cardiac disease mediated by alpha-adrenergic reflex arches between the esophagus and the coronary arteries. This observation has not been confirmed in humans, but it is a plausible explanation for the observations made by Roesler and by Kramer and Hollander.[16,17]

Vagally mediated esophagocardiac and esophagobronchial reflexes occur in humans.[19] In a large series of patients receiving intraesophageal perfusion of O.I N hydrochloric acid, there was a significant decrease in airway resistance (forced expiratory volume in 1 sec, FEV_1) and heart rate. The pretreatment of subjects given atropine, 0.6 mg IM, abolished both parameters, indicating the presence of a cholinergic, vagally mediated reflex between the esophagus and heart/bronchus mediated by acid receptors in the esophageal mucosa.[19]

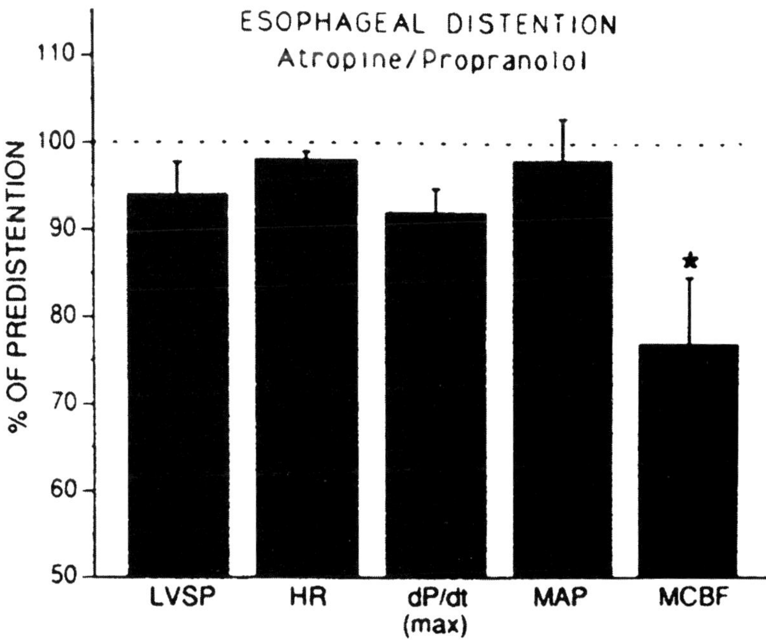

Figure 6.2. Mean steady-state values during esophageal distention after muscarinic and nonselective beta-adrenergic blockage. The values are expressed as a percentage of predistention. Vertical bars are standard errors of the mean. Note that there was a significant decrease in circumflex coronary blood flow compared to its predistention value. Abbreviations: dP/dt = maximal rate of left ventricular pressure rise; HR = heart rate, LVSP = left ventricular systolic pressure, MAP = mean arterial pressure, MCBF = mean circumflex blood flow. From Gayheart PA, Gwirtz PA, Bravenec JS, et al. An α-adrenergic coronary constriction during esophageal distention in the dog. *J Cardiovasc Pharm* 17:747–753, 1991. Reprinted with permission of author and publisher.

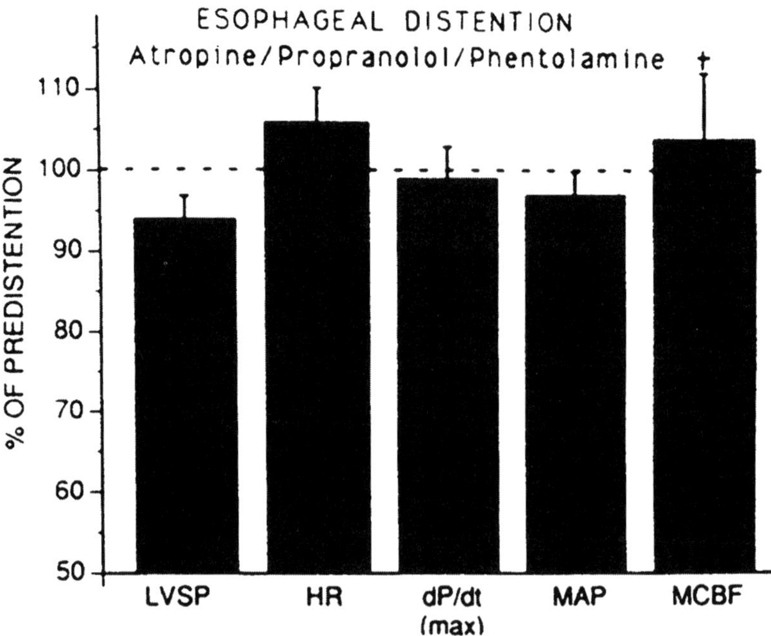

Figure 6.3. Mean steady-state values during esophageal distention after muscarinic and nonselective beta-adrenergic blockage, as well as after intracoronary alpha-adrenergic blockade with phentolamine. The values are expressed as a percentage of predistention. Vertical bars are standard errors of the mean. Note that mean circumflex blood flow was not significantly reduced compared to its predistention value. The dagger indicates p,0.05 when the response of a variable after phentolamine administration was compared to that before phentolamine administration. Abbreviations: as in Figure 6.2. From Gayheart PA, Gwirtz PA, Bravenec JS, et al. An α-adrenergic coronary constriction during esophageal distention in the dog. *J Cardiovasc Pharm* 17:747–753, 1991. Reprinted with permission of author and publisher.

Cardioesophageal reflexes have been studied in only a preliminary manner. In our laboratory, we performed simultaneous esophageal manometry on a series of patients undergoing cardiac catheterization. Seventeen percent developed diffuse esophageal spasm during ventriculography. All of these individuals met the criteria for Syndrome X. An additional 12% of patients developed nonperistaltic esophageal contractions after injection of the left main coronary artery. In a small number of patients undergoing balloon angioplasty, motility abnormalities and gastroesophageal reflux were noted. This small series suggests that there may indeed be cardioesophageal reflexes present in humans. Might it be possible that the patients observed by Roesler and by Kramer and Hollander actually had ischemic cardiac disease and developed diffuse esophageal spasm with dysphagia as a result of a cardioesophageal reflux? Further studies are needed to answer this question.

NATURAL HISTORY OF THE DISEASE

The natural history of noncardiac chest pain is generally quite benign. Patients with severe GERD may develop ulcerations, strictures, Barrett's esophagus, and laryngitis. Motor disorders of the esophagus cause no long-term sequelae except the increased risk of squamous cell carcinoma in patients with achalasia. Musculoskeletal etiologies of noncardiac chest pain have a benign but symptomatic course.

CURRENT METHODS OF TREATMENT

The treatment of GERD consists of staged therapy. Stage 1 therapy entails elevation of the head of the bed by 6–8 in., providing a gravitational barrier to reflux nocturnally. Cessation of cigarette smoking, weight loss, and dietary therapy (avoidance of coffee, tea, fatty foods, chocolate, peppermint, and onions) are also recommended. Finally, antacids in a liquid formulation are used occasionally for transient symptoms of pyrosis.

Stage 2 therapy consists of histamine 2 receptor antagonists in a twice-daily dosage. It is often necessary to use higher doses of these agents to reduce acidity in patients with pathologic GERD. Alternatively, proton pump inhibitors can be utilized in a standard once-a-day regimen, to be increased if the patients symptoms are not alleviated. Prokinetic agents such as metoclopramide and cisapride may also be used, particularly in patients with historical evidence of delayed gastric emptying and bloating or with objective evidence of gastrointestinal hypomotility.

Stage 3 therapy consists of surgical intervention. Laparoscopic Nissen fundoplication, developed over the last 5 years, is rapidly becoming the surgical treatment of choice. Intermediate-term results are quite promising. However, expertise in this modality is still lacking in many centers, where the preferred surgical approach is the Belsey Mark IV or Hill gastropexy. Theoretically, these operations will reduce the need for long-term, expensive pharmacologic therapy.

The treatment of esophageal motor disorders is quite controversial. Sublingual nitroglycerine is both effective and inexpensive in the treatment of episodic, diffuse esophageal spasm. Longer-acting nitrate derivatives may be used if pain occurs frequently throughout the day. Calcium channel blockers such as nifedipine and diltiazem have been advocated by many. Both drugs cause a dose-dependent decrease in the amplitude of esophageal contractions and reduce pressure in the lower esophageal sphincter, but they do not necessarily change the pattern or severity of chest pain. Anticholinergics such as L-hyoscyamine likewise induce a significant manometric response that does not necessarily coincide with symptom relief. The side effects of anticholinergics are often poorly tolerated. Anxiolytics and antidepressants are often used in patients with appropriate psychiatric disorders. Trazodone induced a significant improvement in well-being after a 6-week double-blind, placebo-controlled trial, but no esophageal manometric changes were found. Consequently, the treatment of the primary psychiatric disorder should be attempted in the hope that esophageal symptoms will diminish as a secondary benefit. Reassurance by both the gastroenterologist and the psychiatrist is considered a major factor in treating patients with chronic chest pain syndromes. However, only a minority of patients respond to such statements.

The use of pneumatic dilation and Maloney bougies in patients with nutcracker esophagus and achalasia has been advocated for many decades. Unfortunately, except for achalasia, the response is usually transient. Therefore, these methods are generally not recommended. Surgical management of chest pain due to presumed esophageal motor abrasions is controversial. Several large series of patients with esophageal motor abnormalities have undergone long esophagomyotomy, generally with good results.[20] However, these series represent a very select group of patients, and surgery has not been universally accepted as a standard of care.[20]

REFERENCES

1. Osler W: *Principles and Practice of Medicine.* New York, Appleton, 1892.
2. Katz PO, Dalton CB, Richter JE, et al: Esophageal testing in patients with noncardiac chest pain or dysphagia. *Ann Intern Med* 106:593–597, 1987.
3. Barist CF, Castell DO, Richter JE: Graded esophageal balloon distention—a new provocative test for noncardiac chest pain. *Dig Dis Sci* 31:1292–1298, 1986.

4. Lam HGT, Breumelhof R, Van Berge Henegouwen GP, et al: Temporal relationships between episodes of noncardiac chest pain and abnormal oesophageal function. *Gut* 35:733–736, 1994.

5. Deschner WK, Maher KA, Cattau EL, et al: Intraesophageal balloon distention versus drug provocation in the evaluation of noncardiac chest pain. *Am J Gastroenterol* 85:938–943, 1990.

6. Gignoux C, Bost R, Hostein J, et al: Role of upper esophageal reflux and belch reflex dysfunction in noncardiac chest pain. *Dig Dis Sci* 38:1909–1914, 1993.

7. Vam HGT, Breumelhof R, Roelofs JMM, et al: What is the optimal time window in symptom analysis of 24 hour esophageal pressure and pH data? *Dig Dis Sci* 39:402–409, 1994.

8. Stein HJ, Demeester TR: Indications, technique and clinical use of ambulatory 24 hour esophageal motility monitoring in a surgical practice. *Ann Surg* 217:128–137, 1993.

9. Richter JE, Barism CF, Castell DO: Abnormal sensory perception in patients with esophageal chest pain. *Gastroenterology* 91:845–852, 1986.

10. Mellow MH, Simpson AG, Watt L, et al: Esophageal acid perfusion in coronary artery disease: Induction of myocardial ischemia. *Gastroenterology* 85:306–312, 1983.

11. Breumelhof R, Nadorp JHSM, Akkermans LMA, et al: Analysis of 24 hour esophageal pressure and pH data in unselected patients with noncardiac chest pain. *Gastroenterology* 99:1257–1264, 1990.

12. Lam HGT, Dekker W, Kan G, et al: Acute noncardiac chest pain in a coronary care unit: Evaluations by 24 hour pressure and pH recording of the esophagus. *Gastroenterology* 102:453–460, 1992.

13. Gignoux C, Bonaz B, Wolf JE, et al: Air in the esophagus may be the culprit in angina-like chest pain. *J Gastrointest Motil* 2:142, 1990.

14. Sengupta JN, Kauvar D, Goyal RK: Characteristics of vagal esophageal tension sensitive afferent fibers in the opossum. *J Neurophysiol* 61:1001–1010, 1989.

15. Cannon RO, Benjamin SB: Chest pain as a consequence of abnormal visceral nociception. *Dig Dis Sci* 38:193–196, 1993.

16. Kramer P. Hollander W: Comparison of experimental esophageal pain with clinical pain of angina pectoris and esophageal disease. *Gastroenterology* 29:719–741, 1955.

17. Roesler H: Esophageal reflux origin of myocardiac infarction. *Am J Med Sci* 240:159–162, 1960.

18. Gayheart PA, Gwirtz PA, Bravenec JS, et al: An α-Adrenergic coronary construction during esophageal distention in the dog. *J Cardiovasc Pharm* 17:747–753, 1991.

19. Wright RA, Miller SA, Corsello B: Acid induced esophago-bronchial-cardiac reflexes in humans. *Gastroenterology* 99:71–73, 1990.

20. Jamieson WR, Miyagishima RT, Carr DM, et al: Surgical management of primary motor disorders of the esophagus. *Am J Surg* 148:36–45, 1984.

Cardiac Involvement with Liver Disease

Laszlo J.K. Makk, M.D.
Richard A. Wright, M.D.

PRESENTING MANIFESTATIONS

History

Patients with significant liver disease affecting cardiovascular function will usually complain of fatigue, altered mental status, gastrointestinal bleeding, abdominal pain, and anorexia.

Physical Examination

Patients with chronic liver disease commonly manifest with spider angioma, palmar erythema, gynecomastia, testicular atrophy, ascites, hepatosplenomegaly, gastrointestinal bleeding, and hepatic encephalopathy.

Laboratory Evaluation

Laboratory evaluation frequently reveals abnormal alanine aminotransferase, aspartate aminotransferase, bilirubin, alkaline phosphatase, gamma glutamyl transpeptidase (GGTP), and prothrombin time. Thrombocytopenia is common in patients with hypersplenism as a result of portal hypertension.

DIAGNOSTIC CRITERIA

The physical findings of jaundice, hepatosplenomegaly, ascites, and encephalopathy are sufficient to make a diagnosis of liver disease. Laboratory evaluation, paracentesis, and computed tomography scan of the abdomen are valuable in selected patients. Liver biopsy is usually not necessary and can be hazardous in patients with thrombocytopenia and coagulopathy.

DIFFERENTIAL DIAGNOSIS

The physical history, physical findings, and laboratory evaluation, as described above, can lead to a diagnosis of liver disease with certainty. The major differential diagnosis depends on the etiology of the liver disease, whether it be alcohol induced; viral hepatitis; toxins; autoimmune diseases such as primary biliary cirrhosis, primary sclerosing cholangitis, or lupoid hepatitis; or congenital hepatopathies (Wilson's disease, hemochromatosis).

PATHOPHYSIOLOGY

Cardiovascular Changes with Cirrhosis

In humans, the liver receives 25% of the cardiac output in spite of being only 2% of the body weight. A variety of mechanisms regulating blood flow can be altered in various disease states of the liver. End-stage liver disease has many hemodynamic consequences that affect all major organ systems. In this era of increasing numbers of hepatic transplants, it is important that the clinicians involved in the care of these patients understand the hemodynamic perturbations of liver disease.

Over 40 years ago, the hemodynamic consequences of cirrhosis were first described. These included vasodilation, attenuated arterial pressure, and increased cardiac output and organ flow.[1] Currently there are a variety of theories regarding the pathogenesis of these conditions.

It is thought that in the setting of cirrhosis, there is peripheral arterial vasodilation which could be an expression of microvascular anatomic changes, such as portal blood escaping through collaterals and/or functional changes such as intrahepatic shunts created by hepatocellular necrosis,[2] leading to renal sodium and water retention. Splanchnic vasodilation occurs early in cirrhosis and leads to volume expansion.[3] There is a tendency toward hyponatremia and a concomitant increase in aldosterone, renin, and norepinephrine.[4]

A variety of mediators have been postulated to play a part in the vasodilation of cirrhosis. Glucagon has been found to be elevated in cirrhotic patients. When glucagon antiserum is given to these patients, splanchnic blood flow is reduced.[5] Octreotide, a somatostatin analogue, has been found to inhibit glucagon release and produce systemic and splanchnic vasoconstriction. Other vasodilators are also inhibited by octreotide, such as vasoactive intestinal polypeptide, calcitonin gene-related peptide, and substance P.[6] It is thought that endogenous opiates may contribute to vasodilation because administration of naloxone (a narcotic antagonist) to cirrhotics has been found to enhance sodium and water excretion after a water load.[7] In portal vein ligated rats, it has been an increase in the tumor necrosis factor (TNF) alpha level has been found. When antitumor TNF alpha is given, it prevents the hyperdynamic cardiovascular state that occurs in the portal vein ligated rat model.[8]

Bacterial translocation from the gut is increased in rats with cirrhosis and portal vein ligation. It is thought that perhaps local endotoxins in this setting stimulate macrophages to increase the production of TNF alpha and other cytokines.[2] In cirrhotic patients, mononuclear cells produce large quantities of TNF alpha in response to endotoxin. This reaction is thought to result from endotoxin priming of these cells.[9] Cirrhotic rats are highly sensitive to the systemic hypoperfusion effects of endotoxin. This reaction may be mediated in part by platelet-activating factor. In cirrhotic rats, platelet activating factor antagonists attenuate renal hypoperfusion from endotoxin.[10]

Atrial natriuretic factor (ANF), a hormone that causes natriuresis and vasodilation, is often elevated in cirrhotics.[11] In these patients there is an increase in both total blood volume and ANF levels.[12] A significant elevation in the ANF level can be seen in response to a sodium load, with a fraction of it excreted, suggesting renal resistance to ANF in cirrhotic patients.[11] In addition, infusion of ANF in cirrhotics does not lead to natriuresis.[13] Perhaps with more severe sodium retention there is down regulation of ANF receptors.[12] Hepatic sinusoidal pressures have been found to correlate with plasma ANF levels, which suggests a tendency toward sodium retention with increased sinusoidal pressure.[14] It is postulated that increased sinusoidal pressure, which occurs early in cirrhosis, leads to renal sodium retention, which in turn leads to ANF elevation with natriuresis. With the eventual development of ascites, which occurs outside the thoracic compartment and hence is not a signal to increase ANF, there is a perceived underfilling due to decreased effective plasma volume secondary to splanchnic pooling. This latter condition leads to elevation of aldosterone, angiotensin II, and norepinephrine.[11]

Many investigators believe that there is no underfilling in patients with cirrhosis. Patients have been found to have an increased left ventricular diameter at end systole and end diastole, with increased fractional shortening. In addition, the increased cardiac output in cirrhosis is affected by increased ventricular filling during diastole.[15]

Cirrhotic laboratory animals have been found to be hyporeactive to the vasoconstrictive effects of norepinephrine, vasopressin, potassium chloride, and methoxamine.[16] Nitric oxide blockade reverses hyperactivity to methoxamine in rats with portal vein stenosis. This suggests that in cirrhosis there is an overproduction of nitric oxide.[17] In rats with bile duct ligation there is a blunted pressor response to norepinephrine, tyramine, angiotensin I, angiotensin II, and isoproterenol.[18]

Patients with cirrhosis have elevated norepinephrine levels even in the absence of sodium retention. Plasma renin activity is commonly viewed as a reflection of effective vascular volume. In cirrhotics, plasma renin activity is similar to those with and without norepinephrine elevation. In one series, systolic blood pressure, diastolic blood pressure, mean arterial pressure, pulse pressure, systemic vascular resistance, and blood volume were virtually identical in patients irrespective of norepinephrine levels.[19] One confounding variable is that caffeine levels parallel norepinephrine levels, and the former is a sympathetic nervous system stimulant. The elevation in norepinephrine levels may be secondary to the reduced hepatic clearance of caffeine.[19] In one study, patients with ascites tended to have higher norepinephrine levels than those without ascites.[20] Generally, patients with ascites tend to have worse liver disease than those without it. Perhaps the elevated norepinephrine levels reflect a worsening hyper-

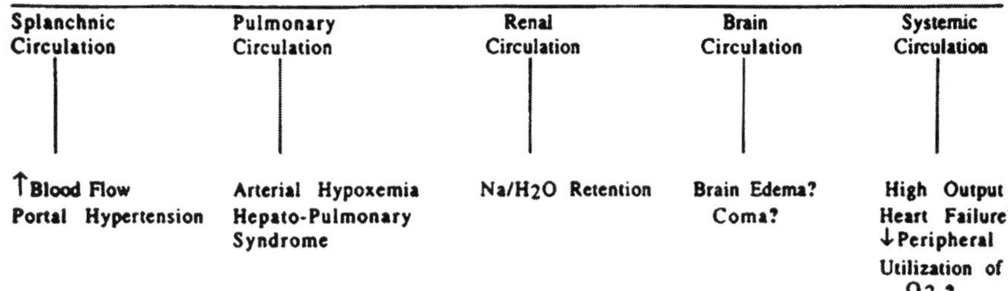

Figure 6.4. Vasodilatation and hyperdynamic circulation in liver disease. From Groszmann R. Hyperdynamic Circulation of Liver Disease Forty Years Later: Pathophysiology. *Hepatology* 20:1359–1363, 1994. Reprinted with permission of author and publisher.

dynamic state or reduced caffeine clearance. Hence norepinephrine elevation is associated with more significant hepatic dysfunction.

Ventricular function appears to be affected by liver disease. In an isolated rat heart model, a perfusate of venous effluent from postischemic or postanoxic livers resulted in a tendency toward bradycardia, reduced coronary flow, and increased coronary vascular resistance.[21] Thus a plasma-borne factor may lead to ventricular depression. Myocardial performance has been shown to be impaired in cirrhosis.[22] In rats with portal vein stenosis, beta-adrenergic atrial chronotropic and ventricular inotropic responses are diminished.[23]

The circulatory abnormalities in cirrhosis, the hyperdynamic state, lead to a variety of consequences in various systems (Figure 6.4). Splanchnic circulatory effects of portal hypertension can lead to the formation of collaterals, ascites, and the dreaded complication of variceal hemorrhage. Pulmonary circulatory changes can lead to the hepatopulmonary syndrome, which consists of pulmonary arteriovenous shunting in the pulmonary microvasculature. The kidneys tend to retain sodium and water.[2] It is thought that dilation of cerebral vasculature increases the capillary surface area for absorption of luminal gut–generated compounds such as ammonia, which can lead to hepatic encephalopathy.[23] Beta-adrenergic blockers have been used to treat portal hypertension. Perhaps there is also a favorable result secondary to beta blockage in its reduction of the hyperdynamic state of cirrhosis.[24]

Cardiovascular Abnormalities Associated with Complications Secondary to Portal Hypertension

Patients with cirrhosis and ascites tend to have evidence of central hypervolemia and a hyperdynamic circulation. Even in those without ascites, there is still an increased central blood volume without significant vasodilation, suggesting that vasodilation is not solely responsible for the increased central blood volume.[25] In one investigation, hemodynamic parameters were compared in cirrhotics with no ascites, disappearance of ascites, appearance of ascites, and persistent ascites over a period of time. Analysis of the systolic blood pressure, diastolic blood pressure, and mean arterial pressure revealed no significant differences among the patient groups.[26] In addition, patients with ascites had a larger blood volume and greater left ventricular size than those without ascites, but this finding was not statistically significant. Blood pressure and systemic vascular resistance were similar among these groups.[27]

Therapy for ascites usually entails diuretic therapy. In patients refractory to the latter, it is often necessary to perform a large-volume paracentesis. There is controversy regarding the safety of this procedure. Fears of significant adverse hemodynamic consequences from removing a large amount of fluid are not supported by the literature. In fact, large-volume paracentesis is very safe.[28–31] One study evaluated the hemodynamic and humoral consequences of this procedure in 12 subjects with tense ascites. The volume removed was 10.7 ± 4.4 L at a rate of 25 mL/min. The hemodynamic consequences included a decrease in

129

intra-abdominal, intrathoracic, right atrial, and pulmonary pressures, a slight decrease in mean arterial pressure and systemic vascular resistance, and an increase in cardiac output and heart volumes but no change in heart rate. Plasma renin activity and aldosterone levels decreased. These hemodynamic and humoral changes persisted for 24 hr. Most of these cardiovascular changes appear to be beneficial.[32]

Another therapeutic modality for the treatment of ascites is the placement of a peritoneovenous shunt. This shifts ascitic fluid from the peritoneal space into the systemic circulation. Usually these devices have a one-way valve that prevents retrograde venous flow into the peritoneum. Studies have shown that after placement of such a device there is a sixfold increase in ANF, which is thought to promote the diuresis of fluid.[33]

HEMODYNAMIC CONSEQUENCES OF PORTOSYSTEMIC SHUNTS

Surgical therapy for portal hypertension includes the creation of portosystemic shunts. Investigators reviewed portocaval shunts and found postoperatively that patients had an increase in cardiac index, a significant decrease in systemic vascular resistance, and an increase in pulmonary artery occlusion pressure. There was no change in heart rate or blood pressure.[33] Cardiac output appeared to be more accentuated after a mesocaval shunt than after a splenorenal shunt.[34] Survivors of shunt surgery tended to have better preoperative cardiac contractility and an elevated cardiac index postoperatively.[35] Results of portosystemic shunting that portended a worse prognosis include a high central blood volume, a higher mean systolic ejection rate, an above-normal cardiac index (that failed to rise after surgery), very high total peripheral resistance, and cardiac output that failed to rise after extubation.[36]

The Budd Chiari syndrome is a rare form of portal hypertension secondary to occlusion of the hepatic veins. Hemodynamically, the cardiac output and pulmonary capillary wedge pressure are in the upper range of normal, the cardiac index is in the lower range of normal, and the systemic vascular resistance is normal. Surgical therapy for this condition involves the creation of a mesoatrial shunt. Postoperatively, these patients have an increase in right atrial pressure and pulmonary capillary wedge pressure, a slight increase in mean aortic pressure, and a decrease in systemic vascular resistance.[37]

Transjugular intrahepatic portosystemic shunting (TIPS) is a fairly recent modality utilized to treat varices and ascites secondary to portal hypertension. Basically, this procedure involves passing a needle through the inferior vena cava to make a tract through the hepatic parenchyma into the portal vein. A balloon is used to dilate this tract; then an expandable wire wall stent is placed. This procedure is often used as a bridge to minimize variceal bleeding until a liver transplant is possible. As noted above, cirrhosis leads to a hyperdynamic cardiovascular state. This hyperdynamic state is rapidly and significantly worsened by TIPS. In one series, 1 of 12 patients had cardiac decompensation after TIPS. Thus this procedure should be employed only in patients with good cardiac reserve.[38]

HEPATOPULMONARY SYNDROME

The hepatopulmonary syndrome is characterized by the abnormal arterial oxygen, hepatic dysfunction, and pulmonary vascular dilation[39] (Figure 6.5). In a Mayo Clinic series of 145 orthotopic liver transplant patients, 11% had alveolar oxygen pressure (PaO$_2$) less than 70 mm Hg, and only one was denied a liver transplant.[40] There is precapillary dilation where relative hyperperfusion (Va/Q) is low. This dilation progress to overt shunting.[41] There is a spectrum of vascular changes with this condition: vascular dilation at the precapillary level close to the gas exchange units, large arteriovenous communications, and possibly intracardiac shunts. Supplemental oxygen can improve arterial oxygen, but this is attenuated because of significant pulmonary shunts. Hemodynamically, there is increased cardiac output, diminished systemic vascular resistance, and low pulmonary systolic and diastolic pressures. Basi-

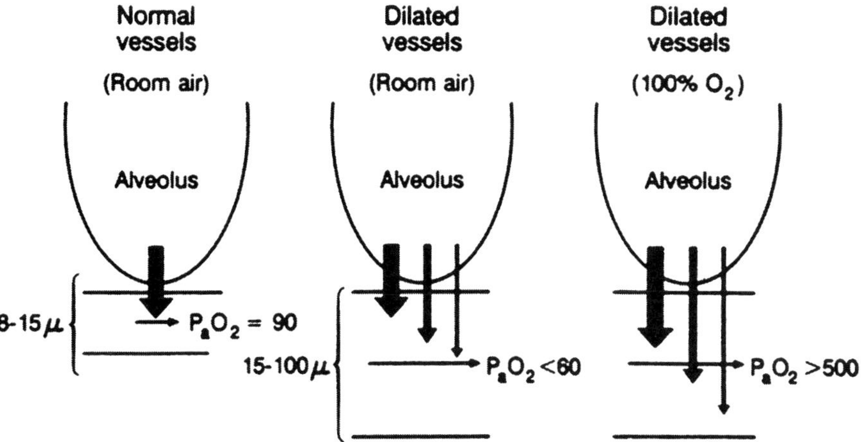

Figure 6.5. Schematic of pulmonary vascular abnormality suspected in the hepatopulmonary syndrome. This presumes that abnormal vessels are present at the precapillary level and exist close to gas exchange units in the lung, thereby participating in diffusion of oxygen molecules from the alveolus. Some vascular dilations or communications may not be in proximity to gas exchange units, or may have vascular wall that preclude the transfer oxygen molecules into venous blood flow. From Krowka MJ, Cortese DA: Hepatopulmonary syndrome: An evolving perspective in the era of liver transplantation *Mayo Clin Proc* 1987, 62:164–173. Reprinted with permission from author and publisher.

cally, there is relative pulmonary hypotension with severe hypoxia. The PaO_2 is worse when the patient is standing (orthodeoxia).[42] If the PaO_2 is greater than 500 mm Hg with 100% face mask oxygen, then there is no shunt. A PaO_2 greater than 300 mm Hg with 100% oxygen does not exclude a significant shunt. The chest roentgenogram typically shows bibasilar mottling, which may be mistaken for interstitial disease.[40]

A variety of diagnostic modalities are employed in evaluating the hepatopulmonary syndrome. The test of choice is contrast-enhanced echocardiography. The contrast is indocyanine green dye, which appears as microbubbles that become trapped in the capillary beds. If there is an intracardiac shunt, there will be immediate opacification of the left atrium. With dilated pulmonary vessels, there will be opacification of the left atrium within three to six ventricular contractions.[43] Contrast-enhanced echocardiography is more sensitive than Technetium-99-labeled, macroaggregated albumin scanning.[42] In a series of 40 consecutive liver transplant patients, 13.2% had evidence of intrapulmonary vascular dilations. Not all of them were hypoxemic, suggesting that there is subclinical dilation of pulmonic vessels.[44]

Various agents have been tried in the treatment of intravascular pulmonary dilation, including estrogens, cyclooxygenase inhibitors, and beta blockers, with no success.[45] Almitrine bimesyulate appears to alter V/Q relationships in the lung. In a series of five patients, one had significant improvement in PaO_2. Currently, this drug is not available in the United States.[46] Octreotide has been tried in one case, with some improvement in PaO_2. One study evaluated a somatostatin analogue used for 4 days in seven patients and noted no improvement in PaO_2.[47] Orthotopic liver transplantation can reverse the hypoxia-associated hepatopulmonary syndrome.[48] Patients with persistent hypoxia after liver transplantation may have such a severely hyperdynamic state that there is delayed closure of the intravascular pulmonary dilations. In a series of nine children with pretransplant hypoxia, liver transplantation seemed to be of benefit, especially in those with preoperative PaO_2 above 60 mm Hg.[49] Some advocate avoiding hepatic transplantation in patients with a PaO_2 below 50 mm Hg.[50] Certainly patients with a preoperative PaO_2 below 50 mm Hg need further evaluation. A contrast-enhanced echocardiogram and PaO_2 measurement with 100% inspired oxygen are recommended. Patients with a PaO_2 below 70 mm Hg who can easily increase their oxygen saturation with 100% inspired oxygen will likely fare well with liver transplantation.[42]

AUTONOMIC DYSFUNCTION IN CIRRHOSIS

Patients with cirrhosis of the liver often have evidence of autonomic dysfunction. One series reported evidence of vagal neuropathy in 45% of patients with cirrhosis, with a similar incidence in alcoholic and non-alcoholic patients, and with a worse prognosis in patients with neuropathy than those with normal autonomic function.[51] Another series reported at least one or more abnormalities with cardiovascular reflex testing in 60% of patients. Autonomic dysfunction in cirrhotics tends to parallel degree of hepatic disease severity. There were similar prevalences of autonomic dysfunction in patients with liver disease of all etiologies, which suggests that perhaps cirrhosis itself plays a role in development of autonomic dysfunction.[52] Patients with cirrhosis tend to have a prolonged corrected QT interval, which does parallel degree of autonomic dysfunction.[53] Patients with cirrhosis also tend to have an impairment in sodium and water excretion, which tends to occur with greater frequency in those with autonomic dysfunction than those with normal autonomic function. Cirrhotics also had higher atrial natriuretic peptide levels with vagal dysfunction. In addition, cirrhotics with vagal dysfunction given a water load tended to have higher levels of noradrenaline, antidiuretic hormone and renin.[54] Cardiovascular responsiveness to isotonic exercise is almost intact in compensated cirrhotics. These patients do require supernormal activation of sympathadrenergic and renin-angiotensin systems to maintain cardiovascular homeostasis.[55] A series of patients with primary biliary cirrhosis found cardiovascular autonomic abnormalities in 63% of patients, compared with 7.1% of controls. Two thirds of the patients with cardiovascular autonomic nervous system abnormalities had peripheral neurophysiologic abnormalities.[56]

HEMODYNAMIC CONSEQUENCES OF ORTHOTOPIC LIVER TRANSPLANTATION

Hepatic transplantation is an increasingly utilized therapeutic modality for end stage liver disease. A variety of hemodynamic changes occur during the transplant period. In a series of 21 patients with end-stage liver disease, 75% had increased cardiac output and reduced systemic vascular resistance. After liver transplantation, the cardiac output decreased significantly by 64 hr and the systemic vascular resistance increased significantly by 48 hr.[57] A longer follow-up period, 2 years after liver transplantation in another series, demonstrated persistence of the high cardiac output associated with the hyperdynamic state of cirrhosis.[58] The pulmonary capillary wedge pressure increased from baseline at 32 hr and was significantly elevated at 96 hr. The pulmonary artery pressure followed this trend, but the pulmonary vascular resistance did not change.[57] Others have reported an increase in pulmonary vascular resistance after liver transplantation.[59] However, the systemic blood pressure did not change significantly. At a posttransplant follow-up period of 96 hr, there was no significant difference between survivors and nonsurvivors in terms of hemodynamic patterns.[57] Others have reported that patients with an increasing cardiac output had a worse prognosis.[60] During the anhepatic phase of hepatic transplantation there can be a variety of unstable hemodynamic consequences. In a porcine hepatectomy model, the animals survived for 12 hr without a liver. Interestingly, these animals were hemodynamically stable, suggesting that the absence of the liver per se does not cause the hemodynamic alterations, which may be a function of preexisting liver disease.[61] A postperfusion syndrome has been described in liver transplant patients after the implanted liver begins perfusion, consisting of diminished mean arterial pressure and systemic vascular resistance; increased pulmonary artery pressure, pulmonary artery occlusion pressure, and central venous pressure; and the presence of bradyarrhythmias.[62]

MISCELLANEOUS CONDITIONS IN END-STAGE LIVER DISEASE THAT AFFECT THE CARDIOVASCULAR SYSTEM

The Watson-Alagille syndrome, also known as *arteriohepatic dysplasia,* is an autosomal dominant condition that has congenital cardiovascular abnormalities, with a 12–14% incidence of cirrhosis and a 5% mortality from hepatic involvement. Clinically this entity involves growth retardation, dysmorphic facies, neonatal cholestasis, mental retardation, skeletal abnormalities, and xanthomas.[63] A significant proportion of these patients have peripheral pulmonary stenosis. Other cardiac defects include pulmonary valve stenosis, atrial septal defects, pulmonary venous stenosis, bicuspid aortic valve, and coarctation of the aorta. Patients without heart disease can benefit from liver transplantation. In the setting of severe heart disease in this condition, heart, lung, and liver transplants may be the only viable option.[64]

Hepatocellular carcinoma has been reported to have a 1–4% incidence of cardiac metastasis. Typically, this involves extension of the tumor through the inferior vena, with formation of a tumor thrombus in the right atrium. Clinically, patients can have a pulmonary embolus and heart failure. In rare cases, patients have achieved significant improvement after resection.[65] In one interesting case, a patient presented 3 years after orthotopic liver transplant with an apparent pericardial effusion on radionuclide angiocardiography. Further evaluation demonstrated the lesion to be hepatocellular carcinoma; there was no evidence of tumor in the implanted liver.[65]

NATURAL HISTORY OF THE DISEASE

The natural history of the cardiovascular manifestations of liver disease are closely related to the natural history of the liver disease itself. The major prognostic factor in alcoholic liver disease is cessation of alcohol use. Wilson disease and hemochromatosis, if untreated, commonly result in cirrhosis and hepatic failure. The course of viral hepatitis is variable but can be predicted by seriologic test results. The course and progression of primary biliary cirrhosis and primary sclerosing cholangitis vary from patient to patient but can be predicted based on bilirubin and prothrombin time.

CURRENT METHODS OF TREATMENT

Treatment of chronic end-stage liver disease consists of corticosteroid therapy in selected patients with alcoholic hepatitis, alpha interferon for patients with hepatitis B and C, and liver transplantation in appropriate candidates. Patients with spontaneous bacterial peritonitis with sensitive organisms will usually respond to third-generation cephalosporins. The prognosis has improved with liver transplantation, which is the only cure for most types of chronic liver disease.

REFERENCES

1. Kowalski HJ, Abelmann WH: The cardiac output at rest in Laennec's cirrhosis. *J Clin Invest* 32:1025–1033, 1953.
2. Abelmann WH: Hyperdynamic circulation of liver disease 40 years later: Pathophysiology and clinical consequences. *Hepatology* 20:1359–1363, 1994.
3. Schrier RW, Arroyo V, Bernardi M, et al: Peripheral arterial vasodilation hypothesis: A proposal for the initiation of renal sodium and water retention in cirrhosis. *Hepatology* 8:1151–1157, 1988.
4. Schrier RW: An odyssey into the milieu interieur: Pondering the enigmas. *J Am Soc Nephrol* 2:1549–1559, 1992.
5. Benoit JN, Granger DN: Splanchnic hemodynamics in chronic portal hypertension. *Semin Liver Dis* 6:287–298, 1986.
6. Albillos A, Colombato LA, Lee FY, et al: Chronic octreotide treatment ameliorates peripheral vasodilation and prevents sodium retention in portal hypertensive rats. *Gastroenterology* 104:568–572, 1993.
7. Leehey DJ, Gallapudi P, Deakin A, et al: Naloxone increases water and electrolyte excretion after water loading in patients with cirrhosis and ascites. *J Lab Clin Med* 118:484–491, 1991.
8. Lopez-Talavera JC, Merrill W, Groszmann RJ: Treatment with anti-tumor necrosis factor alpha polyclonal antibodies prevents the development of the hyperdynamic circulation and reduces portal pressure in portal-hypertensive rats (abstract). *Hepatology* 1993;18:140A.

9. Khorts A, Stahnke L, McClain C, et al: Circulating tumor necrosis factor, interleukin-1 and interleukin-6 concentration in chronic alcoholic patients. *Hepatology* 13:267–276, 1991.

10. Kleber G, Braillon A, Gaudin C, et al: Hemodynamic effects of endotoxin and platelet activating factor in cirrhotic rats. *Gastroenterology* 103:282–288, 1992.

11. Warner LC, Campbell PJ, Morali GA, et al: The response of atrial natriuretic factor and sodium excretion to dietary sodium challenges in patients with chronic liver disease. *Hepatology* 12:460–466, 1990.

12. Rector WG, Adair O, Hossack KF, et al: Atrial volume in cirrhosis: Relationship to blood volume and plasma concentration of atrial natriuretic factor. *Gastroenterology* 99:766–770, 1990.

13. Warner L, Leung WM, Logan A, et al: A comparison in natriuretic (UNaV) responses between head out water immersion: Infusion of atrial natriuretic factor and peritoneovenous shunting in cirrhotic patients with massive ascites (abstract). *Hepatology* 8:1246, 1988.

14. Unikowsky B, Wexler MJ, Levy M: Dogs with experimental cirrhosis of the liver but without intrahepatic hypertension do not retain sodium or form ascites. *J Clin Invest* 72:1594–1604, 1983.

15. Lewis FW, Adiar O, Rector WG: Arterial vasodilation is not the cause of increased cardiac output in cirrhosis. *Gastroenterology* 102:1024–1029, 1992.

16. Sieber CC, Groszmann RJ: Nitric oxide mediates in vitro hyperactivity to vasopressors in mesenteric vessels of portal hypertensive rats. *Gastroenterology* 103:235–239, 1992.

17. Lee FY, Albillos A, Colombato LA, et al: The role of nitric oxide in the vascular hyporesponsivenesss to methoxamine in portal-hypertensive rats. *Hepatology* 16:1043–1048, 1992.

18. Bomzon A, Weinbroum A, Kamenetz L: Systemic hypotension and pressor responsiveness in cholestasis—a study in conscious 3-day bile duct ligated rates. *J Hepatol* 11:70–76, 1990.

19. Rector WG, Robertson AD: Prevalence and determinants of elevated plasma norepinephrine concentration in compensated cirrhosis. *Am J Gastroenterol* 89:2049–2053, 1994.

20. Lewis FW, Cohen JA, Rector WG: Autonomic dysfunction in alcoholic cirrhosis: Relationship to indicators of synthetic activation and the occurrence of renal sodium retention. *Am J Gastroenterol* 86:553–559, 1991.

21. Pretto EA: Cardiac function after hepatic ischemia-anoxia reperfusion injury: A new experimental model. *Crit Care Med* 19:1188–1194, 1991.

22. Cohn JN: Hepatocirculatory failure. *Med Clin North Am* 59:955–962, 1975.

23. Lockwood AH, Yap EWH, Wong W: Cerebral ammonia metabolism in patients with severe liver disease and minimal hepatic encephalopathy. *J Cerebr Blood Flow Metab* 11:337–341, 1991.

24. Sarin SK, Groszmann RJ, Mosca PG, et al: Propanolol ameliorates the development of portal-systemic shunting in a chronic murine schistosomiasis model of portal hypertension. *J Clin Invest* 87:1032–1036, 1991.

25. Wong F, Liu P, Tobe S, et al: Central blood volume in cirrhosis: Measurement of radionuclide angiography. *Hepatology* 19:312–321, 1994.

26. Rector WG, Robertson AD, Lewis FW: Arterial underfilling does not cause sodium retention in cirrhosis. *Am J Med* 95:286–295, 1993.

27. Lewis FW, Adair O, Rector WG: Arterial vasodilation is not the cause of increased cardiac output in cirrhosis. *Gastroenterology* 102:1024–1029, 1992.

28. Gines P, Arroyo V, Quintere E, et al: Comparison of paracentesis and diuretics in the treatment of cirrhotics with tense ascites: Results of a randomized study. *Gastroenterology* 93:234, 1987.

29. Pinto PC, Amerian J, Reynolds TB: Large volume paracentesis in nonedematous patients with tense ascites: Its effect on intravascular volume. *Hepatology* 8:207, 1988.

30. Runyon BA: Paracentesis of ascitic fluid: A safe procedure. *Arch Intern Med* 146:2259–2261, 1986.

31. Tito L, Gines P, Arroyo V, et al: Total paracentesis associated with intravenous albumin management of patients with cirrhosis and ascites. *Gastroenterology* 98:148–151, 1990.

32. Pozzi N, Osculati G, Boari G, et al: Time course of circulatory and humoral effects of rapid total paracentesis in cirrhotic patients with tense, refractory ascites. *Gastroenterology* 1994;106:709–720, 1994.

33. Gelman S, Aldrete JS, Halpern N: Hemodynamics during portacaval shunt surgery in humans. *Anesth Analg* 61:185–186, 1982.

34. Reichle FA, Owen OE: Hemodynamic patterns in human hepatic cirrhosis—a prospective randomized study of the hemodynamic sequelae of distal splenorenal (Warren) and mesocaval shunts. *Ann Surg* 190:523–533, 1979.

35. Waxman K, Shoeman WC: Physiologic determinants of operative survival after portocaval shunt. *Ann Surg* 197:72–78, 1982.

36. Del Guercio LRM, Commaraswamy RP, Feins NR, et al: Pulmonary arteriovenous admixture and the hyperdynamic cardiovascular state in surgery for portal hypertension. *Surgery* 56:57–74, 1964.

37. Beattie C, Sitzmann JV, Cameron JL: Mesoatrial shunt hemodynamics. *Surgery* 104:1–9, 1988.

38. Azoulay D, Casting D, Dennison A, et al: Transjugular intrahepatic portosystemic shunt worsens the hyperdynamic circulatory state of the cirrhotic patient: Preliminary report of a prospective study. *Hepatology* 19:129–132, 1994.

39. Agusti AGN, Roca J, Bosch J, et al: The lung in patients with cirrhosis. *J Hepatol* 10:251–257, 1990.

40. Krowka MJ, Cortese DA: Pulmonary aspects of liver disease and liver transplantation. *Clin Chest Med* 10:593–616, 1989.

41. Eriksson LS, Soderman C, Ericzon BG, et al: Hypoxemia cured by liver transplantation. *Transplant Proc* 22:172–173, 1990.

42. Krowka MJ, Cortese DA: Hepatopulmonary syndrome: An evolving perspective in the era of liver transplantation (editorial). *Hepatology* 11:138–142, 1990.

43. Hind CRK, Wong CM: Detection of pulmonary arteriovenous fistulae in patients with cirrhosis by contrast two-dimensional echocardiography. *Gut* 22:1042–1045. 1981.

44. Krowka MJ, Tajik AJ, Dickson ER, et al: Intrapulmonary vascular dilatations (IVPD) in liver transplant candidates: Screening by two-dimensional contrast enhanced echocardiography (abstract). *Chest* 96(Suppl):164S, 1989.

45. Sherlock S: *Disorders of the Liver and Biliary System*, ed 8. Oxford: Blackwell Scientific, 1989, pp 82–85.

46. Krowka MJ, Cortese DA: Severe hypoxemia associated with liver disease: Mayo Clinic experience of experimental use of almitrine bismesylate. *Mayo Clin Proc* 1987;54:164–173, 1987.

47. Krowka MJ, Dickson ER, Cortese DA: Hepatopulmonary syndrome: clinical observations and lack of therapeutic response to somatostatin analogue. *Chest* 104:515–521, 1993.

48. Scott V, Miro V, Kang Y, et al: Reversibility of the hepatopulmonary syndrome by orthotopic. *Liver Transplant* 1993;25:1787–1788, 1993.

49. Hobeika J, Houssin D, Bernard O, et al: Orthotopic liver transplantation in children with chronic liver disease and severe hypoxemia. *Transplantation* 57:224–228, 1994.

50. Van Thiel DH, Schade RR, Gavaler JB, et al: Medical aspects of liver transplantation. *Hepatology* 4(Suppl):79–83, 1984.

51. Hendrickse MT, Thuluvath PJ, Triger DR: Natural history of autonomic neuropathy in chronic liver disease. *Lancet* 339:1462–1464, 1992.

52. Dillon JF, Plevris JN, Nolan J, et al: Autonomic function in cirrhosis assessed by cardiovascular reflex tests and 24-hour heart rate variability. *Am J Gastroenterol* 9:1544–1547, 1994.

53. Kempler P: Autonomic neuropathy and prolongation of QT interval in liver disease. *Lancet* 340:318, 1992.

54. Hendrickse MT, Triger DR: Vagal dysfunction and impaired urinary sodium and water excretion in cirrhosis. *Am J Gastroenterol* 89:750–756, 1994.

55. Iwao T, Toyonaga A, Ikegami M, et al: Cardiovascular responsiveness after exercise in cirrhotic patients: Study on sympathoadrenergic and renin-angiotensin systems. *Am J Gastroenterol* 89:1043–1046, 1994.

56. Hendrickse MT, Triger DR: Autonomic and peripheral neuropathy in primary biliary cirrhosis. *J Hepatol* 1993;19:401–407, 1993.

57. Glauser FL: Systemic hemodynamic and cardiac function changes in patients undergoing orthotopic liver transplantation. *Chest* 98:1210–1215, 1990.

58. Henderson JM, Mackay GJ, Hooks M, et al: High cardiac output of advanced liver disease persists after orthotopic liver transplantation. *Hepatology* 15:258–262, 1992.

59. Eriksson LS, Soderman C, Ericzon GB, et al: Normalization of ventilation/perfusion relationships

after liver transplantation in patients with decompensated cirrhosis: Evidence for a hepatopulmonary syndrome. *Hepatology* 12:1350–1357, 1990.

60. Waxman K, Shoemaker WC: Physiologic determinants of operative survival after portocaval shunt. *Ann Surg* 197:72–78, 1983.
61. Thompson JF, Bell R, Bookallil MJ, et al: Effects of total hepatectomy: Studies in a porcine model. *Aust NZ Surg* 64:560–564, 1994.
62. Aggarwal S, Kang Y, Pinsky M: Post-reperfusion syndrome: cardiovascular collapse following hepatic reperfusion during liver transplantation. *Transplant Proc* 19(Suppl 3):54–55, 1987.
63. Alagille D, Odievre M, Gautier M, et al: Hepatic ductular hypoplasia associated with characteristic facies, vertebral malformations, retarded physical, mental and sexual developments, and cardiac murmur. *J Pediatr* 86:63–71, 1975.
64. Tzakis A, Reyes J, Tepetes K, et al: Liver transplantation for Alagille's syndrome. *Arch Surg* 128:337–339, 1993.
65. Shyo KG, Chiang FT, Kuan P, et al: Cardiac metastasis of hepatocellular carcinoma mimicking pericardial effusion on radionuclide angiography. *Chest* 101:261–262, 1992.

Nutritional Conditions that Affect the Cardiovascular System

Laszlo J.K. Makk, M.D.
Richard A. Wright, M.D.

PRESENTING MANIFESTATIONS

History

Patients with dumping syndrome complain of postprandial bloating, diarrhea, palpations, diaphoresis, and hypotension. Reseeding syndrome can present with syncope, arrhythmias, and sudden cardiac death.

Physical Examination

Physical examination may reveal evidence of malnutrition, a prior gastric operation, loss of subcutaneous fat, and increased muscle mass.

Laboratory Evaluation

Hypoalbuminemia, hypoglycemia, hyperglycemia, hypophosphatemia, and electrolyte imbalance are found.

DIAGNOSTIC CRITERIA

Patients with dumping syndrome, by definition, have undergone a gastrectomy or pyloroplasty with vagotomy. Reseeding syndrome occurs in a malnourished patient, whatever the etiology.

DIFFERENTIAL DIAGNOSIS

Differential diagnosis in dumping syndrome consists of malignancies such as carcinoid, VIP-omas, and other malignant and nonmalignant tumors that secrete vasoactive substances.

PATHOPHYSIOLOGY

There are numerous nutritional conditions that affect the heart. Of historical interest is the finding of high-output cardiac failure in the setting of thiamine deficiency. Atherosclerosis associated with hypercholesterolemia has been well documented. Following is a review of a few nutritional entities that affect the cardiovascular system.

The dumping syndrome is a significant cause of morbidity following gastric surgery in which the pylorus is removed or ablated.[1] There is accelerated gastric emptying, with corresponding diarrhea and a variety of cardiovascular manifestations.[2] There is a significant decrease in mean plasma volume, although this is similar to the condition in nondumpers in response to a hypertonic glucose load into the duodenum.[3] Atrial natriuretic peptide, which is elevated in hypervolemic states, is decreased after a meal in dumping syndrome.[4] A significant increase in glucose and enteroglucagon levels was demonstrated in patients with dumping syndrome when a hypertonic glucose load was instilled into the duodenum. Vasoactive intestinal peptide levels rise and fall with a hypertonic load, but to a similar extent in dumpers and nondumpers. In the cardiovascular system, patients with dumping syndrome tend to have an increase in heart rate and a decrease in pulsatility index, indicating peripheral vasodilation in response to a meal.[3] The cardiac symptoms can be somewhat pronounced in some patients.

In the reseeding syndrome, there is severe hypophosphatemia in the setting of nutritional repletion. In the starvation state, patients become catabolic. Many electrolytes are depleted via the kidneys after breakdown of various cells. With reseeding, there is a net influx of electrolytes and nutrients into cells, and previously normal levels of electrolytes decrease quickly. Significantly low levels of phosphate, potassium, and magnesium occur.[5] This scenario can lead to various arrhythmias. With severe phosphate depletion, there is a decrease in adenosine triphosphate levels, which leads to reduced sarcomere contractility.[6] In starved-refed swine, hypophosphatemia leads to the myofibrillar fragmentation found at autopsy.[7] A series of three patients taking large doses of phosphate-binding antacids had congestive heart failure secondary to hypophosphatemia.[8] It is also thought that sodium fluxes with reseeding are associated with sudden cardiac death.[8] In starved patients before reseeding, there is a decrease in total heart volume, end-diastolic volume, and left ventricular mass. After reseeding, the left ventricular volume decreases to baseline but the ventricular mass remains diminished, which leads to congestive heart failure.[9] In one series of patients receiving enteral feeding, 20–25% had evidence of overhydration.[10] Patients with anorexia nervosa, in addition to the above cardiovascular changes, have a reduced cardiovascular response to exercise,[11] as well as QT prolongation.[12] Conditions thought to place a patient at highest risk for hypophosphatemia include alcoholism, chronic weight loss, hyperglycemia, an exogenous insulin requirement, chronic antacid use, and diuretic therapy. Patients who are being refed and who have a significant increase in pulse rate may have some cardiac insufficiency and warrant a decrease in caloric feeding rate, with close monitoring. Patients thought to be at risk for reseeding syndrome should have their serum electrolytes followed carefully during the first week of nutritional repletion.[5]

NATURAL HISTORY OF THE DISEASE

Patients with dumping syndrome have diarrhea, weight loss, and the complications thereof. Nutritional deficiencies can lead to opportunistic infection, inanition, and electrolyte imbalance.

CURRENT METHODS OF TREATMENT

Dumping syndrome is treated by dietary manipulation. The patient consumes solid and liquid foods separately and avoids hyperosmolar liquid formulations. Repeating syndrome is treated by phosphate supplements and careful monitoring of electrolytes.

MISCELLANEOUS CONSIDERATIONS

In the past, an association between aortic valvular disease and angiodysplasia of the right colon was thought to exist. However, a recent prospective, controlled evaluation showed no such association. The two phenomena are probably independent, with no clear-cut association.[13,14]

There is a strong association between *Streptococcus bovis,* bacteremia/endocarditis, and colon cancer. Patients with bacteremia secondary to this organism should undergo a colonoscopy to determine whether a cecal carcinoma is present. There is a fivefold increase in colon cancers and villous adenomas in patients presenting with *Strep. bovis* or bacteremia.[15]

Kwashiorkor and marasmus can result in decreased cardiac output, presumably secondary to wasting of the cardiac muscle. Hypoalbuminemia can result in decreased oncotic pressure, leading to a partially decreased plasma volume. This may result in decreased cardiac output and diminished tissue perfusion.

REFERENCES

1. Ralphs DNL: The dumping syndrome. *Br J Clin Pract* 35:291–293, 1981.
2. Ralphs DNL, Thomson JPS, Haynes S, et al: The relationship between the rate of gastric emptying and the dumping syndrome. *Br J Surg* 65:637–641, 1979.
3. Snook JA, Wells AD, Prytherch DR, et al: Studies on the pathogenesis of the early dumping syndrome induced by intraduodenal instillation of hypertonic glucose. *Gut* 30:1716–1720, 1989.
4. Tulassay Z, Tulassay T, Gupta R, et al: Atrial natriuretic peptide in dumping syndrome. *Digestion* 54:44–47, 1993.
5. Solomon SM, Kirby DF: The refeeding syndrome: A review. *J Parenter Enteral Nutr* 14:90–96, 1990.
6. O'Connor LR, Wheeler WS, Bethune JE: Effect of hypophosphatemia on myocardial performance in man. *N Engl J Med* 297:901–903, 1977.
7. Smith GS, Smith JL, Mameesh MS, et al: Hypertension and cardiovascular abnormalities in starved-refed swine. *Nutrition* 82:173–182, 1964.
8. Patrick J: Death during recovery from severe malnutrition and its possible relationship to sodium pump activity in the leukocyte. *Br Med J* 1:1051–1054, 1977.
9. Heymsfield SB, Bethel RA, Ansley JD, et al: Cardiac abnormalities in chectic patients before and during nutritional repletion. *Am Heart J* 95:584–594, 1978.
10. Heymsfield SB, Bethel RA, Ansley JD, et al: Enteral hyperalimentation: An alternative to central venous hyperalimentation. *Ann Intern Med* 90:63–71, 1979.
11. Moodie DS: Anorexia and the heart: Results of studies to assess effects. *Postgrad Med* 81:46–61, 1987.
12. Isner JM, Roberts WC, Heymsfield SB, et al: Anorexia nervosa and sudden death. *Ann Intern Med* 102:49–52, 1985.
13. Bhutani MS, Gupta SC, Markert RJ, et al: A prospective controlled evaluation of endoscopic detection of angiodysplasia and its association with aortic valvular disease. *Gastrointest Endosc* 42;398–402, 1995.
14. Gostout CJ: Angiodysplasia and aortic valve disease: Let's close the book on this association. *Gastrointest Endosc* 42:491–493, 1995.
15. Klein RS, Recco RA, Catalano MT, et al: Association of *Streptococcus bovis* with carcinoma of the colon. *N Engl J Med* 297:800–803, 1977.

Cardiovascular Involvement with Pulmonary Diseases

F. Charles Hiller, M.D.
Section Editor

Chronic Obstructive Pulmonary Disease

Marcia L. Erbland, M.D.

PRESENTING MANIFESTATIONS

Chronic obstructive pulmonary disease (COPD) is the fifth leading cause of death in the United States, and chronic cigarette smoking is the primary cause. Typically, patients are middle-aged or older at diagnosis, have smoked for many years, and complain of progressive dyspnea on exertion.

DIAGNOSTIC CRITERIA

Terminology in obstructive lung diseases is problematic; however, in the United States, COPD refers primarily to the diseases known as *emphysema* and *chronic obstructive bronchitis*. Morphologically, emphysema and chronic obstructive bronchitis are recognized by enlargement and destruction of alveolar units, and by inflammatory and fibrotic changes in distal airways, respectively. On spirometry, these patients exhibit reduced expiratory airflow, as measured by the forced expiratory volume in 1 sec (FEV_1) and FEV_1/FVC (FVC = forced vital capacity), that is mostly irreversible after bronchodilation. In advanced COPD, severe emphysema is almost always present, and there may be characteristic signs of hyperinflation on physical exam and chest radiography.

DIFFERENTIAL DIAGNOSIS

The main diagnostic dilemma occurs in certain patients who have features of both COPD and asthma. Most experts recognize asthma and COPD as separate diseases, but in some patients this distinction is difficult. Some asthma patients may develop nearly irreversible airflow obstruction that is similar in severity to that seen in advanced COPD; conversely, many COPD patients have a modest degree of reversibility in airflow obstruction. Isolated bullous lung lesions are not considered diagnostic of COPD, as they may be present without the airflow obstruction seen in typical emphysema. Other lung diseases that are associated with airflow obstruction but have specific diagnostic criteria, such as cystic fibrosis, silicosis, or some cases of sarcoidosis, are not grouped with COPD.

139

PATHOPHYSIOLOGY

The most common and most important cardiovascular complication of COPD is the development of chronic pulmonary hypertension, with subsequent changes in right ventricular structure and function known as *cor pulmonale*. Cor pulmonale encompasses a spectrum of cardiac abnormalities, including right ventricular hypertrophy and dilatation, limitations on the maximum output of the right ventricle, and overt right ventricular failure. In the United States, COPD is the leading cause of this form of heart disease.

A number of studies point to chronic hypoxemia as the primary risk factor for pulmonary hypertension in COPD. While reversible hypoxic vasoconstriction plays a role, unrelieved hypoxia also leads to structural changes in the pulmonary arteries, so that the increased vascular resistance is no longer completely reversible when the hypoxia is corrected. Acidosis also causes pulmonary vasoconstriction. In patients with marked emphysema, the cross-sectional area of the pulmonary vascular bed is also anatomically reduced. Together these abnormalities increase the pulmonary vascular resistance in COPD.

In most COPD patients, cardiac output is normal to increased at rest, and can increase further during exercise and during periods of respiratory decompensation. Patients with pulmonary hypertension may not display right ventricular dysfunction at rest, but output will not increase normally with exercise. Therefore, right ventricular dysfunction may be considered to be present when disease results in output levels which are inadequate to meet demands. The cardiac impact of COPD will depend on the interaction of the hypoxic stimulus, individual variations in ventricular response to pulmonary hypertension, and demands imposed by illness or activity.

Pulmonary hypertension and right ventricular hypertrophy and dilation may lead to specific abnormalities on physical examination, the chest radiograph, and the electrocardiogram. However, in patients with COPD, increased lung volumes often reduce the reliability of the usual signs of right or left ventricular dysfunction. Edema, long considered a classic sign of right ventricular failure in patients with COPD, should be interpreted with caution. Although it is still a poor prognostic sign, there is growing evidence that chronic edema in these patients is more closely related to hypercapnia than to right ventricular dysfunction. When indicated, a number of other noninvasive techniques can be used to evaluate cardiac function. Because lung tissue conducts ultrasound poorly, echocardiography may not yield adequate images in COPD patients who have hyperinflated lungs and an increased retrosternal air space. Nevertheless, two-dimensional echocardiography can give useful information in many patients with COPD. Radionuclide measurement of right ventricular function, using either the first-pass or equilibrium-gated blood pool technique, is not affected by hyperinflation and is a useful alternative to echocardiography. While not all patients need definitive evaluation of right ventricular function, an accurate diagnosis is especially helpful in two circumstances. First, worsening symptoms and gas exchange may be due to a variety of causes, including worsening lung function, right ventricular failure, left ventricular and coronary disease, or even pulmonary emboli. If the clinical picture is unclear, additional testing may be needed to determine appropriate therapy. Second, if cor pulmonale is suspected but blood gas abnormalities are borderline for home oxygen guidelines, tests of right ventricular function may be useful to decide whether home oxygen might be beneficial and to confirm the presence of right ventricular dysfunction for third-party payment of home oxygen.

The cardiovascular impact of acute respiratory illness in patients with COPD is based on the effects of acute hypoxemia and respiratory acidosis, the potentially adverse hemodynamic effects of mechanical ventilation, and the increased frequency of cardiac arrhythmias. Pulmonary vascular resistance and pulmonary hypertension increase when hypoxemia and respiratory acidosis occur in acute exacerbations in COPD. Hypoxemia should be corrected promptly with supplemental oxygen as needed.

COPD patients who require intubation and mechanical ventilation will need increased expiratory time due to reduced expiratory flow rates. These patients may be at risk for dynamic hyperinflation, with a resulting increase in intrathoracic pressure known as *intrinsic positive end-expiratory pressure (PEEP).* Intrinsic PEEP may cause hypotension due to its effect on ventricular filling. In most COPD patients who require mechanical ventilation, respiratory rate and tidal volume can be easily adjusted to allow adequate expiratory time and minimize intrinsic PEEP. Strategies for monitoring and minimizing intrinsic PEEP have been described.

Most clinically important cardiac arrhythmias in COPD occur during acute respiratory illness. During acute exacerbations, supraventricular arrhythmias predominate and may occur in 50% of hospitalized COPD patients. The exact etiology of cardiac arrhythmias in this setting is not clear, as experimental hypoxia and hypercapnia have not been shown to be arrhythmogenic. There is some debate over how closely arrhythmias are related to the use of various drugs in COPD. Multifocal atrial tachycardia (MAT) is common in COPD. MAT appears to be unrelated to the use of digoxin, but it has been linked to theophylline. Because hypoxemic COPD patients are highly dependent on cardiac output to maintain oxygen delivery, cardiac arrhythmias are poorly tolerated during periods of worsening gas exchange. Mortality is high when arrhythmias accompany acute illness in COPD.

NATURAL HISTORY OF THE DISEASE

While many patients with COPD die prematurely, the prognosis depends on several factors. Mortality is most closely related to age and degree of airflow obstruction. FEV_1 will continue to decline to decline at an accelerated rate if the patient continues to smoke. Smoking cessation, however, causes the rate of decline to return to that of nonsmokers. Smokers who quit when airflow obstruction is only mild or moderate may then have a normal life expectancy; patients who quit when the disease is severe will live longer on average than similar patients who continue to smoke. In the British home oxygen study, 67% of untreated hypoxemic COPD patients died within 5 years, but the prognosis in similar patients is significantly better now with the widespread use of continuous oxygen therapy. While some deaths can be directly attributable to respiratory failure from COPD, these patients are especially susceptible to sudden death or death during an acute illness. The exact cause may be unclear.

CURRENT METHODS OF TREATMENT

Smoking cessation should be the cornerstone of therapy for every patient diagnosed with COPD. The life expectancy of COPD patients is improved after smoking cessation even in those with advanced disease. Although cor pulmonale in COPD correlates more closely with the degree of hypoxemia than with FEV_1, significant hypoxemia is unusual unless the FEV_1 is moderately to severely reduced. Currently, smoking cessation is the only intervention known to reduce the rate of decline of FEV_1 in smokers with COPD.

Chronic home oxygen therapy is currently the mainstay of prevention and treatment of cor pulmonale in COPD patients. Two large clinical trials have shown that supplemental oxygen prolongs life in COPD patients with chronic resting hypoxemia. There is some evidence that at least part of this benefit may occur via a reduction in pulmonary artery pressures, but the exact mechanism by which oxygen therapy improves mortality may be more complex. The risk of cor pulmonale is greatest in patients who have persistent hypoxemia while awake and at rest and who have recovered from any acute respiratory illness. A smaller number of patients with lesser degrees of resting hypoxemia may have marked nocturnal desaturation and may in effect experience chronic hypoxemia. Patients with COPD may coincidentally develop sleep apnea, and if baseline blood gas levels are already deranged, even mild to moderate sleep apnea may cause severe desaturation.

Arterial blood gas determinations or screening pulse oximetry are the only reliable means of assessing hypoxemia. Any COPD patient whose FEV_1 or FEV_1/FVC is less than 50%

should have an initial measurement and periodic reassessment. The best survival was seen when oxygen was given continuously, defined as 18 hr or more per day, at flow rates adequate to achieve arterial oxygen pressure (PaO_2) in the range of 60–80 mm Hg while awake and at rest. Home oxygen prescriptions should follow these criteria in order to achieve similar benefits. Usually flow rates of 1–2 L/min at rest, increasing by 1 L/min during sleep and exercise, will be sufficient, but flow rates up to 4 L/min may be necessary. Patients with resting hypoxemia should not be advised to limit their oxygen use to hours of sleep or as needed.

More rarely, a patient with severe COPD will develop cor pulmonale despite near-normal resting values for PaO_2. In these patients, the primary mechanism of the pulmonary hypertension is the tremendous loss of capillary surface area due to advanced emphysema. Clinically, such patients have dyspnea, hyperinflation, and a marked reduction in FEV_1 and diffusing capacity and may desaturate with mild exertion. It is not known whether oxygen can improve mortality in this group of patients, but some will derive symptomatic benefit from home oxygen.

Various drugs have been used in attempts to improve hypoxemia, pulmonary vascular resistance, or cardiac output. With the exception of judicious use of diuretics, none of the usual pharmacologic therapy for left ventricular failure is effective in managing cor pulmonale.

Bronchodilators are the foundation of symptomatic treatment in COPD and may improve baseline PaO_2. The most widely used and recommended bronchodilators for COPD are inhaled intermediate-acting beta-adrenergic agents, inhaled ipratropium bromide, and, to a lesser degree, theophylline. Theophylline has been shown to improve the right ventricular ejection fraction, but as with other drug therapy in COPD, it has been difficult to correlate physiologic improvements measured in the laboratory with symptomatic improvements.

Almitrine is not currently recommended for patients with COPD. While almitrine has been shown to improve blood gases in patients with COPD, it appears to improve ventilation-perfusion via increased hypoxic pulmonary vasoconstriction and has been associated with a rise in pulmonary artery pressure at rest and during exercise.

Vasodilators, particularly hydralazine and nifedipine, have been studied in COPD patients with cor pulmonale but at present are not recommended. A primary problem is that the long-term effects have not been studied and are therefore unknown. In addition, the complex acute effects of vasodilators on cardiopulmonary function make it difficult to assess the response and to predict which responses might produce a favorable outcome.

Digoxin is not indicated for isolated right ventricular failure. When COPD patients underwent hemodynamic assessment with and without digoxin, only those with evidence of left ventricular failure had any improvement.

Diuretics, while often used to treat the edema in COPD patients, should be supplanted by oxygen therapy and treatment of the underlying pulmonary disease. Vigorous diuresis is contraindicated in cor pulmonale because volume depletion may worsen cardiac output of the preload-dependent right ventricle.

Phlebotomy has been shown to produce acute improvement in hemodynamics in polycythemic COPD patients with cor pulmonale, but it has not produced long-term benefits. Phlebotomy may, on occasion, be helpful in the initial management of a patient who presents with severe right heart failure and a markedly increased hematocrit. If polycythemia persists with oxygen therapy, it may be fruitful to assess the adequacy of, or compliance with, oxygen therapy and smoking cessation.

End-stage COPD is among the indications for lung transplantation. As a practical matter, the average middle-aged to elderly patient with COPD is not a candidate for lung transplantation under current transplant center restrictions on age and concurrent medical illness. In contrast, patients who have alpha-1 antitrypsin deficiency and have smoked cigarettes may develop severe emphysema as early as the third or fourth decade of life and may have no other significant medical problems. Initially, double-lung transplantation was considered the preferred procedure for COPD, but more recently, single-lung transplantation has been successful and is gaining favor. Currently, the choice of procedure depends on a variety of patient factors, as well as the experience of the transplant center.

REFERENCES

1. Anthonisen NR: Prognosis in chronic obstructive pulmonary disease: Results from multicenter clinical trials. *Am Rev Respir Dis* 140:S95–S99, 1989.
2. Chronic cor pulmonale: Report of an expert committee. *Circulation* 27:594–615, 1963.
3. Dockery EW, Speizer FE, Ferris BG Jr, et al: Cumulative and reversible effects of lifetime smoking on simple tests of lung function in adults. *Am Rev Respir Dis* 137:286–292, 1988.
4. Fletcher C, Peto R, Tinker C, et al: *The Natural History of Chronic Bronchitis and Emphysema. An Eight Year Study of Early Chronic Obstructive Lung Disease in Working Men in London.* Oxford: Oxford University Press, 1976.
5. Hale KA, Ewing SL, Gosnell BA, et al: Lung disease in long-term cigarette smokers with and without chronic air-flow obstruction. *Am Rev Respir Dis* 130:716–721, 1984.
6. MacNee W: Pathophysiology of cor pulmonale in chronic obstructive pulmonary disease. *Am J Respir Crit Care Med* 150:833–852, 1158–1168, 1994.
7. Magee F, Wright JL, Wiggs BR, et al: Pulmonary vascular structure and function in chronic obstructive pulmonary disease. *Thorax* 43:183–189, 1988.
8. Matthay RA, Niederman MS, Wiedemann HP: Cardiovascular–pulmonary interaction in chronic obstructive pulmonary disease with special reference to the pathogenesis and management of cor pulmonale. *Med Clin North Am* 74:571–618, 1990.
9. Medical Research Council Working Party: Long-term domiciliary oxygen therapy in chronic hypoxic cor pulmonale complicating chronic bronchitis and emphysema. *Lancet* 1:681–686, 1981.
10. Nocturnal Oxygen Therapy Trial Group: Continuous or nocturnal oxygen therapy in hypoxemic chronic obstructive lung disease: A clinical trial. *Ann Intern Med* 93:391–398, 1980.
11. Pepe PE, Marini JJ: Occult positive end-respiratory pressure in mechanically ventilated patients with airflow obstruction. *Am Rev Respir Dis* 126:166–170, 1982.
12. Thurlbeck WM: Pathology of chronic airflow obstruction. *Chest* 97:6–10(Suppl), 1990.
13. Weitzenblum E, Loisceau A, Hirth C, et al: Long-term course of pulmonary arterial pressure in patients with chronic obstructive pulmonary disease. *Am Rev Respir Dis* 130:993–998, 1984.

Cystic Fibrosis

Paula J. Anderson, M.D.

PRESENTING MANIFESTATIONS

Cystic fibrosis (CF) is one of the most common lethal genetic defects in Caucasians, occurring in 1 out of every 2500 births.[1] Pulmonary disease is by far the leading cause of morbidity and mortality in CF and is characterized by recurrent suppurative pulmonary infections resulting in the development of bronchiectasis. Classically obstructive and progressive, the pulmonary disease in CF leads to hypoxemia and eventual respiratory failure. Patients present with cough productive of purulent and sometimes bloody sputum. Dyspnea, wheezing, weight loss, and sinusitis are also common. Nonrespiratory manifestations include pancreatic insufficiency with malabsorption, intestinal obstruction, and infertility. Physical exam may reveal hyperexpansion of the chest, with rhonchi, crackles, or wheezes heard on auscultation. Clubbing of the digits is common and does not correlate with the degree of pulmonary impairment. Sputum culture typically shows colonization with *Staphylococcus aureus* and *Pseudomonas aeruginosa,* and the chest radiograph may show bronchiectasis with dilated airways, increased interstitial markings, and air trapping.

DIAGNOSTIC CRITERIA

The basic defect in CF is an abnormality in the regulation of the chloride ion channel in epithelial cells which causes impaired chloride secretion and increased sodium reabsorption in the respiratory epithelium.[2] The same defect causes an excessive salt concentration in the sweat, and the sweat chloride test remains the gold standard for diagnosis. More than 98% of CF patients have sweat chloride concentrations greater than 60 mEq/L. Elevated sweat chloride levels and either chronic pulmonary disease or pancreatic insufficiency are the major diagnostic criteria. In 1989, the gene responsible for the disease was mapped to the long arm of chromosome 7 and cloned.[3] The abnormal portion that causes CF functions in the cell as a cAMP-regulated chloride channel has been labeled the *cystic fibrosis transmembrane regulator (CFTR)*. DNA analysis may replace the sweat chloride test in the future.

DIFFERENTIAL DIAGNOSIS

Differential diagnostic considerations include bronchiectasis, infection with fungus or tuberculosis, immunoglobulin deficiencies, immotile cilia syndrome, allergic bronchopulmonary aspergillosis, eosinophilic granuloma, sarcoidosis, and lymphoma.

PATHOPHYSIOLOGY

Studies indicate that chloride channels in the heart are the same as the CFTR chloride channels found in airway epithelium.[4] It is not known whether functional alterations in cardiac CFTR chloride channels are present in patients with CF. Cardiac disease in CF manifests primarily as right ventricular dysfunction secondary to cor pulmonale.[5] In CF, cor pulmonale is caused by chronic pulmonary hypertension. Many factors may contribute to elevated pulmonary artery pressures, the most important of which is chronic hypoxemia. Ventilation/perfusion abnormalities caused by inflammatory infiltrates, bronchial obstruction, and air trapping result in poor gas exchange. Mediators such as prostaglandins and thromboxane which are released from areas of chronic pulmonary inflammation may also contribute to pulmonary hypertension.[6] These mediators appear to be associated with the presence of nonendotoxin bacterial toxins such as *S. aureus* alphatoxin and *P. aeruginosa* cytotoxin.

Other factors which may increase pulmonary artery pressures include bronchopulmonary vascular anastomoses and peripheral blood vessel loss, both of which are consequences of chronic suppurative infection and lung destruction. Late in the course of CF, hypercapnia may exert a direct vasoconstrictive effect due to molar CO_2. The site of pulmonary vasoconstriction is in the small pulmonary arteries associated with terminal and respiratory bronchioles; they respond to increased pressures by the muscularization of the arterial media in sites that are normally nonmuscular. The right ventricle responds to this increased resistance in the pulmonary vasculature by right ventricular wall hypertrophy and dilatation, with eventual failure. Left ventricular dysfunction is uncommon in CF. Rarely, it is seen in patients with secondary amyloidosis or in older CF patients with atherosclerotic coronary artery disease. There is also evidence that left ventricular function may be mechanically impaired by massive right ventricular enlargement in chronic cor pulmonale or by expiratory airflow limitation.

The clinical diagnosis of cor pulmonale in CF is difficult to substantiate since dyspnea, cyanosis, tachypnea, and tachycardia may be due to pulmonary disease. Findings on cardiac examination, such as an abnormal right ventricular impulse and accentuation of the second pulmonary sound, may be masked by the presence of overlying hyperexpanded lungs. Edema may be due to right heart failure or hypoproteinemia secondary to malnutrition. Diagnostic confirmation by electrocardiography and chest radiography is also difficult, since changes may be absent in the presence of advanced cor pulmonale. Variance electrocardiography, a procedure for detection of variability in the electrical expression of the depolarization phase, shows that the electrical variability index is increased in CF and correlates with atrial oxygen pressure (PaO_2) and forced expiratory volume in 1 sec (FEV_1).[7] Radionuclide techniques have also been used successfully to examine cardiac performance in CF but have the disadvantage of involving exposure to radioactivity.[8]

M-mode echocardiography is useful for the diagnosis of cor pulmonale in CF, particularly the use of systolic time intervals. However, hyperinflated lungs and large respiratory variations in patients with advanced disease may impair the quality of the exam. Major advances have been possible with Doppler echocardiography for the noninvasive prediction of right ventricular pressures. Data using pulsed Doppler echocardiography acceleration time showed a significant correlation between high pulmonary artery pressure and low acceleration time. The relationship between diagnostic test results and the clinical status of pulmonary disease may be variable in patients with CF. A two-dimensional and Doppler echocardiographic study found a poor correlation between right ventricular ejection fraction and clinical score in a group of patients with mild to moderate disease.[9] This result is corroborated by a radionuclide study which showed only a moderate decrease in right ventricular ejection fraction in patients with severe lung disease, while some patients with terminal lung disease had normal contractility.[8] It appears that right ventricular function may be maintained in many patients with moderately severe pulmonary impairment.

NATURAL HISTORY OF THE DISEASE

In the 1940s, median survival of patients with CF was approximately 1 year, with death from respiratory failure due to infection and pancreatic insufficiency. Over the past 50 years, the median age at death in CF patients has risen from 1 to 29 years due to improved antibiotic therapy and nutritional support. Increased survival may make the nonpulmonary complications of CF more frequent and significant for all patients.

CURRENT METHODS OF TREATMENT

The goal of therapy of cor pulmonale in CF is to correct the hypoxemia and lower the elevated pulmonary artery pressures. Supplemental oxygen is the mainstay of therapy since it is directed at the primary underlying cause of pulmonary hypertension. Criteria for oxygen therapy in CF have not been clearly established, but general recommendations are that supplemental oxygen be added if the PaO_2 in the awake patient on room air is less than 60 mm Hg, since there is often nocturnal desaturation to lower levels. Supplemental oxygen also minimizes oxygen desaturation and reduces ventilatory and cardiovascular work during exercise. Oxygen therapy may be more difficult to institute in young patients with CF than in those with other hypoxemic lung diseases such as COPD because of the underlying stigma of oxygen use and because of the implication that oxygen therapy signifies the imminence of death.

Other potential therapies for cor pulmonale in CF include diuretic, digoxin, theophylline, and vasodilators. Diuretics may be required for symptomatic relief of edema but must be used judiciously. Since hypoproteinemia may contribute to edema, there is some risk of using diuretics inappropriately. Although there is some rationale for the use of digoxin and/or theophylline in CF with cor pulmonale, there is no evidence that either of these drugs offers benefits. Studies using vasodilators for the treatment of pulmonary hypertension are limited in CF, and the results are inconclusive.

Heart-lung or bilateral sequential lung transplantation may be the only option for patients with end-stage cardiopulmonary disease. The first successful heart-lung transplantation for a patient with CF was performed in 1985, and the first successful double-lung transplantation was performed in 1988.[10] In 1987, the first "domino transplant" was performed, during which a CF patient received a heart-lung transplant and his heart was transplanted into another patient. If a heart is to be used in a domino procedure, normal valves and left ventricular function are required; mild to moderate tricuspid regurgitation and right ventricular dysfunction are acceptable. In these domino donor hearts, right ventricular dysfunction resolves with removal of the diseased lungs. Also, impaired right ventricular function in patients with secondary pulmonary hypertension improves rapidly following double-lung transplantation, allowing lung transplantation without replacement of the heart in patients with pulmonary hypertension.

REFERENCES

1. Fiel SB: Clinical management of pulmonary disease in cystic fibrosis. *Lancet* 341:1070–1076, 1993.
2. Cutting GR: Pathophysiology of pulmonary disease in cystic fibrosis. *Semin Respir Crit Care Med* 15:364–374, 1994.
3. Riordan JR, Rommens JM, Kerem B, et al: Identification of the cystic fibrosis gene: Cloning and characterization of complementary DNA. *Science* 245:1066–1069, 1989.
4. Levesque PC, Padraig JH, Hume JR, et al: Expression of cystic fibrosis transmembrane regulator Cl-channels in heart. *Circ Res* 711:1002–1007, 1992.
5. Gotz ML, Burghuber OC, Salzer-Muhar U, et al: Cor pulmonale in cystic fibrosis. *J R Soc Med* 82(Suppl 16):26–31, 1989.
6. Seeger W, Suttorp N: Role of membrane lipids in the pulmonary vascular abnormalities caused by bacterial toxins. *Am Rev Respir Dis* 136:426–466, 1987.
7. Freyschuss U, Hjelte L, Johannesson M, et al: Signal variance electrocardiogram: A test for early detection of myocardial involvement in cystic fibrosis? *Clin Sci* 87:103–107, 1994.
8. Piepsz A, Ham HR, Millet E, et al: Determination of right ventricular ejection fraction in children with cystic fibrosis. *Pediatr Pulmon* 3:24–28, 1987.
9. Panidis IP, Jian-Fang R, Holsclaw DW, et al: Cardiac function in patients with cystic fibrosis: Evaluation by two-dimensional and Doppler echocardiography. *J Am Coll Cardiol* 1985;6:701–706, 1985.
10. Tamm M, Higenbottam T: Heart-lung and lung transplantation for cystic fibrosis: World experience. *Semin Respir Crit Care Med* 15:414–425, 1994.

Interstitial Lung Disease

James Rish, M.D.

PRESENTING MANIFESTATIONS

Interstitial lung diseases (ILD) represent a large group of chronic heterogeneous disorders which share a common histologic theme and culminate in fibrosis of the alveolar interstitium. These disorders not only affect the alveolar interstitium but also involve the alveolar epithelial and endothelial cells.[1]

History

The clinical presentation of patients with ILD varies with the responsible etiology, but typically patients present with an insidious onset of dyspnea and an occasional nonproductive cough.

Physical examination most commonly shows tachypnea, bibasilar end-inspiratory dry rales, digital clubbing, and an increased resting heart rate.[2,3] Signs of advanced disease associated with pulmonary hypertension and cor pulmonale include an accentuated P_2, right-sided S_3, right heart precordial lift, and elevated jugular venous pressure.[2]

Laboratory Evaluation

The chest radiograph is normal in approximately 10% of patients with ILD. However, when it is abnormal, there are four characteristic radiographic patterns: "ground glass," reticular, nodular, and reticulonodular.[4] As the disease progresses, a honeycomb pattern may develop.

In early disease, resting gas exchange may be normal. However, hypoxemia and widening of the alveolar-arterial oxygen gradient frequently occur with exercise.[5] With disease progression, arterial hypoxemia occurs at rest and is associated with hyperventilation with a compensated respiratory alkalosis and a reduced single-breath diffusing capacity for carbon monoxide $(D_L CO)$.[1] This impairment in diffusion was once thought to be the predominant mechanism of hypoxemia, but only during exercise, when capillary transit time is decreased, does diffusion limitation occur. The major mechanism responsible for arterial hypoxemia is ventilation-perfusion mismatching, which occurs as a result of progressive loss of alveolar-capillary units.[6]

Lung volume alterations are dependent upon the stage of disease and the coexistence of obstructive lung disease.[7] Typically, a restrictive ventilatory defect with decreased vital capacity and total lung capacity but with a normal FEV_1/FVC ratio is present in the middle to advanced stages of disease.[6] While the FEV_1 may be low, the normal FEV_1/FVC indicates the absence of obstructive disease. However, the ventilatory defect is variable, depending on the specific disease entity.

Diagnostic Criteria

Interstitial lung disease is a syndrome of pulmonary fibrosis and is associated with a reticulonodular pattern on the chest x-ray.

Differential Diagnosis

Interstitial lung disease encompasses a heterogeneous group of disorders. These can generally be divided into two broad categories: those of known etiology and those of unknown etiology. Known causes of ILD include occupational and environmental inhalants, drugs such as various antineoplastic agents, nitrofurantoin, and amiodarone, poisons, radiation, infectious diseases, metabolic abnormalities, and chronic pulmonary edema. Those of unknown etiology are a large, complex, heterogeneous group of disorders including idiopathic pulmonary fibrosis, interstitial disease associated with the collagen-vascular diseases, sarcoidosis, histiocytosis X, lymphangioleiomyomatosis, lymphocytic infiltrative disorders, pulmonary hemorrhage syndromes, vasculitides, veno-occlusive disease, and chronic eosinophilic pneumonias.[1–3]

Pathophysiology

Despite the etiology of ILD, these groups of diseases all have some common histologic features. The initial injury is an inflammatory process involving the alveoli (alveolitis) or interstitium. Poorly defined stimuli cause accumulation of inflammatory and immune effector cells within the alveolar and/or interstitial space.[6] The predominant inflammatory cell present within the alveoli varies, depending upon the etiology of the ILD.[1] These cells are capable of altering the normal cellular and connective tissue elements of the lung.[6] This lesion is believed to be reversible as long as the normal basement membrane scaffolding is intact to direct the placement of new parenchymal cells by the remaining epithelial and endothelial cells.[1,6] As the alveolitis becomes chronic and sustained, the alveolar structures are irreversibly damaged, and these areas of pulmonary parenchyma are replaced by fibrous tissue. End-stage ILD is characterized by cystic parenchymal lesions, fibrotic replacement of alveoli, and small airway distortion and dilation.[1]

Pulmonary hypertension (PH) is common in patients with advanced ILD. This results mainly from derangement in pulmonary vascular resistance rather than from reduced cardiac output.[5] The mechanisms of PH in ILD are multifactorial and involve both anatomic and physiologic factors.[5,6] Anatomic alterations are of undisputed importance in the development of PH. These alterations include tissue destruction with loss of pulmonary blood vessels due to the interstitial process, decreased pulmonary vascular bed distensibility, and obstructive pulmonary vascular lesions such as intimal thickening and medial hypertrophy.[5,6] However, in certain collagen vascular ILDs such as scleroderma and rheumatoid lung disease, PH can occur independently of the destructive interstitial fibrotic process.[6] One important cause of PH is pulmonary vasoconstriction mediated by alveolar hypoxia.[5,6,8] As a general rule, changes in pulmonary hemodynamics parallel changes in arterial blood gases, with PH occurring initially with exercise and subsequently at rest.[5,6] Transient right ventricular dysfunction can occur with exercise-induced PH, and can result in exercise limitation characterized by a low maximum oxygen uptake ($\dot{V}O_2$max) and low anaerobic threshold. With the onset of sustained resting PH, patients can develop chronic cor pulmonale.[2] The chronic cor pulmonale that develops in ILD once resting PH and chronic hypoxemia occur is mechanistically similar to the cor pulmonale seen with the various ILDs discussed.

Natural History of the Disease

Though the course of chronic ILD is variable, the typical course is slowly progressive, with death ensuing after 4–5 years from the pulmonary disease itself or its complications.[2]

CURRENT METHODS OF TREATMENT

Treatment involves an aggressive search for and removal of the etiologic agent if possible, prevention of disease progression, and providing supportive care. Although corticosteroids are commonly tried in ILD, they are usually not very successful, whether dealing with idiopathic ILD related to collagen vascular diseases, occupational lung diseases, or most others, the possible exception being the ILD associated with eosinophilic pneumonia. Supplemental oxygen is indicated in patients with a resting or exercise PaO_2 <55 mm Hg or in the presence of PH or cor pulmonale.[7]

REFERENCES

1. Crystal RG, Gadek JE, Ferrans VJ, et al: Interstitial lung disease: Current concepts of pathogenesis, staging and therapy. *Am J Med* 70:542–568, 1981.
2. Mortenson RL, Panos RJ, King TE Jr: Idiopathic pulmonary fibrosis. In Bone RC, Dantzker DR, George RB, et al (eds): *Pulmonary and Critical Care Medicine.* St Louis, Mosby, M3, 1993, pp 1–46.
3. Spiro SG, Dowdeswell IRG, Clark TJM: An analysis of submaximal exercise responses in patients with sarcoidosis and fibrosing alveolitis. *Br J Dis Chest* 75:169–180, 1981.
4. Fulmer JD: Interstitial lung disease. In Stein JH (ed): *Internal Medicine,* ed 4. Boston, Little, Brown, 1994, pp 1681–1692.
5. Weitzenblum E, Ehrhart M, Rasaholinjanahary J, et al: Pulmonary hemodynamics in idiopathic pulmonary fibrosis and other interstitial pulmonary diseases. *Respiration* 44:118–127, 1983.
6. Jackson LK, Fulmer JD: Structural-functional features of the interstitial lung diseases. In Fishman AP (ed): *Pulmonary Diseases and Disorders,* ed 2. New York, McGraw-Hill, 1988, pp 739–754.

7. Fulmer JD, Katzenstein AA: The interstitial lung diseases. In Bone RC, Dantzker DR, George RB, et al (eds): *Pulmonary and Critical Care Medicine*, St Louis, Mosby, M1, 1993, pp 1–15.

8. Lupi-Herrera E, Sandoyal J, Bialostozky D, et al: Extrinsic allergic alveolitis caused by pigeon breeding at a high altitude (2,240 m): Hemodynamic behavior of pulmonary circulation. *Am Rev Respir Dis* 124:602–607, 1981.

Myocardial Sarcoidosis

Gary L. Templeton, M.D.

Sarcoidosis is a multisystem disease that most commonly affects the lungs. In retrospective autopsy studies, cardiac involvement is observed in about one-fourth of patients but clinical evidence of myocardial involvement is present in only five percent.

PRESENTING MANIFESTATIONS

HISTORY

Patients with sarcoidosis can present with a variety of symptoms. Some of them are non-specific, such as fever, fatigue, malaise, weight loss, and occasionally night sweats. Others are related to the organ systems that are involved, such as dyspnea, dry cough, and chest pain in persons with pulmonary disease or rash in persons with cutaneous involvement. All tissues of the heart can be affected in sarcoidosis, and symptoms are related to the location and extent of the lesions. Unfortunately, patients with cardiac involvement are frequently asymptomatic, and when symptoms are present, they are nonspecific.

PHYSICAL EXAMINATION

The physical exam of a patient suspected of having sarcoidosis should be directed toward finding evidence of involvement of other organ systems, including lymphadenopathy, hepatomegaly, splenomegaly, or pulmonary findings. Cardiac signs, such as murmurs and rubs, are sometimes present but are not specific for sarcoidosis.

LABORATORY EVALUATION

Sarcoidosis most commonly presents as a pulmonary disease and is typically classified based upon changes seen on chest x-ray. In stage 0 disease, the x-ray is clear. Stage I sarcoid is defined as bilateral hilar lymphadenopathy only, while in stage II disease, the x-ray shows bilateral hilar lymphadenopathy and parenchymal infiltration. The x-ray of patients with stage III disease shows parenchymal infiltration only. In stage IV disease, there is irreversible fibrosis and bullae formation.[1]

Electrocardiographic changes are common in sarcoid patients but are nonspecific. In patients known to have sarcoidosis, special attention should be paid to any conduction abnormalities because many of the cardiac symptoms result from involvement of the conduction system. The most common clinical presentation of cardiac sarcoidosis is complete heart block. other dysrhythmias include first-degree atrioventricular block, intraventricular conduction delays, and ventricular tachycardia. Supraventricular arrhythmias are less common but include atrial ectopy, paroxysmal atrial tachycardia, atrial flutter, and atrial fibrillation.

An echocardiogram can be useful for the diagnosis of pericardial disease and wall motion abnormalities. Myocardial perfusion imaging with thallium-201 has been studied as a possible tool to use in diagnosing myocardial sarcoidosis. Early reports with small patient populations were encouraging, but other investigators have suggested that the test is too sensitive and too nonspecific to be used in sarcoid patients without cardiac symptoms.[2] Due to the diffuse nature of the disease, myocardial biopsy is not helpful in making the diagnosis.

DIAGNOSTIC CRITERIA

Sarcoidosis should be considered whenever noncaseating granulomas are seen on a tissue biopsy.

DIFFERENTIAL DIAGNOSIS

The patient should not be given the diagnosis of sarcoidosis until other diseases that cause noncaseating granulomas are excluded. These diseases include tuberculosis, berylliosis, zirconiosis, tuberculous leprosy, cutaneous leishmaniasis, and deep fungal infection.[3]

PATHOPHYSIOLOGY

The basic lesion of sarcoidosis is a noncaseating granuloma made up of epithelioid cells with pale-staining nuclei. Multinucleated giant cells are commonly observed in the granuloma. The lungs are involved in 90% of patients with sarcoidosis. The lymph nodes, spleen, and liver are frequently also involved.[1]

Sarcoidosis can result in cardiac disease either through an indirect mechanism, whereby extensive pulmonary fibrosis leads to cor pulmonale, or via direct infiltration of noncaseating granulomas into cardiac structures. Noncaseating granulomas have been reported in the epicardium, the pericardium, the myocardium, the cardiac conduction system, and the heart valves.[1,3,4] Congestive heart failure may occur as the result of granulomatous infiltration of the myocardium. Occasionally, after healing and scarring occurs, a ventricular aneurysm may develop. Additionally, if papillary muscles become involved, the mitral and tricuspid valves may become insufficient. Aortic valve dysfunction is rare and is most common in patients with congenital valve abnormalities.[3,4] The exact incidence pericardial sarcoidosis is unknown. Clinical pericarditis is rare, but asymptomatic pericardial effusions have been reported in patients with other manifestations of sarcoid. Large pericardial effusions with cardiac tamponade have also been reported.[3] Constrictive pericarditis is very rare.[1]

NATURAL HISTORY OF THE DISEASE

The natural history of sarcoidosis varies greatly among patients. In acute cases, patients will have more generalized symptoms, and the chest x-ray will show only bilateral hilar lymph node enlargement and occasionally pulmonary infiltrates. These lesions will frequently resolve spontaneously over 12 to 18 months. However, sarcoidosis can also be more insidious, with multisystem involvement and slow progression to pulmonary fibrosis followed by the development of cor pulmonale.

CURRENT METHODS OF TREATMENT

Aside from routine therapy for specific cardiac manifestation (antiarrhythmic medications, pacemaker placement, and treatment of heart failure), most experts agree that corticosteroid therapy is the preferred treatment for patients with sarcoidosis who are symptomatic or have signs of active disease.[1,3] There is no consensus as to the optimum dose or duration of therapy because the natural history of sarcoidosis with frequent spontaneous remissions makes controlled clinical trials difficult.[1] Improvement in electrocardiographic abnormalities, left ventricular function, and perfusion defects as measured by thallium-201 testing have been reported with steroid therapy.[3] However, one report suggested that the risk of ventricular aneurysm is increased in patients treated with steroids.[5] Cardiac transplantation has been used as a last resort in a limited number of patients with severe, irreversible cardiac sarcoidosis.

REFERENCES

1. Sharma OP: Sarcoidosis. *Disease-a-Month* 26:471–535, 1990.
2. Kenney EL, Caldwell JW: Do thallium myocardial perfusion scan abnormalities predict survival in sarcoid patients without cardiac symptoms? *Angiology* 41:573–576, 1990.
3. Shammas RL, Movahed A: Sarcoidosis of the heart. *Clin Cardiol* 16:462–472, 1993.
4. Sharma OP, Maheshwari A, Thaker K: Myocardial sarcoidosis. *Chest* 103:253–258, 1993.
5. Roberts WC, McAllister HA Jr, Ferrans VJ: Sarcoidosis of the heart. *Am J Med* 63:86–108, 1977.

Primary Pulmonary Hypertension

F. Charles Hiller, M.D.

PRESENTING MANIFESTATIONS

History

Clinical manifestations of severe pulmonary hypertension are mainly those related to right ventricular failure, namely, exertional dyspnea and fluid retention. In the later stages, dyspnea at rest is also seen. Syncope is sometimes associated with exertion and can be an early sign. Angina is fairly common. Cough, hemoptysis, and hoarseness are sometimes seen.[1] Death is usually caused by progressive right ventricular failure or sudden death.[2] Suggested causes of sudden death are arrhythmias, pulmonary embolism, massive pulmonary hemorrhage, and right ventricular ischemia.[3]

Physical Examination

Inspection and palpation of the anterior chest may reveal an active precordium. A loud P_2 sound is often heard. The second sound may be split during exhalation as well as inspiration, which is abnormal. A right ventricular S_3 and/or S_4 sound may be heard in half of the cases. Pulmonic ejection murmurs and tricuspid regurgitation murmurs are relatively common, while pulmonic regurgitation murmurs are heard less often. Hepatomegaly is seen in right ventricular failure, and a pulsatile liver is palpated in tricuspid regurgitation. Ascites and peripheral edema develop as the disease progresses. Examination of the lung fields is usually unremarkable.

The evaluation of patients with suspected pulmonary hypertension begins with a careful history and physical examination. Pulmonary hypertension, especially primary pulmonary hypertension (PPH), is often missed because it is not considered in the initial evaluation of a relatively young, otherwise healthy woman whose only complaint is dyspnea on exertion. Physical findings are a prominent P_2, a right ventricular heave, a palpable systolic impulse of the pulmonary artery, a pulmonic ejection murmur, a tricuspid regurgitation murmur, right ventricular S_4 and/or S_3, a pulmonic regurgitation murmur, hepatomegaly, edema and ascites, and cyanosis.[1] Physical findings are relatively modest in the early stages of the disease, making discovery often difficult. Clubbing is rare in PPH.

Laboratory Evaluation

Diagnostic workup begins with the electrocardiogram and ends with right (and sometimes left) heart catheterization to measure pulmonary artery pressures and in some cases for contrast studies of the pulmonary circulation. The electrocardiogram shows right axis deviation and right ventricular hypertrophy. An electrocardiogram may also be useful in patients with known PPH who have deteriorated, since an atrial tachyarrhythmia which is ordinarily not expected to cause significant symptoms may markedly impair cardiac output and cause severe systemic hypotension.[1] The chest radiograph may show prominence of the pulmonary arteries with pruning of the peripheral pulmonary circulation. The chest film is occasionally normal. Thin section computed tomography may be indicated in some cases if there is any question about the pulmonary parenchyma. This technique is useful when there is a question about the presence of occult interstitial lung disease as a cause of pulmonary hypertension.[4] Echocardiography is used to determine the size and functional state of the right atrium and ventricle, and Doppler studies can be used to estimate pulmonary artery pressure.[5,6] Pulmonic and tricuspid valve insufficiency resulting from pulmonary hypertension may be seen, and some congenital heart diseases as a cause of pulmonary hypertension may be evaluated.

Since occular pulmonary emboli are always a possible cause of pulmonary hypertension, they must always be sought. A ventilation-perfusion lung scan should always be done, and if it is normal, it can be considered sufficient to rule out pulmonary embolism. A low probability scan can also be considered sufficient to eliminate pulmonary embolism if there are no other clinical indicators for this disease. However, if there are other clinical indicators, such as any evidence of venous disease, leg trauma, or unilateral leg swelling, a pulmonary angiogram (as well as appropriate venous studies) should be considered. An angiogram should be performed by an expert in the radiographic study of the pulmonary circulation. This angiogram may be part of the initial right heart catheterization.

Pulmonary function testing should always be performed, including spirometry, lung volumes, and carbon monoxide diffusion testing to rule out pulmonary parenchymal and airways diseases. Arterial blood gas determinations are essential since hypoxemia contributes to further constriction of the pulmonary circulation. Pulmonary hypertension is sometimes a cause of dyspnea which is difficult to explain. In this setting, especially in patients whose physical findings are not clearly diagnostic, pulmonary exercise testing with measurement of oxygen consumption and serial arterial blood gases from an indwelling arterial catheter can be useful. Pulmonary hypertension limits cardiac output and thereby limits maximum exercise tolerance. Exercise testing is usually abnormal in patients who have pulmonary hypertension.

Right heart catheterization is required in all cases of suspected pulmonary hypertension when no obvious cause such as chronic obstructive pulmonary disease (COPD) is identified. This establishes the severity of the hypertension and helps evaluate for right-to-left shunts or valvular heart disease. Left heart catheterization may also be useful in selected cases. It is important to determine that left ventricular filling pressure is normal or near-normal to ensure that pulmonary hypertension is not caused by left ventricular failure. Pulmonary veno-occlu-

TABLE 7.1. Pulmonary Hemodynamics at Sea Level in Normal Adults

Pulmonary artery pressure (mm Hg)	
Systolic pressure	18–25
Diastolic pressure	6–10
Mean	12–16
Capillary wedge pressure (mm Hg)	6–10
Pulmonary vascular resistance (dynes/sec/cm^{-5}	60–120
Cardiac index (L/min/m^2)	2.6–4.2

Modified from Olivari MT: Primary pulmonary hypertension. *Am J Med Sci* 302:185–198, 1991. Reprinted with permission from author and publisher.

sive disease is characterized by a gradient between the left ventricular end-diastolic pressure and the pulmonary capillary wedge pressure. Another goal of right heart catheterization is to determine the responsiveness of the pulmonary circulation to vasodilators such as prostacyclin.[7] Those patients who are responsive may benefit from vasodilators, as discussed below.

DIAGNOSTIC CRITERIA

Pulmonary hypertension is defined as a mean pulmonary arterial pressure (PAP) greater than 25 mm Hg (normal, 8–15 mm Hg) or 30 mm Hg during exercise.[1,3] Pulmonary hypertension is considered severe if the mean PAP exceeds 40 mm Hg. Table 7.1 lists normal pulmonary hemodynamics at sea level.

PATHOPHYSIOLOGY

Pulmonary hypertension may be primary (PPH) or secondary, i.e., attributable to some other disease process. Secondary pulmonary hypertension may be the result of a variety of clinical conditions, including a number of pulmonary or cardiovascular diseases, and may complicate the course and management of the primary disorder. It may also result from hematologic, infectious, and inflammatory conditions not solely involving the cardiorespiratory system, or it may occur in the absence of an identifiable precipitating disorder. Fewer than 5% of patients with pulmonary hypertension have PPH.[1] Because PPH is so uncommon, it is important to be aware of, and rule out, disease states that can cause secondary pulmonary hypertension before making a diagnosis of PPH. Causes of secondary pulmonary hypertension are listed in Table 7.2.[1,3] Some of these are discussed in other sections of this chapter.

DIFFERENTIAL DIAGNOSIS

Primary pulmonary hypertension is idiopathic by definition and is caused by some intrinsic abnormality of the pulmonary vasculature. The defect(s) usually involve the pulmonary arteries, which have well-characterized pathologic abnormalities, the original descriptions of which were used to characterize the pulmonary vascular abnormalities seen in congenital heart disease.[8] Primary pulmonary hypertension is reported to be familial in some cases.[4,9] In adults, the male:female ratio is 1:3.

    Pulmonary veno-occlusive disease (PVOD) is another disease intrinsic to the pulmonary circulation which causes pulmonary hypertension. The disease is caused by an idiopathic, obstructive, thrombotic process of the pulmonary veins and venules.[3] An even more uncommon entity, pulmonary capillary hemangiomatosis, is caused by proliferation of microvessels

TABLE 7.2. Causes of Secondary Pulmonary Hypertension

Cardiac disease
  Increased pulmonary flow (ventricular septal defect, patent ductus arteriosus, atrial septal defect)
  Resistance to pulmonary venous drainage
    Left ventricular failure (cardiomyopathy, valvular disease, coronary disease)
    Reduced left ventricular compliance (hypertension)
    Mitral stenosis
    Left atrial myxoma, cortriatriatum
Diseases of the lung and ventilation
  Pulmonary parenchymal diseases
    Chronic obstructive pulmonary disease
    Pulmonary fibrosis (idiopathic interstitial fibrosis and others)
    Granulomatous lung diseases (sarcoidosis, berylliosis)
    Cystic fibrosis
  Respiratory drive and neuromusculoskeletal disorders
    Sleep apnea syndromes
    Obesity-hypoventilation syndromes
    Neuromuscular diseases (myasthenia, poliomyelitis, and others)
    Thoracic cage deformities (kyphoscoliosis)
  Pulmonary vascular diseases
    Pulmonary thromboembolism
    Peripheral pulmonary artery stenosis
    Persistent fetal circulation
    Mediastinal fibrosis
Systemic diseases affecting the pulmonary circulation
  Collagen vascular diseases
  Sickle cell anemia
  Schistosomiasis, filariasis
  Portal hypertension
  Takayasu's disease (with pulmonary arteritis)
Drugs (medicinal and illicit) and chemicals
  Anorexic agents
  L-Tryptophan (contaminated)
  Crack cocaine
Intravenous drug abuse (talc contamination)
  Anorexic agents
  Toxic rapeseed oil
  Aminorex fumarate
  Bush tea (crotalaria)
Miscellaneous
  Residence at high altitude
  Human immunodeficiency virus (HIV) infection

Modified from Olivari MT: Primary pulmonary hypertension. *Am J Med Sci* 302:185–198, 1991; and Rubin LJ: Primary pulmonary hypertension. *Chest* 104:236–250, 1993. Reprinted with permission from author and publisher.

into the peribronchial/perivascular interstitium, lung parenchyma, and pleura.[10] There is involvement of pulmonary veins and hypertrophy of pulmonary arteries. The microvessels tend to bleed, resulting in hemoptysis.

    Secondary pulmonary hypertension caused by obstructive lung diseases and pulmonary thromboembolism has been discussed elsewhere in this chapter. Any cause of chronic hypoxemia, if of sufficient magnitude, causes pulmonary vasoconstriction. As the alveolar oxygen tension falls below 50 mm Hg, the pulmonary artery pressure rises rapidly. For this reason, correction of hypoxemia is important in all patients with hypoxemia, regardless of the cause; supplemental oxygen is used when the atrial oxygen pressure (PaO_2) is below 55 mm Hg.

Of the numerous causes of secondary pulmonary hypertension, a few merit brief comment because they are relatively common. The pulmonary hypertension associated with cardiac disease is well known. Pulmonary hypertension can result from defects causing high flow in the pulmonary circulation such as right-to-left shunting associated with atrial or ventricular septal defects. Obstructions to left heart emptying such as mitral stenosis can also cause pulmonary hypertension. Left ventricular failure with systolic dysfunction is a well-recognized cause of secondary pulmonary hypertension.[11] In patients with dilated cardiomyopathy, the magnitude of the pulmonary hypertension is a predictor of morbidity and mortality.[12] Severe pulmonary hypertension caused by diastolic left ventricular dysfunction has also been described.[13]

Secondary pulmonary hypertension has been reported following chemotherapy with agents such as carmustine, bleomycin, cyclophosphamide, etoposide, and mitomycin C.[14,15] A few cases of pulmonary hypertension have been seen in smokers of crack cocaine.[16] Intravenous drug users sometimes inject talc, which is a common contaminant in street drugs and causes vascular occlusion.

Pulmonary hypertension has been described in association with portal hypertension.[17,18] The pulmonary hypertension is thought to be related to the portal hypertension rather than to cirrhosis.[3] There is evidence to indicate that HIV positivity is associated with pulmonary hypertension in a few cases.[19]

PATHOPHYSIOLOGY

The right ventricle bears the brunt of the elevated pressure in the pulmonary circulation. When the heart and lungs are normal, right ventricular output can increase up to fivefold without any increase in pulmonary artery pressure. This is possible because of the low resistance of the distensible normal pulmonary circulation and recruitment of that portion of the pulmonary circulation which is underperfused at rest. When pressure in the pulmonary circulation increases for a prolonged period for any reason, the right ventricle hypertrophies. The magnitude of pulmonary hypertension which can be tolerated depends upon the prior status of the right ventricle and the rapidity with which the hypertension occurs. If pulmonary hypertension occurs relatively slowly, right ventricular hypertrophy can be sufficient to sustain, for a limited time, systolic pressures as high as systemic pressures. If the pulmonary circulatory abnormality occurs suddenly, as can happen with massive pulmonary embolism, so that the cross-sectional area of the pulmonary circulation is rapidly reduced, right ventricular compensatory hypertrophy cannot occur rapidly enough, and the ventricle fails. With more chronic pulmonary hypertension and compensatory right ventricular hypertrophy, higher pressures can be maintained, but eventually failure occurs. When this happens, cardiac output cannot be maintained, initially during exercise and finally at rest. Fluid retention and edema occur, and eventually tricuspid insufficiency may result. The liver may be enlarged because of passive congestion, and it may be pulsatile because of tricuspid insufficiency. Severe right ventricular hypertension can increase left ventricular end-diastolic pressure and decrease left ventricular filling. This may result in modest increases in left ventricular end-diastolic pressure and decreased left ventricular filling.[3]

NATURAL HISTORY OF THE DISEASE

The prognosis in PPH depends upon the hemodynamic status of the pulmonary circulation. Mean survival is 2–3 years after the onset of symptoms, and survival beyond 2 years is unlikely once right ventricular failure develops.[1]

CURRENT METHODS OF TREATMENT

Therapy of PPH is symptomatic and palliative. There is no cure for PPH. Secondary pulmonary hypertension is managed by treatment of the underlying disease. Adequate oxygenation is critical in all patients with pulmonary hypertension. Supplemental oxygen in hypoxemic patients with pulmonary hypertension relieves hypoxemia-induced vasoconstriction in the pulmonary circulation. Pregnancy in women with PPH presents a significant risk of mortality for the mother and fetus, so women with PPH should be strongly urged to avoid pregnancy. Left ventricular failure is treated with diuretics, but care must be taken to avoid excessive diuresis. Intravascular volume must be adequate to maximize left ventricular filling in the face of compromised pulmonary circulation and right heart function. The efficacy of digitalis in right heart disease associated with pulmonary hypertension is controversial and generally should be avoided.

Evidence supports the long-term use of anticoagulation in patients with PPH.[20,21] The usual approach is to use coumadin to achieve a prothrombin time about 1.3 times control levels. Heparin may be used to achieve a partial thromboplastin time of about 1.3 times control levels in patients in whom bleeding presents an increased risk, so that anticoagulation might need rapid easy reversal.

Patients who respond to vasodilators during right heart catheterization should be treated with calcium channel blockers to reduce the pressure in the pulmonary circulation. There is good evidence that vasodilators prolong survival in patients with primary pulmonary hypertension and may help prolong survival until a suitable donor can be found for transplantation.[22] Nifedipine and diltiazem are agents of choice; verapamil is not recommended, since it has relatively greater negative inotropic effects.[3] The usual complications of calcium channel blockers including reduced cardiac output, systemic hypotension, and peripheral edema are seen in these patients, so that dose titration is necessary. Sometimes arterial hypoxemia worsens when vasodilators are used, a complication caused by the opening of some parts of the pulmonary circulation not adequately oxygenated, so that there is pulmonary shunting. The peripheral edema which may be seen with calcium channel blockers may be caused by their negative inotropic effect on the heart, their renal salt and water retention properties, or both. There are also some patients with secondary pulmonary hypertension in COPD who may benefit from calcium channel blockers if therapy with supplemental oxygen and bronchodilators has been maximized.[23] Other new vasodilator techniques are being studied in the research setting. Continuous intravenous infusion of prostacyclin has been tried, using indwelling catheters and portable infusion pumps.[24] Recent evidence indicates improved survival in patients with severe PPH.[25] Prostacyclin is now available for use.

Atrial septostomy can provide temporary relief in patients with severe pulmonary hypertension and right heart failure.[26] The procedure is experimental and should be used only when investigational protocols are in place.

Lung transplantation, single or double, and heart-lung transplantation are the only long-term solutions for PPH. Patients who are New York Heart Association Class III and Class IV functionally should be referred to transplant centers for evaluation. Patients who have very advanced disease with liver damage from passive hepatic congestion and ascites are poor candidates for transplantation because they have high postoperative mortality.[3] Consequently, patients should be urged to seek transplantation assessment before they reach end-stage disease.

The recent release by the U.S. Food and Drug Administration of the anorexic agent dexfenfluramine makes it essential that physicians be especially aware of the risk for pulmonary hypertension in those taking this agent.[27] The risk (odds ratio) for pulmonary hypertension in those using dexfenfluramine more than three months in a year was 23.1 (6.9–77.7) (95% confidence interval).[27]

REFERENCES

1. Olivari MT: Primary pulmonary hypertension. *Am J Med Sci* 302:185–198, 1991.

2. Moser KM, Page ST, Ashburn WI, et al: Perfusion lung scans provide a guide to which patients with apparent primary pulmonary hypertension merit angiography. *West J Med* 148:167–170, 1988.

3. Rubin LJ: Primary pulmonary hypertension. *Chest* 104:236–250, 1993.

4. Rich S, Dantzker DR, Ayres SM, et al: Primary pulmonary hypertension; a national prospective study. *Ann Intern Med* 107:216–223, 1987.

5. Masuyama T, Kodama K, Kitabatake A, et al: Continuous-wave Doppler echocardiographic detection of pulmonary regurgitation and its application to noninvasive estimation of pulmonary artery pressure. *Circulation* 74:484–494, 1986.

6. Martin-Duran R, Larman M, Trugeda A, et al: Comparison of Doppler-determined elevated pulmonary arterial pressure with pressure measured at cardiac catheterization. *Am J Cardiol* 57:859–863, 1986.

7. Rubin LJ, Groves BM, Reeves JT, et al: Prostacyclin-induced pulmonary vasodilation in primary pulmonary hypertension. *Circulation* 66:334–338, 1982.

8. Heath D, Edwards JE: The pathology of hypertensive pulmonary vascular disease: A description of six grades of structural changes in the pulmonary arteries with special reference to congenital cardiac septal defects. *Circulation* 18:533–547, 1958.

9. Loyd JE, Primm RK, Newman JH: Familial primary pulmonary hypertension: Clinical patterns. *Am Rev Respir Dis* 129:194–197, 1984.

10. Wagegvoort CA, Beetsra A, Spijker J: Capillary hemangiomatosis of the lung. *Histopathology* 2:401–406, 1978.

11. Cody RJ, Kubo SH: Assessment of the right and left heart interactions: Application of resistance ratio in chronic congestive heart failure. In Fisk RL (ed): *The Right Heart.* Philadelphia: WB Saunders, pp 133–144, 1986.

12. Abramson SV, Burke JF, Kelly JJ Jr, et al: Pulmonary hypertension predicts mortality and morbidity in patients with dilated cardiomyopathy. *Ann Intern Med* 116:888–895, 1992.

13. Willens HJ, Kessler KM: Severe pulmonary hypertension associated with diastolic left ventricular dysfunction. *Chest* 103:1877–1883, 1993.

14. Ellis DA, Capewell SJ: Pulmonary veno-occlusive disease after chemotherapy. *Thorax* 41:415–416, 1986.

15. Lombard CM, Churg A, Winokur S: Pulmonary veno-occlusive disease following therapy for malignant neoplasms. *Chest* 92:871–876, 1987.

16. Russell LA, Spehlmann JE, Clarke M, et al: Pulmonary hypertension in female crack users (abstract). *Am Rev Respir Dis* 145(Suppl):A717, 1992.

17. McDonnell PJ, Toye PA, Hutchins GM: Primary pulmonary hypertension and cirrhosis: Are they related? *Am Rev Respir Dis* 127:437–441, 1983.

18. Hadengue A, Behayoun MK, Lebrec D, et al: Pulmonary hypertension complicating portal hypertension: Prevalence and relation of splanchnic hemodynamics. *Gastroenterology* 100:520–528, 1991.

19. Speich R, Jenni R, Opravil M, et al: Primary pulmonary hypertension in HIV infection. *Chest* 100:1268–1271, 1991.

20. Fuster V, Steele PM, Edwards WD, et al: Primary pulmonary hypertension: Natural history and the importance of thrombosis. *Circulation* 70:580–587, 1984.

21. Rich S, Kaufmann E, Levy PS: The effect of high doses of calcium channel blockers on survival in primary pulmonary hypertension. *N Engl J Med* 327:76–81, 1992.

22. Peacock A: Vasodilators in pulmonary hypertension. *Thorax* 48:1196–1199, 1993.

23. Salvaterra CG, Rubin LJ: Investigation and management of pulmonary hypertension in chronic obstructive pulmonary disease. *Am Rev Respir Dis* 148:1414–1417, 1993.

24. Rubin LJ, Mendoza J, Hood M, et al: Treatment of primary pulmonary hypertension with continuous intravenous prostacyclin (epoprostenol). *Ann Intern Med* 112:485–491, 1990.

25. Barst RJ, Rubin LJ, Long WA, et al: A comparison of continuous intravenous epoprostenol (prostacyclin) with conventional therapy for primary pulmonary hypertension. *N Engl J Med* 334:296–301, 1996.
26. Kerstein D, Garofano RP, Hsu DT, et al: Efficacy of blade balloon atrial septostomy in advanced pulmonary vascular disease (abstract). *Am Rev Respir Dis* 145:A717, 1992.
27. Abenhaim L, Moride Y, Brenot F, et al: Appetite suppressant drugs and the risk of primary pulmonary hypertension. *N Engl J Med* 335:609–16, 1996.

Pulmonary Embolism

Kirkland C. Nolan, M.D.
J. David Talley, M.D.

PRESENTING MANIFESTATIONS

History

Patients with a pulmonary embolus frequently present with dyspnea. An acute rise in pulmonary artery pressure may cause chest discomfort. Pluritis suggests pulmonary infarction. Lightheadedness, dizziness, and syncope suggest massive pulmonary embolus with hemodynamic collapse.

Physical Examination

Findings on physical examination are related to the possible source of the emboli, pulmonary hypertension with secondary acute right ventricular failure, and systemic arterial hypotension due to left ventricular failure. Deep venous thrombosis is a suggestive finding. Features suggesting right ventricular failure include a prominent "a" wave in the jugular venous pressure waveform, a loud and delayed "snap" in the pulmonary component of the second heart sound, a right ventricular S_3 and S_4, and signs of venous hypertension including an enlarged, tender liver and peripheral venous engorgement. Systemic hypotension and a left ventricular S_3 are seen with a massive pulmonary embolus.

Laboratory Evaluation

There are many possible findings on the routine chest x-ray in patients with acute pulmonary embolism. While a completely normal chest x-ray is unusual, the vast majority of the findings are nonspecific and are seen with a variety of disorders.[1] Possible findings include atelectasis, parenchymal areas of increased opacity, vascular redistribution, a pleural effusion, an elevated hemidiaphragm, and hilar enlargement. A few of the radiographic findings in acute pulmonary embolism are unusual and noteworthy (Figure 7.1). These abnormalities include oligemia (Westermark's sign),[2] a prominent central pulmonary artery (Fleischner's sign),[3] lines or opacities compatible with pulmonary infarction (Fleischner's lines), a pleural-based area of increased opacity (Hampton's hump),[4] a diminutive pulmonary artery on the involved side (knuckle sign),[5] and rapid tapering of the right pulmonary artery (sausage sign).[6]

The S1, Q3, T3 pattern seen on the electrocardiogram suggests acute right ventricular strain. Decreased oxygen content and saturation are common findings.

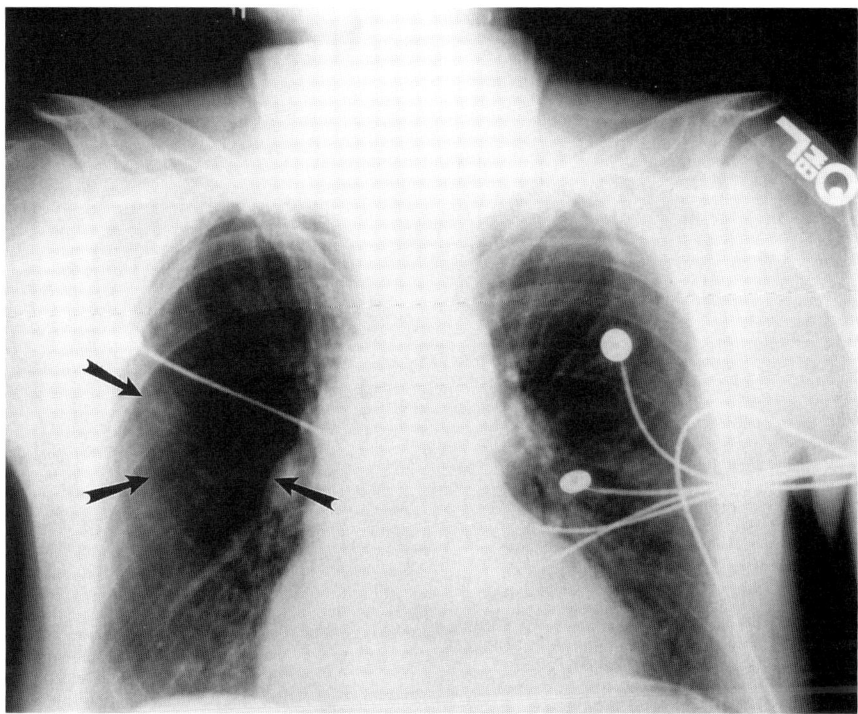

Figure 7.1. Portable upright chest x-ray of a patient with an acute pulmonary embolism of the right lung. The arrows show an area of relative hyperlucency (Westermark's sign). This radiographic finding is seen occasionally in patients with a pulmonary embolism; it is highly specific for the disease. (From Velusamy M, Patel N, Talley JD. The chest x-ray in the diagnosis of acute pulmonary embolism: Westermark's sign. *J Arkansas Med Society* 91:501–502, 1995. Reprinted with permission of the author and publisher.)

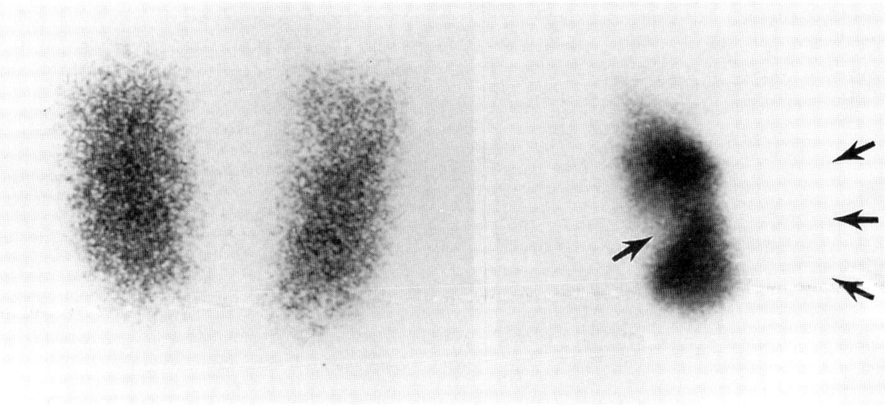

Figure 7.2. Ventilation-perfusion scan of a patient with an acute pulmonary embolism of the right lung. The anterior view of the perfusion lung scan (left panel) shows nearly complete absence of blood flow to the right lung (large arrows) compared with the left lung. There is also a moderately large wedge-shaped defect in the upper lobe of the left lung (small arrows). (From Velusamy M, Patel N, Talley JD. The chest x-ray in the diagnosis of acute pulmonary embolism: Westermark's sign. *J Arkansas Med Society* 91:501–502, 1995. Reprinted with permission of the author and publisher.)

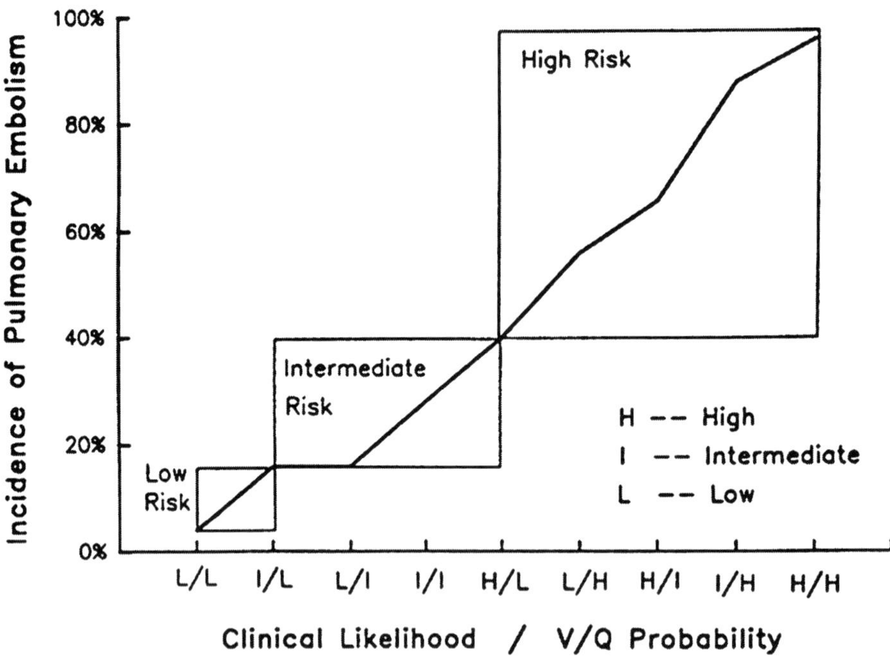

Figure 7.3. Heightened clinical suspicion is necessary to diagnose a pulmonary embolus. Importantly, patients with a low-probability ventilation-perfusion scan may have as much as a 16% chance of having a pulmonary embolus. Clinical judgment in conjunction with the lung scan improves diagnostic accuracy. (From Bone RC. The low-probability lung scan: A potentially lethal reading. *Arch Intern Med* 153:2621–2622, 1993. Copyright 1993, American Medical Association Reprinted with permission of the author and publisher.)

DIAGNOSTIC CRITERIA

The pathognomonic findings in pulmonary embolus is angiographic confirmation of an embolus in a pulmonary artery. Less invasive methods are less specific and sensitive than pulmonary angiography. In fact, a "low-probability" lung scan (ventilation-perfusion) is associated with an angiographically defined pulmonary embolus in 16% of all scanned patients.[7] The classic finding on a lung scan is ventilation without perfusion (a ventilation-perfusion mismatch) (Figure 7.2). A high index of clinical suspicion must be maintained to properly diagnose a patient with a pulmonary embolus (Figure 7.3).

DIFFERENTIAL DIAGNOSIS

Diseases or conditions which may mimic the history, physical examination, and laboratory findings of pulmonary embolus include sarcoidosis, sickle cell disease, pulmonary veno-occlusive disease, pulmonary arteriovenous fistula, schistosomiasis, vasculitis, chronic interstitial lung disease, left-to-right shunting, and elevated left ventricular end-diastolic pressure.[8]

PATHOPHYSIOLOGY

In animal models, once an embolus lodges within the pulmonary artery system, the pulmonary artery pressure increases.[9] Generally this is a transient increase, with the pressure returning to baseline within 10 min. This elevation in pressure is not a localized phenomenon but occurs throughout the pulmonary artery system. While the pulmonary artery pressure increases, the mean pulmonary wedge pressure and mean pulmonary venous pressure do not change in the initial stage of pulmonary embolism.

Patients with pulmonary embolus may be divided into two groups: those with and without underlying cardiopulmonary disease.[10] Many of the same effects documented in animal modes have also been documented in humans without underlying cardiopulmonary disease. The most consistent finding is a decrease in the partial pressure of oxygen.[10] The amount of hypoxia tends to be linearly dependent upon the amount of pulmonary vascular obstruction. Other hemodynamic findings that occur with pulmonary embolus in patients without prior cardiopulmonary disease include an increase in mean pulmonary artery mean pressure and right atrial mean pressure. The cardiac index in this group of patients is usually normal or elevated.[10]

In comparison with patients without prior cardiopulmonary disease, patients with cardiopulmonary disease tend to have higher pulmonary artery mean pressure, total pulmonary vascular resistance, and cardiac index despite having less angiographic obstruction.[10] Therefore, the amount of obstruction does not correlate linearly with the pulmonary artery pressure. Pulmonary mean pressure does seem to correlate with the pulmonary capillary wedge pressure in this group of patients.

In animals, when one of the two main pulmonary arteries is externally occluded with a clamp, pulmonary artery pressure does not change significantly. Yet when one of the pulmonary arteries is occluded by a large embolus, pulmonary hypertension ensues, with elevation of right ventricle and right atrial pressures.[11] It is therefore theorized that some factor must be released by the pulmonary embolus, causing pulmonary hypertension to develop. In support of this theory is that if, after embolization, aqueous extract of rabbit lung is injected into a second normal animal, signs of pulmonary embolism are produced in the second animal without an embolus.[12] Serotonin is the chemical considered most likely to be responsible. Serotonin is a very potent pulmonary vasoconstrictor. It constricts the arteriolar system directly by stimulating the smooth muscle system.[13] The constricting ability of serotonin is not reduced by the application of 100% oxygen.[14] Chemicals like histamine, acetylcholine, epinephrine, and norepinephrine are not potent pulmonary vasoconstrictors.

The mechanism for systemic hypotension caused by massive pulmonary embolus is as follows: Once the clot is lodged in the pulmonary artery, the pulmonary artery pressure begins to rise. This rise causes the right ventricle pressure to rise. With the rise in right ventricle pressure, the septum to right ventricle free wall diameter increases.[15] The increasing right ventricle diameter pushes the septum, so that the septum to left ventricle free wall diameter begins to decrease.[15] The left ventricle anteroposterior diameter does not change with the bulging of the septum. This results in a decrease of the left ventricle area index, left ventricle area stroke work, and left ventricle end-diastolic pressure, with eventual systemic hypotension.

NATURAL HISTORY OF THE DISEASE

Approximately 600,000 individuals suffer a pulmonary embolus in the United States each year.[16] It is the primary cause of death in over 100,000 patients each year and is a contributing cause of death in another 100,000 patients. It is through complete cardiovascular collapse from massive pulmonary embolus that these patients die.

CURRENT METHODS OF TREATMENT

Thrombolytic therapy is indicated for massive pulmonary embolism that results in cardiovascular collapse. Unlike heparin, urokinase will decrease pulmonary artery pressure acutely, right ventricular systolic and diastolic pressures, right atrial pressure, and total pulmonary vascular resistance.[17] These effects apply to patients with massive pulmonary emboli but not to those with submassive emboli.

REFERENCES

1. McDonald IG, Hirsh J, Hale GS, et al: Major pulmonary embolism, a correlation of clinical findings, haemodynamics, pulmonary angiography, and pathological physiology. *Br Heart J* 34:356–364, 1972.
2. Westermark N: On the roentgen diagnosis of lung embolism: Brief review of the incidence, pathology and clinical symptoms of lung embolism. *Acta Radiol (Stockh)* 19:357–372, 1938.
3. Fleischner FG: Unilateral pulmonary embolism with increased compensatory circulation through the unoccluded lung. *Radiology* 73:591–597, 1959.
4. Hampton AO, Castlman B: Correlation of postmortem chest teleroentgenograms with autopsy findings: With special reference to pulmonary embolism and infarction. *AJR* 43:305–326, 1940.
5. Torrance DJ: *The Chest Film in Massive Pulmonary Embolism.* Springfield, IL, Charles C Thomas, 1963.
6. Palla A, Donnamaria V, Petruzzzelli S, et al: Enlargement of the right descending pulmonary artery in pulmonary embolism. *AJR* 141:513–517, 1983.
7. The PIOPED investigators: Value of the ventilation/perfusion scan in acute pulmonary embolism: Results of the Prospective Investigation of Pulmonary Embolism Diagnosis (PIOPED). *JAMA* 263:2753–2759, 1990.
8. Goldhaber SZ: Strategies for diagnosis. In Goldhaber SZ (ed): *Pulmonary Embolism and Deep Venous Thrombosis.* Philadelphia: WB Saunders, 1985, pp 79–97.
9. Parmley LF, North RL, Ott BS: Hemodynamic alterations of acute pulmonary thromboembolism. *Circ Res* 11:450–465, 1962.
10. McIntyre KM, Sasahara AA: The hemodynamic response to pulmonary embolism. In Mobin-Uddin K (ed): *Pulmonary Thromboembolism.* Springfield, IL, Charles C Thomas, 1975, pp 116–131.
11. Gibbon JH, Churchill ED: The physiology of massive pulmonary embolism. An experimental study of the changes produced by obstruction to the flow of blood through the pulmonary artery and its lobar branches. *Ann Surg* 104:811–822, 1936.
12. Miselli L: Humoral mechanisms in palliogenesis of pulmonary embolism. *Rass Ital Chir Med (Genoia)* 6:307–311, 1957.
13. Rose JC, Lazaro EJ: Pulmonary vascular responses to serotonin and effects of certain serotonin antagonists. *Circ Res* 6:283–288, 1958.
14. Rudolph AM, Paul MH: Pulmonary and systemic vascular response to continuous infusion of 5-hydroxytryptamine (serotonin) in the dog. *Am J Physiol* 189:263–268, 1957.
15. Belenkie B, Danie R, Smith ER, et al: Ventricular interaction during experimental acute pulmonary embolism. *Circulation* 78:3, 1752–1761, 1988.
16. Dalen JE, Alpert JS: Natural history of pulmonary embolism. In Sasahara AA, Sonnenblick EH, Lesch M (eds): *Pulmonary Embolism.* New York, Grune & Stratton, 1975, pp 77–88.
17. Urokinase Pulmonary Embolism Trial: A cooperative study. *Circulation* 47(Suppl 2):1–108, 1973.

Pulmonary Vasculitis

Tyrone T. Lee, M.D.

PRESENTING MANIFESTATIONS

Vasculitis is defined as an inflammatory process involving blood vessels that can lead to destruction of the vessels and ischemic damage to the organs supplied by these vessels.[1] The presentation of pulmonary vasculitis varies from one disease to another. Wegener's granulomatosis is a disseminated vasculitis characterized by cavitary or noncavitary pulmonary nodules along with oral and renal involvement. The presence of anti nuclear cytoplasmic antibody is a highly specific and moderately sensitive marker for Wegener's granulomatosis. Churg-Strauss syndrome is characterized by the presence of asthma, a history of atopy, and eosinophilia in conjunction with a systemic necrotizing vasculitis.[2] Peripheral eosinophilia exceeding 10% on a white blood cell differential is seen in the Churg-Strauss syndrome. Takayasu's arteritis presents with pulmonary infiltrates, headache, cranial neuropathies, and other nonspecific features including fever, malaise, weight loss, arthralgias, and an elevated erythrocyte sedimentation rate.[1] Behçet's syndrome is a multisystemic disorder presenting with recurrent oral and genital ulcerations, as well as uveitis often leading to blindness.[3,4] Hypersensitivity vasculitis generally presents with pulmonary infiltrates, along with multiorgan systemic involvement including the skin, kidney joints, gastrointestinal tract, and central nervous system.[5] Vasculitis associated with connective tissue diseases presents with pulmonary nodules or infiltrates, skin rash, arthritis, and ocular manifestations. Antinuclear antibodies and rheumatoid factor are often positive.

DIAGNOSTIC CRITERIA

The diagnosis of Wegener's granulomatosis by American College of Rheumatology criteria requires any two of these four findings: (1) painful or painless oral ulcers or a purulent or bloody nasal discharge; (2) chest x-ray showing the presence of nodules, fixed infiltrates, or cavities; (3) microhematuria or red cell casts in urine sediment; and (4) histologic changes showing granulomatous inflammation within the wall of an artery or in the perivascular or extravascular area.[6] The American College of Rheumatology developed six criteria for the diagnosis of Churg-Strauss syndrome in a patient with documented vasculitis: (1) asthma, (2) eosinophilia exceeding 10% on a white blood cell differential, (3) mononeuropathy (including multiplex) or polyneuropathy, (4) nonfixed infiltrate on a chest x-ray, (5) paranasal sinus abnormality, and (6) biopsy containing a blood vessel with extravascular eosinophilia. The diagnosis of Takayasu's arteritis requires histologic confirmation on temporal artery biopsy. Behçet's disease, hypertension, vasculitis, and vasculitis associated with connective tissue diseases are, for the most part, clinical diagnoses based on presentation and serologic tests.[7]

DIFFERENTIAL DIAGNOSIS

The differential diagnosis of pulmonary vasculitis includes granulomatous vasculitis (Wegener's granulomatosis and Churg-Strauss syndrome), Takayasu's arteritis, Behçet's disease, and the hypersensitivity vasculitides including Henoch-Schönlein purpura, mixed cryoglobulinemia, and vasculitis associated with connective tissue diseases.

PATHOPHYSIOLOGY

Cardiac involvement occurs in approximately 15% of patients with Wegener's granulomatosis and includes dilated congestive cardiomyopathy, myocardial infarction, mitral or aortic valvulitis, acute myocarditis, and pericarditis.[8] Cardiac manifestations of Churg-Strauss syndrome include acute pericarditis, constrictive pericarditis, cardiac failure, and myocardial infarction. Also, widespread myocardial damage may result from vasculitis of the coronary arteries, and myocardium may be replaced by granulomas and scar tissue.[9] Cardiac manifestations of Takayasu's arteritis include aortic regurgitation, aortic aneurysms, cardiomegaly, and cardiac failure secondary to aortic or pulmonary hypertension.[10] The association of Behçet's disease, hypersensitivity vasculitis, and vasculitis secondary to connective tissue diseases is less pronounced.[1]

NATURAL HISTORY OF THE DISEASE

The natural history of pulmonary vasculitis consists of slowly to rapidly progressive disease resulting in organ system dysfunction and failure followed by death, especially if the disease is untreated.

CURRENT METHODS OF TREATMENT

Treatment of pulmonary vasculitis usually includes the use of prednisone, with or without cyclophosphamide.[1,11]

REFERENCES

1. Leavitt RY, Fauci AS: Pulmonary vasculitis. *Am Rev Resp Dis* 134:149–166, 1986.
2. Churg J, Strauss L: Allergic granulomatosis, allergic angiitis, and pericardia nodosa. *Am J Pathol* 27:277–301, 1951.
3. O'Duffy JD, Carney JA, Doedhar S: Behçet's disease. *Ann Intern Med* 75:561–570, 1971.
4. Chajek T, Fainaru M: Behçet's disease: Report of 41 cases and a review of the literature. *Medicine (Balt)* 54:179–196, 1975.
5. Sams WA Jr: Human hypersensitivity angiitis, an immune complex disease. *J Invest Dermatol* 85(Suppl): 144–148, 1985.
6. Leavitt RY, Fauci AS, Bloch DA: The American College of Rheumatology 1990 criteria for the classification of Wegener's granulomatosis. *Arthritis Rheum* 33:1101–1107, 1990.
7. Masi AT, Hunder GG, Lie JT, et al: The American College of Rheumatology 1990 criteria for the classification of Churg-Strauss syndrome (allergic granulomatosis and angiitis). *Arthritis Rheum* 33:1094–1100, 1990.
8. Specks U, DeRemee RA: Granulomatous vasculitis: Wegener's granulomatosis and Churg-Strauss syndrome. *Rheum Dis Clin North Am* 16:377–397, 1990.
9. Lanhan JG, Elkon KB, Pusey CD, et al: Systemic vasculitis with asthma and eosinophilia: A clinical approach to the Churg-Strauss syndrome. *Medicine (Balt)* 63:65–80, 1984.
10. Hall S, Barr W, Lie JT, et al: Takayasu's arteritis: A study of 32 North American patients. *Medicine (Balt)* 64:89–99, 1985.
11. Fauci AS, Haynes BF, Katz P, et al: Wegener's granulomatosis: Prospective clinical and therapeutic experience with 85 patients for 21 years. *Ann Intern Med* 98:76–85, 1983.

— VIII —
Cardiovascular Involvement with Diseases Related to Hematology and Oncology

J. David Talley, M.D.
Section Editor

Amyloidosis

Muthu Velusamy, M.D.
J. David Talley, M.D.

PRESENTING MANIFESTATIONS

History

Patients may complain of chest discomfort, dizziness, nausea, diaphoresis, and shortness of breath. The family history is important, especially regarding the possibility of Jewish, Swedish, or Portuguese ancestry.

Physical Examination

Typically, the patient with amyloidosis is lethargic and icteric due to hepatic involvement. Autonomic dysfunction may cause orthostatic hypotension. Systolic murmurs of tricuspid and mitral regurgitation may be heard; however, a third heart sound is frequently absent.[1]

Laboratory Evaluation

Mild cardiomegaly and pulmonary vascular congestion may be seen on the chest x-ray. The electrocardiogram may show abnormalities in atrioventricular and intraventricular conduction, Q waves consistent with an old myocardial infraction, and low-voltage QRS complexes. Echocardiography may show symmetric left ventricular hypertrophy, small to normal cavity dimensions, decreased systolic contraction, and the characteristic diffuse, hyperrefractile "granular sparkling" appearance of the amyloid deposits. Quantitative texture analysis of the myocardium may be helpful in differentiating infiltrative disorders and myocardial hypertrophy.[2,3] Cardiac catheterization confirms the findings of right and left ventricular dysfunction seen on echocardiography. Hemodynamic features of restrictive heart disease have been noted in both ventricles.[4,5]

Endomyocardial biopsy may show degenerated and fibrosed endomyocardium, with subendocardial, perivascular, and interstitial apple-green birefringent amyloid deposits after staining with Congo red (Figure 8.1).

DIAGNOSTIC CRITERIA

Amyloidosis is the extracellular deposition of the insoluble fibrous protein amyloid in one or more sites of the body. Definitive diagnosis of cardiac involvement requires an endomyocar-

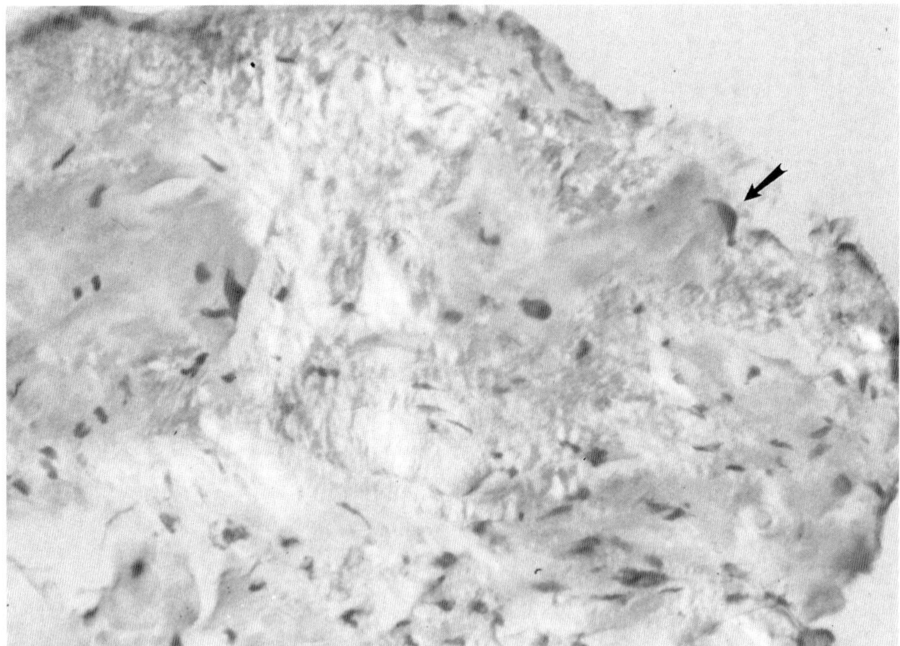

Figure 8.1. Photomicrograph of an endomyocardial biopsy specimen showing amyloid deposits (arrows). (Courtesy of James A. Waldron, Jr, M.D.) From Velusamy M, Lawhorn SL, Talley JD. Primary cardiac amyloidosis. J Arkansas Med Society 91:398–399, 1995. Reprinted with permission of author and publisher.

dial biopsy showing apple-green birefringent amyloid deposits. Electron microscopy and immunohistochemical staining may show light chains in the endomyocardial specimen (light chain deposition disease).

DIFFERENTIAL DIAGNOSIS

Amyloid heart disease should be differentiated from other forms of restrictive cardiomyopathy. The diastolic dysfunction resembles constrictive pericarditis.

PATHOPHYSIOLOGY

Primary cardiac amyloidosis is a rare infiltrative disorder. Virchow described it in 1854 based on the color of the fibrils after staining with iodine and sulfuric acid.[6] Excessive production or deposition of polypeptide molecules (amyloid fibrils) interferes with normal tissue. Amyloid deposits are seen as an apple-green birefringence with Congo red under the polarized light microscope. The most sensitive method of diagnosis is electron microscopy, in which the amyloid deposits are seen as rigid, linear, nonbranching, aggregated fibrils 7.5 to 10 nm wide with variable length. Light chain deposition disease occurs most frequently in association with multiple myeloma, and is characterized by rapidly progressive renal disease, cardiac involvement manifested by congestive heart failure and restrictive cardiomyopathy, hepatic disease, and polyneuropathy.[7]

There are three types of systemic amyloidosis: secondary, familial, and primary. Secondary amyloidosis may be seen with chronic inflammatory diseases such as granulomatous disease, rheumatoid disease, infections, and malignancy.[8] Familial amyloidosis presents with either progressive neuropathy, cardiomyopathy, or renal dysfunction and is genetically transmitted in an autosomal dominant pattern. Primary amyloidosis includes unrecognized inherited forms, secondary amyloidosis without an identified cause, and amyloid deposits confined to a single organ.[9,10] A defect in the gene responsible for the production of lysozyme protein (found in phagocytic leukocytes and tears) has been linked to the production of amyloid protein.[11]

Fractionation of amyloid fibrils has allowed chemical identification and categorization of the major protein components. These components include the minor "P" pentagonal component, which is identical in all types of amyloidosis and the major fibrillar insoluble component, which varies among the various types of amyloidosis. Secondary amyloidosis and amyloidosis associated with familial Mediterranean fever consist of the amyloid A (AA) protein. In primary amyloidosis and in amyloidosis associated with the plasma cell dyscrasias, the amyloid fibril consists of the protein AL. There are three distinctly different forms of senile amyloidosis: SSA1 (isolated atrial involvement), SSA2 (confined to the aorta), and SSA3 (generalized deposition in the lungs, liver, kidneys, and myocardium). In familial amyloidosis the amyloid fibrils consist of transthyretin (prealbumin).[12]

There are multiple cardiac manifestations of amyloidosis. The abnormal protein is deposited extracellularly within the interstitium and eventually replaces the myocardial cells. It is also found in the intima and media of the coronary arteries. The usual symptoms are congestive heart failure and arrhythmia. These physiologic features reflect diffuse myocardial involvement. Vascular involvement may cause myocardial ischemia.

NATURAL HISTORY OF THE DISEASE

The outlook of patients with amyloidosis is dismal. In a Mayo Clinic series of 229 cases, median survival was 12 months and less than one quarter of the patients were alive at 3 years. The median survival of patients with cardiac failure was only 6 months from the time of onset of symptoms. The extent of interstitial amyloid did not correlate well with survival, although patients with vascular deposition had a better prognosis than those with interstitial involvement.[13]

CURRENT METHODS OF TREATMENT

Treatment of Amyloidosis

The treatment of amyloidosis is generally unsatisfactory. Symptomatic relief and control of the secondary cause, if present, are the mainstays of treatment. The response to prednisone and melphalan has been disappointing. The use of alkylating agents in primary systemic amyloidosis is promising.[14] Colchicine is helpful in familial Mediterranean fever.

Treatment of Cardiovascular Manifestations of Amyloidosis

The concentration of digitalis is elevated in the myocardium due to high protein affinity and therefore may result in a fatal arrhythmia. Heart transplantation has a good immediate outcome; however, the results of a multicenter survey of 10 patients noted reduced late survival. Most of the deaths were due to progressive amyloidosis, including involvement of the allograft.[15] Furthermore, the data suggest that current immunosuppressive protocols do not appear to alter the progression of systemic amyloid deposition. Due to the rapidly progressive nature of the disease, additional procedures such as coronary artery bypass graft surgery should be used sparingly.

REFERENCES

1. Chew C, Ziady GM, Rafael MJ, et al: The functional defect in amyloid heart disease: The "stiff heart" syndrome. *Am J Cardiol* 36:438–444, 1975.
2. Chandrasekaran K, Aylward PE, Fleagle SR, et al: Feasibility of identifying amyloid and hypertrophic cardiomyopathy with the use of computerized quantitative texture analysis of clinical echocardiographic data. *J Am Coll Cardiol* 13:832–840, 1989.
3. Pinamonti B, Picano EM, Ferdeghini EM, et al: Quantitative texture analysis in two-dimensional echocardiography: Application to the diagnosis of myocardial amyloidosis. *J Am Coll Cardiol* 14:666–671, 1989.
4. Klein AL, Hatle LK, Burstow DJ, et al: Comprehensive Doppler assessment of right ventricular diastolic function in cardiac amyloidosis. *J Am Coll Cardiol* 15:99–108, 1990.
5. Klein AL, Hatle LK, Burstow DJ, et al: Doppler characterization of left ventricular diastolic function in cardiac amyloidosis. *J Am Coll Cardiol* 13:1017–1026, 1989.
6. Cohen AS: History of amyloidosis. *J Intern Med* 232:509–510, 1992.
7. McAllister HA, Seger J, Bossart M, et al: Restrictive cardiomyopathy with κ light chain deposits in myocardium as a complication of multiple myeloma. *Arch Pathol Lab Med* 112:1151–1154, 1988.
8. Gertz MA, Kyle RA: Secondary systemic amyloidosis: Response and survival in 64 patients. *Medicine* 70:246–256, 1991.
9. Araki S, Hirai S: Classification of amyloid and amyloidosis. *Intern Med* 32:917–919, 1993.
10. WHO-ICUS Nomenclature Sub-committee: Nomenclature of amyloid and amyloidosis. *WHO Bull* 71:105–108, 1993.
11. Pepys MB, Hawkins PN, Booth DR, et al: Human lysozyme gene mutations cause hereditary systemic amyloidosis. *Nature* 362:553–557, 1993.
12. Jacobson DR, Buxbaum JN: Genetic aspects of amyloidosis. *Adv Hum Genet* 20:69–109, 1991.
13. Kyle RA, Greipp PR: Amyloidosis (AL): Clinical and laboratory features in 229 cases. *Mayo Clinic Proc* 58:665–683, 1983.
14. Gertz MA, Kyle RA, Greipp PR: Response rates and survival in primary systemic amyloidosis. *Blood* 77:257–262, 1991.
15. Hosenpud JD, DeMarco T, Frazier OH, et al: Progression of systemic disease and reduced long-term survival in patients with cardiac amyloidosis undergoing heart transplantation: Follow-up results of a multicenter survey. *Circulation* 84:III-338–III-343, 1991.

Carcinoid Syndrome

J. David Talley, M.D.

PRESENTING MANIFESTATIONS

History

Patients with the carcinoid syndrome characteristically present with flushing, especially after eating. Characteristics of the flushing may pinpoint the diagnosis of the tumors. Pulmonary carcinoid produces a long-lasting flush associated with hypotension, facial edema, lacrimation, and sweating. Carcinoid tumors of the stomach and ileum cause flushing of the head and neck.[1] Diarrhea, asthma, wheezing, rash, and arthritis are other common presenting symp-

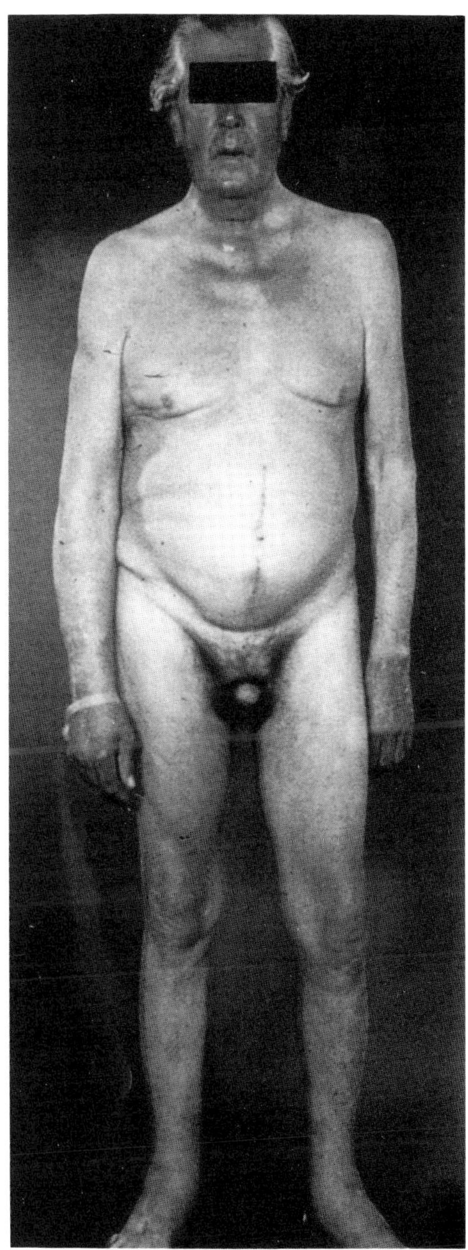

Figure 8.2. The characteristic plethora located on the head and neck of a patient with carcinoid syndrome. From Shapiro LM, Fox KM. *Color Atlas of Physical Signs in Cardiovascular Disease,* Chicago, IL: Year Book Medical Publishers, Inc. 1989: pg. 14. Reprinted with permission of author and publisher.

toms. Due to a deficiency of nicotinic acid production, patients may present with pellagra-like symptoms.

Physical Examination

Patients with carcinoid syndrome have plethora (Figure 8.2). Carcinoid tumors which have metastasized to the right side of the heart show the characteristic CV wave and systolic murmur of tricuspid regurgitation. The systolic murmur of pulmonary stenosis may be heard. With progressive cardiac involvement, right heart failure and peripheral edema may be seen.

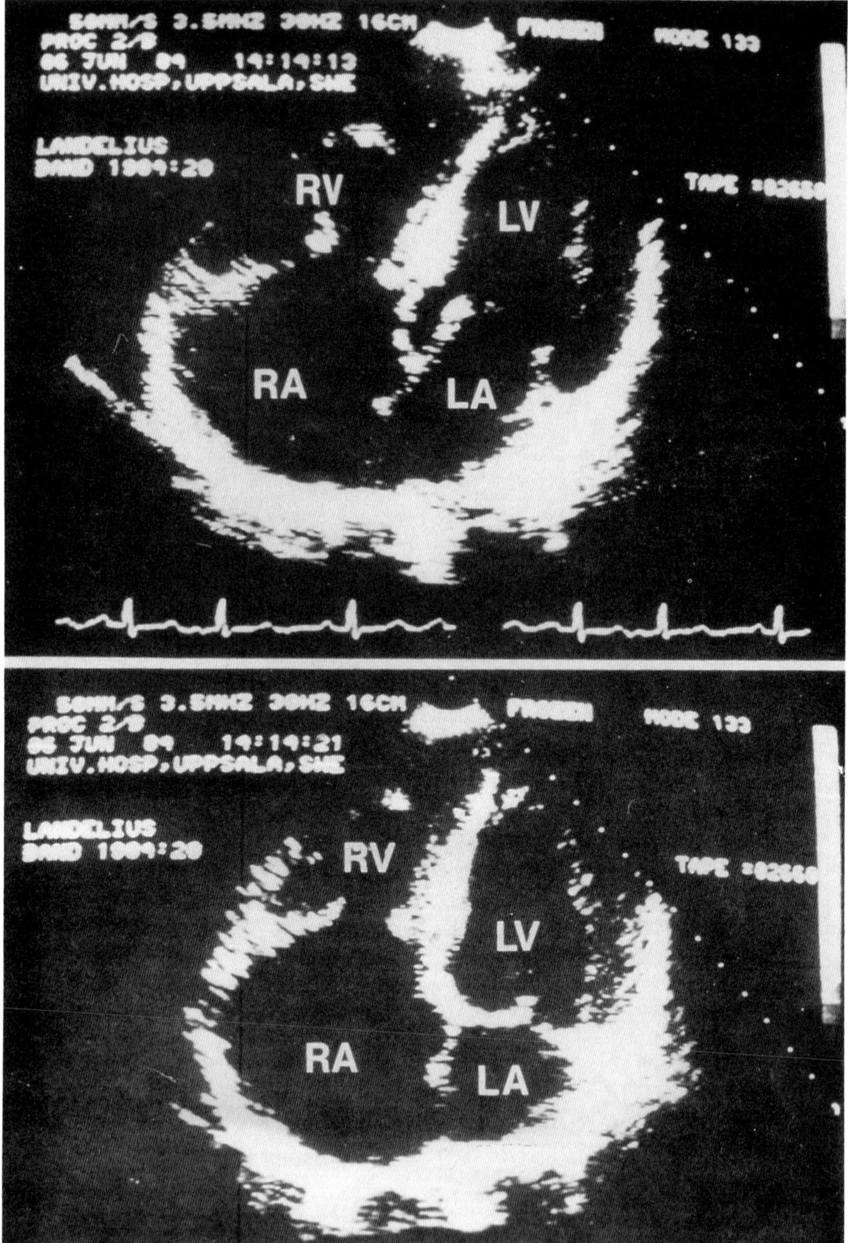

Figure 8.3. Apical 4 chamber echocardiogram showing fixation of the tricuspid valve leaflets. Upper frame, diastole (mitral valve, on right, leaflets open), lower frame, systole (mitral valve, on right, leaflets closed).

Laboratory Evaluation

5-Hydroxytryptophan (serotonin) is metabolized by the aromatic amino acid decarboxylase to yield 5-hydroxyindoleacetic acid, which can be easily measured in the urine. A level of 5-hydroxyindoleacetic acid greater than 150 μmol/24 hr in the urine is characteristic of carcinoid syndrome.[2] Occasionally, carcinoid tumors located in the stomach and bronchial tree do not contain the decarboxylase; therefore, 5-hydroxytryptophan is measured directly in the urine.[3]

On chest x-ray examination, there may be right atrial and ventricular enlargement. The electrocardiogram may show low voltage, but other changes are nonspecific unless there is enlargement of the right atrium or ventricle. The echocardiogram may show evidence of a mass in the right heart, with plaques on the tricuspid or pulmonary valve (Figure 8.3). Evidence of tricuspid regurgitation and pulmonary stenosis may be seen on Doppler examination.[4]

DIAGNOSTIC CRITERIA

Flushing, diarrhea, and an elevated level of 5-hydroxyindoleacetic acid confirm the diagnosis.

DIFFERENTIAL DIAGNOSIS

The differential diagnosis of flushing is presented in Table 8.1.

PATHOPHYSIOLOGY

Carcinoid tumors were originally described in 1907.[5] They originate from enterochromaffin cells, which are primitive neuroendocrine cells of the embryonic gut. In patients with carcinoid tumors, tryptophan is diverted from synthesis of protein and nicotinamide to serotonin (5-hydroxytryptamine) production. Serotonin is metabolized by a decarboxylase to 5-hydroxyindoleacetic acid. Excessive levels of serotonin cause diarrhea.[6] Tachykinins may be responsible for the flush reaction. Gastric carcinoid has been associated with long-term H2-receptor antagonist use in animals.[7]

Cardiovascular manifestations relate to excretion of vasoactive substances and deposition of fibrous plaques in the right side of the heart. Vasoactive substances have systemic effects (the carcinoid syndrome) and may reduce peripheral vascular resistance, causing high-output cardiac failure. Serotonin-induced fibrosis may cause constrictive pericarditis and a restrictive cardiomyopathy.[8] In approximately 20% of patients with carcinoid syndrome, glistening fibrous plaques are deposited in the right heart, causing tricuspid regurgitation and

TABLE 8.1. Differential Diagnosis of Flushing

Physiological	*Medications*	*Diseases*
Chinese restaurant syndrome	Alcohol + disulfiram, chlorpropamide	Basophilic chronic granulocytic leukemia
Hot drinks		Carcinoid syndrome
Menopause	Amyl nitrate	Medullary carcinoma of the thyroid
	Bromocriptine	
	Diltiazem	Pancreatic tumors producing vasoactive intestinal peptide
	Levodopa	
	Morphine	
	Nicotinic acid	Renal cell carcinoma
	Nifedipine	Systemic mastocytosis
	Thyrotropin-releasing hormone	

Modified from Maton PN. The carcinoid syndrome. *JAMA* 1988;260:1602–1605. Copyright 1988, American Medical Association. Reprinted with permission of author and publisher.

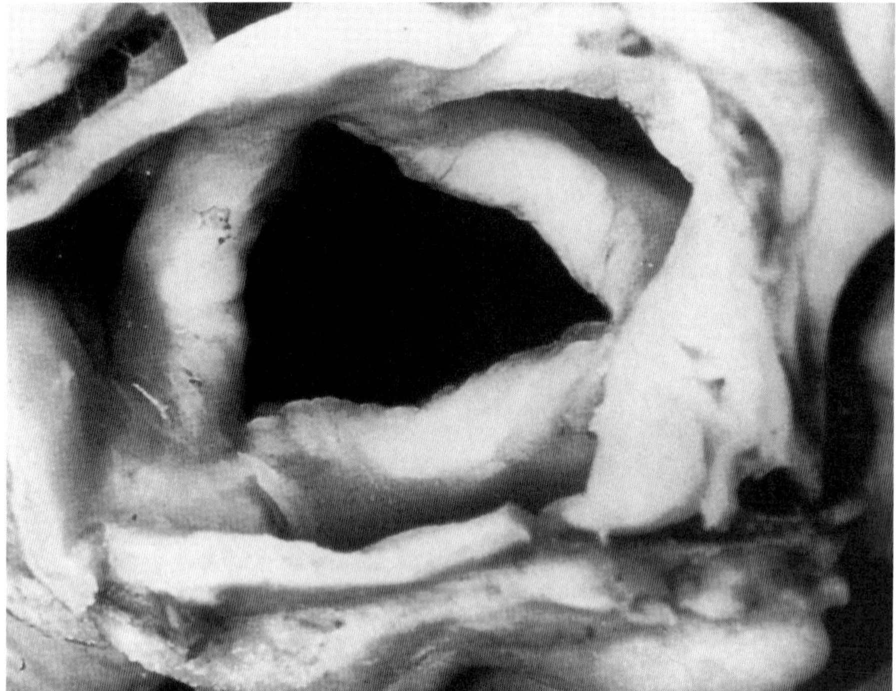

Figure 8.4. Carcinoid plaques causing deformity of the pulmonary valve in a patient with carcinoid heart disease.

pulmonary stenosis (carcinoid heart disease Figure 8.4). Metastatic lesions may be seen in the myocardium.[9]

NATURAL HISTORY

Carcinoid tumors grow slowly, and therefore a prolonged, course is typically seen. In one series, the median survival of patients was 8 years, with the longest survivor living for 12 years. In general, disease extent and prognosis correlates with the level of urinary 5-hydroxyindoleacetic acid excretion.[10]

CURRENT METHODS OF TREATMENT

Treatment of Excess Vasoactive Substances

Somatostatin inhibits the release of certain peptide hormones from normal and neoplastic tissues. A stable analogue of somatostatin with a long half-life (SMS 201-995, octreotide) decreases serotonin release from the tumor. Relief from flushing due to pentagastrin and diarrhea is achieved with this medication.[11,12]

Chemotherapy

Numerous chemotherapeutic regimens have been used, both in isolation and in combination. Typically partial remission are seen; however, long-term results have been disappointing.[13]

Control of Cardiovascular Symptoms

Medications used to control right heart failure include preload-reducing agents (diuretics and nitrates) and digitalis. In carefully selected patients, tricuspid valve replacement and pulmonary valve valvectomy have been used to temporarily relieve symptoms referable to pulmonary stenosis and tricuspid regurgitation.[14,15]

REFERENCES

1. Grahame-Smith, DG: *The Carcinoid Syndrome.* London, Heinemann Medical Books, 1972.
2. Davis Z, Moertel CG, McIlrath DC: The malignant carcinoid syndrome. *Surg Gynecol Obstet* 137:636–644, 1973.
3. Sandler M, Scheuer PJ, Watt PJ: 5-Hydroxytryptophan—secreting bronchial carcinoid tumour. *Lancet* 2:1067–1069, 1961.
4. Lundin L, Norheim I, Landelius J, et al: Carcinoid heart disease: Relationship of circulating vasoactive substances to ultrasound-detected cardiac abnormalities. *Circulation* 77:264–269, 1988.
5. Strickman NE, Hall RJ: Carcinoid heart disease. In Kapoor AS, Reynolds RD (eds): *Cancer and the Heart.* New York, Springer-Verlag, 1986, pp 135–156.
6. Maton PN: The carcinoid syndrome. *JAMA* 260:1602–1605, 1988.
7. Richter JE: Surgery for reflux disease—reflections of a gastroenterologist. *N Engl J Med* 326:825–827, 1992.
8. Rich LL, Lias CP, Nasser WK: Carcinoid pericarditis. *Am J Med* 54:522–527, 1973.
9. Roberts WC, Sjoerdsma A: The cardiac disease associated with the carcinoid syndrome (carcinoid heart disease). *Am J Med* 36:5–34, 1964.
10. Norheim I, Oberg K, Theordorsson-Norheim E: Malignant carcinoid syndrome. *Surg Gynecol Obstet* 137:637–644, 1973.
11. Kvols LK, Moertel CG, O'Connell MJ, et al: Treatment of the malignant carcinoid syndrome: Evaluation of a long-acting somatostatin analogue. *N Engl J Med* 315:663–666, 1986.
12. Öberg K, Norheim I, Theodorsson E, et al: The effects of octreotide on basal and stimulated hormone levels in patients with carcinoid syndrome. *J Clin Endocrinol Metab* 68:796–800, 1989.
13. Moertel CG: An odyssey in the land of small tumors. *J Clin Oncol* 5:1503–1522, 1987.
14. Lundin L, Hansson H-E, Landelius J, et al: Surgical treatment of carcinoid heart disease. *J Thorac Cardiovasc Surg* 100:552–561, 1990.
15. Mullins PA, Hall JA, Shapiro LM: Balloon dilation of tricuspid stenosis caused by carcinoid heart disease. *Br Heart J* 63:249–250, 1990.

Hemochromatosis

J. David Talley, M.D.

PRESENTING MANIFESTATIONS

History

Men are more commonly affected than females. Symptoms occur when patients are 50 to 60 years of age. It is important to elucidate the family history. Primary hemochromatosis is inherited as an autosomal recessive disease.[1,2] Secondary hemochromatosis may develop in patients with severe, chronic anemia who have received more than 100 units of blood transfusions.[3] Fatal congestive heart failure has been reported in patients with hemochromatosis who ingest cocaine and ascorbic acid.[4,5] Rapidly progressive sepsis due to *Vibrio vulnificus* (found in oysters) has been noted in patients with hemochromatosis.[6]

Symptoms of hemochromatosis are related to the site of iron deposition. The classic triad of symptoms is hepatomegaly, diabetes mellitus, and bronze pigmentation.[7] Cardiac symptoms include congestive heart failure and arrhythmias. Other presenting complaints may include abdominal and joint pain, weakness, and frequent infection.

Physical Examination

Bronze pigmentation of the skin is a classic finding in patients with hemochromatosis. Cardiac manifestations include an irregular heart rhythm and signs of congestive heart failure. Iron deposition in the liver causes hepatomegaly.

Laboratory Evaluation

Hyperglycemia and anemia may be seen. The serum iron level may be normal. The transferrin saturation index is high (typically greater than 80%) due to an elevated serum iron level and a low serum transferrin level and low total iron-binding capacity.[8] The serum ferritin level is elevated.

Tissue biopsy specimens stained for iron are diagnostic of hemochromatosis. A liver biopsy specimen will show grossly visible iron deposits, and the hepatic iron concentration can be measured. Calculation of the hepatic iron index (the ratio of the hepatic iron concentration to the age of the patient) and determination of the histologic hepatic iron index (total histologic iron score) confirm the diagnosis and can differentiate homozygous from heterozygous hemochromatosis.[9]

A right ventricular endomyocardial biopsy specimen may show iron deposits in the sarcoplasma of the myocardial cells. However, the distribution of the iron is patchy, and sampling from the same site may miss the involved area.[10]

Cardiomegaly is seen on the chest x-ray. Atrial arrhythmias including premature atrial depolarizations, sick sinus syndrome, and atrial flutter and fibrillation are seen on the electrocardiogram.[11] Heart block, low-voltage complexes, and non-specific T-wave abnormalities may also be seen. Structural and functional abnormalities without evidence of myocardial hypertrophy are seen on echocardiography.[12]

DIAGNOSTIC CRITERIA

The diagnosis of hemochromatosis is confirmed by finding intracellular iron deposits in a biopsy specimen from the liver or endomyocardium.

DIFFERENTIAL DIAGNOSIS

Patients with symptoms and signs of hemochromatosis and laboratory evidence of iron overload have hemochromatosis. The differential diagnosis involves eliminating the various secondary causes of the disease.

PATHOPHYSIOLOGY

Hemochromatosis is due to excessive iron intake or inadequate iron excretion. Excessive iron absorption from the gastrointestinal tract is seen in primary hemochromatosis inherited in an autosomal recessive fashion. The abnormal gene is located on chromosome 6, and the homozygous condition is seen in 3–5/1000 patients. This gene regulates the transferrin receptor on the surface of the epithelial cell in the gastrointestinal tract.[13,14] The heterozygous condition is not associated with excessive iron deposits and may go undetected. Acquired hemochromatosis is seen in anemic patients who have a long-standing need for blood transfusions. Intracellular iron deposits cause release of lysosomal acid hydrolase, resulting in cell death.

The cardiovascular manifestations of hemochromatosis are due to iron deposits in the sarcolemma of the myocytes. The deposits are most prevalent in the epicardial region and in the papillary muscles. The subendocardial region contains an intermediate amount of iron. The smallest amount of iron is seen in the mid-myocardial wall and in the conduction system. The ventricles contain heavier deposits than the atria.[15,16] Early in the course of the disease, iron deposits in the endocardium cause fibrosis and result in diastolic dysfunction. With continued iron deposition and myocardial cell death, systolic function is compromised and ventricular enlargement is seen. Atrial arrhythmias are more common than ventricular arrhythmias, which may be the result of direct iron deposition and increased atrial wall stress. There are conflicting reports about iron overload as a risk factor in the development of coronary artery disease.[17,18]

NATURAL HISTORY OF THE DISEASE

The 8-year survival of patients with hemochromatosis is 80% and is particularly low in patients with cirrhosis.[19] The principal cause of death in patients with hemochromatosis is hepatocellular carcinoma.[20]

CURRENT METHODS OF TREATMENT

Patients with primary hemochromatosis may be treated with phlebotomies, as often as twice a month for years. This therapy is quite effective in reversing the symptoms of congestive heart failure and improving echocardiographic abnormalities, especially if used early in the course of the disease.[21–24] Patients with severe left ventricular dysfunction may not respond to phlebotomy.[25] Cardiac transplantation has been performed in patients with refractory symptoms of congestive heart failure.[26]

Patients with secondary hemochromatosis cannot be treated with phlebotomy. Instead, chelation therapy with deferoxamine mesylate (Desferal) is used to bind iron and promote excretion. This therapy improves the symptoms and signs of hemochromatosis-induced cardiac dysfunction.[27]

REFERENCES

1. Swan WGA, Dewar HA: The heart in hemochromatosis. *Br Heart J* 14:117–124, 1952.
2. Finch SC, Finch CA: Idiopathic hemochromatosis, an iron storage disease. *Medicine* 34:381–430, 1995.
3. Buja LM, Roberts WC: Iron in the heart: Etiology and clinical significance. *Am J Med* 51:209–221, 1971.
4. Goldenberg SP, Zeldis SM: Fatal acute congestive heart failure in a patient with idiopathic hemochromatosis and cocaine use. *Chest* 92:374–375, 1987.

5. McLaran CJ, Bett JHN, Nye JA, et al: Congestive cardiomyopathy and haemochromatosis—rapid progression possibly accelerated by excessive ingestion of ascorbic acid. *Aust NZ J Med* 12:187–188, 1982.

6. Muench KH: Hemochromatosis and infection: Alcohol and iron, oysters and sepsis. *Am J Med* 87: 3-40N–3-43N, 1989.

7. Adams PC, Kertesz AE, Valberg LS: Clinical presentation of hemochromatosis: A changing scene. *Am J Med* 90:445–449, 1991.

8. Bronkovsky HL, Slaker DP, Bills EB, et al: Usefulness and limitations of laboratory and hepatic imaging studies in iron-storage disease. *Gastroenterology* 99:1079–1091, 1990.

9. Deugnier YM, Turlin B, Powell LW, et al: Differentiation between heterozygotes and homozygotes in genetic hemochromatosis by means of a histological hepatic iron index: A study of 192 cases. *Hepatology* 17:30–34, 1993.

10. Olson LJ, Edwards WD, McCall JT, et al: Cardiac iron deposition in idiopathic hemochromatosis: Histologic and analytic assessment of 14 hearts from autopsy. *J Am Coll Cardiol* 10:1239–1243, 1987.

11. Wang T-L, Chen W-J, Liau C-S, et al: Sick sinus syndrome as the early manifestation of cardiac hemochromatosis. *J Electrocardiol* 27:91–96, 1994.

12. Olson LJ, Baldus WP, Tajik AJ: Echocardiographic features of idiopathic hemochromatosis. *Am J Cardiol* 60:885–889, 1987.

13. Milman N, Graudal N, Nielsen LS, et al: An HLA study in 74 Danish haemochromatosis patients and 21 of their families. *Clin Genet* 41:6–11, 1992.

14. Halliday JW: The regulation of iron absorption: One more piece in the puzzle? *Gastroenterology* 102:1071–1073, 1992.

15. Mason JW, O'Connell JB: Clinical merit of endomyocardial biopsy. *Circulation* 79:971–979, 1989.

16. Olson LJ, Edwards WD, Holmes DR Jr, et al: Endomyocardial biopsy in hemochromatosis: Clinico-pathologic correlates in six cases. *J Am Coll Cardiol* 13:116–120, 1989.

17. Miller M, Hutchins GM: Hemochromatosis, multiorgan hemosiderosis, and coronary artery disease. *JAMA* 272:231–233, 1994.

18. Sullivan JL: Heterozygous hemochromatosis as a risk factor for premature myocardial infarction. *Med Hypotheses* 31:1–5, 1990.

19. Adams PC, Speechley M, Kertesz AE: Long-term survival analysis in hereditary hemochromatosis. *Gastroenterology* 101:368–372, 1991.

20. Adams PC, Kertesz AE, Kertesz AE: Long-term survival analysis in hemochromatosis: A changing scene. *Am J Med* 90:445–449, 1991.

21. Easley RM Jr, Schreiner BF Jr, Yu PN: Reversible cardiomyopathy associated with hemochromato-sis.*N Engl J Med* 287:866–867, 1972.

22. Skinner C, Kenmore ACF: Haemochromatosis presenting as congestive cardiomyopathy and responding to venesection. *Br Heart J* 35:466–468, 1973.

23. Dabestani A, Child JS, Henze E, et al: Primary hemochromatosis: Anatomic and physiologic characteristics of the cardiac ventricles and their response to phlebotomy. *Am J Cardiol* 54:153–159, 1984.

24. Candell-Riera J, Lu L, Serés L, et al: Cardiac hemochromatosis: Beneficial effects of iron removal therapy. An echocardiographic study. *Am J Cardiol* 52:824–829, 1983.

25. Westra WH, Hruban RH, Baughman KL, et al: Progressive hemochromatotic cardiomyopathy despite reversal of iron deposition after liver transplantation. *Am J Clin Pathol* 99:39–44, 1993.

26. Jensen PD, Bagger JP, Jensen FT, et al: Heart transplantation in a case of juvenile hereditary haemochromatosis followed up by MRI and endomyocardial biopsies. *Eur J Haematol* 51:199–205, 1993.

27. Wolfe L, Olivieri N, Sallan D, et al: Prevention of cardiac disease by subcutaneous deferoxamine in patients with thalassemia major. *N Engl J Med* 312:1600–1603, 1985.

Hemoglobinopathies
J. David Talley, M.D.

PRESENTING MANIFESTATIONS

History

Two major hemoglobinopathies affect the cardiovascular system: sickle cell disease and thalassemia. Sickle cell disease is a genetic disorder of hemoglobin structure. The family history is important. Approximately 10% of the Afro-American population in the United States are heterozygous for hemoglobin S, and 0.2% are homozygous for hemoglobin SS.[1] Cardiovascular manifestations are related primarily to chronic anemia and secondary hemachromatosis.

Thalassemia is a genetic abnormality of alpha- or beta-chain hemoglobin synthesis. Beta-thalassemia is seen in patients of Mediterranean (Greek or Italian) descent. Alpha-thalassemia is seen in Afro-Americans, especially in combination with sickle cell disease. As with sickle cell disease, the abnormality of hemoglobin synthesis results in chronic anemia and secondary hemochromatosis.

Physical Examination

Anemia is characterized by tachycardia and peripheral vasodilation. The spleen is enlarged due to sequestration, and the liver may be enlarged due to transfusion-related hemochromatosis.

Laboratory Evaluation

Sickle Cell Disease

There is frequently a leukocytosis. The erythrocytes on the peripheral smear are "thin sickle-shaped and crescent-shaped forms." (Figure 8.5).[2] The chest x-ray of patients with sickle cell disease may show wedge-shaped pulmonary infarcts in the lower lobes. Recurrent pulmonary infarction may cause pulmonary hypertension and enlargement of the right ventricle and atrium. On the electrocardiogram, there may be a first-degree heart block, prominent QRS voltage consistent with left ventricular hypertrophy, and low-voltage T waves which may be inverted, diphasic, or notched.[3] On echocardiography, there is evidence of dilated chambers, septal hypertrophy, an elevated left ventricular mass, and normal contractility.[4,5] At cardiac catheterization, the preload (end-diastolic volume index) is elevated and the afterload (systemic vascular resistance) is depressed. The cardiac index is approximately twice that of normal patients. The left ventricular ejection fraction is normal; however, the contractile performance is depressed.[6] Right heart pressures may be elevated in patients with pulmonary hypertension.

Thalassemia

The anemia is hypochromic and microcytic. The red cells in thalassemia are target-shaped and have basophilic stippling. An enlarged heart is seen on the chest x-ray. On the electro-

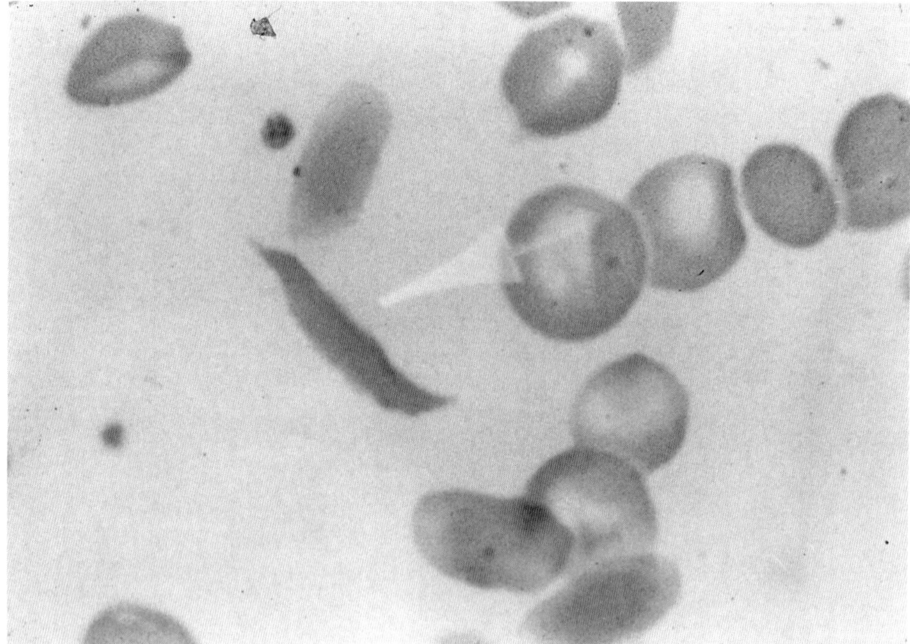

Figure 8.5.   A peripheral blood smear from a patient with sickle cell anemia. The erythrocytes are shaped like a "sickle" or "oat" and the total number is decreased.

cardiogram, voltage changes consistent with left ventricular hypertrophy and nonspecific repolarization abnormalities are seen. Panchamber enlargement, left ventricular hypertrophy, and an increased aortic root dimension are seen on echocardiography.[7] Elevated cardiac output and increased left ventricular diastolic pressure are seen on cardiac catheterization.[8]

DIAGNOSTIC CRITERIA

Characteristic abnormalities on hemoglobin electrophoresis define the presence and phenotype of the hemoglobinopathy.

DIFFERENTIAL DIAGNOSIS

The differential diagnosis of these hemoglobinopathies is facilitated by hemoglobin electrophoresis.

PATHOPHYSIOLOGY

The cardiovascular manifestations of sickle cell disease are primarily related to anemia. The echocardiographic findings of chamber enlargement are related to the duration of the disease and the severity of the anemia. Distinct myocardial abnormalities (sickle cell cardiomyopathy) are not seen. Acute myocardial infarction with normal coronary arteries has been reported.[9]

An association of sickle cell disease with mitral valve prolapse and sudden cardiac death has been noted but has not been confirmed.[10,11] There is an increased occurrence of cerebrovascular accidents.

The cardiovascular findings related to anemia in patients with thalassemia are similar to those of patients with sickle cell disease. Due to the need for frequent transfusions, secondary hemochromatosis and its attendant complications may be seen. Pericarditis is seen in one-half of patients with thalassemia.

NATURAL HISTORY OF THE DISEASE

Infection is the leading cause of death in children with sickle cell disease. The average life expectancy of patients with hemoglobinopathies is approximately 45 years of age.[12]

CURRENT METHODS OF TREATMENT

Patients with thalassemia and sickle cell disease are treated in similar fashion. Transfusion therapy may improve exercise tolerance in patients with sickle cell disease and decrease heart size in children with thalassemia, but these beneficial effects have not been consistently noted.[13] Numerous agents with antiplatelet, anticoagulant, and antisickling properties have been described; however, consistent improvement has not been noted. Complications of transfusion therapy include isoimmunization, hemochromatosis, and infection. The additional volume of the transfusion may increase the volume and viscosity of the plasma and nullify the benefits.

REFERENCES

1. Motulsky AG: Frequency of sickling disorders in U.S. blacks. *N Engl J Med* 288:31–33, 1973.
2. Herrick JB: Peculiar elongated and sickle-shaped red blood corpuscles in a case of severe anemia. *Arch Intern Med* 6:517–521, 1910.
3. Uzsoy NK: Cardiovascular finding in patients with sickle cell anemia. *Am J Cardiol* 13:320–328, 1964.
4. Covitz W, Espeland M, Gallagher D, et al: The heart in sickle cell anemia. The Cooperative Study of Sickle Cell Disease (CSSCD). *Chest* 108:1214–1219, 1995.
5. Simmons BE, Santhanam V, Castaner A, et al: Sickle cell heart disease. Two-dimensional echo and Doppler ultrasonographic findings in the hearts of adult patients with sickle cell anemia. *Arch Intern Med* 148:1526–1528, 1988.
6. Denenberg BS, Criner G, Jones R, et al: Cardiac function in sickle cell anemia. *Am J Cardiol* 51:1674–1678, 1983.
7. Ehlers I H, Levin AR, Klein AA, et al: The cardiac manifestations of thalassemia major: Natural history, noninvasive cardiac diagnostic studies, and results of cardiac catheterization. In Engle MA (ed): *Pediatric Cardiovascular Disease. Cardiovascular Clinics* II. Philadelphia, FA Davis, 1981, p 171–186.
8. Berk PD, Goldberg JD, Donovan PB, et al: Therapeutic recommendations in polycythemia vera based on Polycythemia Vera Study Group protocols. *Semin Hematol* 23:132–143, 1986.
9. Martin CR, Cobb C, Tatter D, et al: Acute myocardial infarction in sickle cell anemia. *Arch Intern Med* 143:830–831, 1983.
10. Rodman T, Close HP, Purnell MK: The oxyhemoglobin dissociation curve in anemia. *Ann Intern Med* 52:295–309, 1960.

11. Ba'Albaki HA, Eckman JR, Ghazzal ZMB, et al: Sickle cell disease and the cardiovascular system. *Emory Univ J Med* 3:163–170, 1989.
12. Powars D: Natural history of sickle cell disease–The first ten years. *Semin Hematol* 12:267–285, 1975.
13. Gaffney JW, Bierman FZ, Donnelly CM, et al: Cardiovascular adaptations to transfusion/chelation therapy of homozygote sickle cell anemia. *Am J Cardiol* 62:121–125, 1988.

Multiple Myeloma

J. David Talley, M.D.

PRESENTING MANIFESTATIONS

History

Patients with multiple myeloma typically present with bone pain due to osteoporosis or lytic lesions. Cardiovascular symptoms may include systolic, diastolic, and high-output congestive heart failure. Patients with high-output cardiac states have tachycardia, peripheral vasodilatation, dyspnea, and orthopnea. In addition to multiple myeloma, these symptoms are seen in hyperthyroidism, beriberi, severe anemia, and with arteriovenous fistulas as in severe liver disease, pregnancy, Paget's disease, fibrous dysplasia, obesity, and carcinoid syndrome.

Physical Examination

Signs of a high-output cardiac output state include tachycardia, jugular venous distension, a hyperdynamic precordium, and peripheral vasodilatation. Findings of an arteriovenous fistula include an abnormally large, asymmetric extremity (Figure 8.6), proximal vessel dilation, and thrill of the continuous murmur. Compression of the arteriovenous fistula causes an initial bradycardia and elevation of both the systolic and diastolic systemic arterial blood pressure (Figure 8.7). A systolic "flow" murmur and a ventricular gallop may be heard.

Laboratory Evaluation

The signs of volume overload with high-output congestive heart failure seen with multiple myeloma and other related conditions are similar. Cardiomegaly, interstitial infiltrates, and pleural effusions may be seen on the chest x-ray. On an electrocardiogram, sinus tachycardia is seen. Panchamber enlargement, pericardial effusion, and signs consistent with cardiac tamponade may be seen on echocardiography.[1,2] Findings at cardiac catheterization include tachycardia, low peripheral vascular resistance, elevated preload of the right- and left-sided cardiac chambers, and high cardiac output.[3]

The endomyocardial biopsy in a patient with multiple myeloma may show evidence of secondary amyloidosis. Light chain deposits (light chain deposition disease) may be seen with electron microscopy and immunohistochemical staining.[4] In patients with multiple myeloma, light chain deposition disease is associated with rapidly progressive renal disease, cardiac

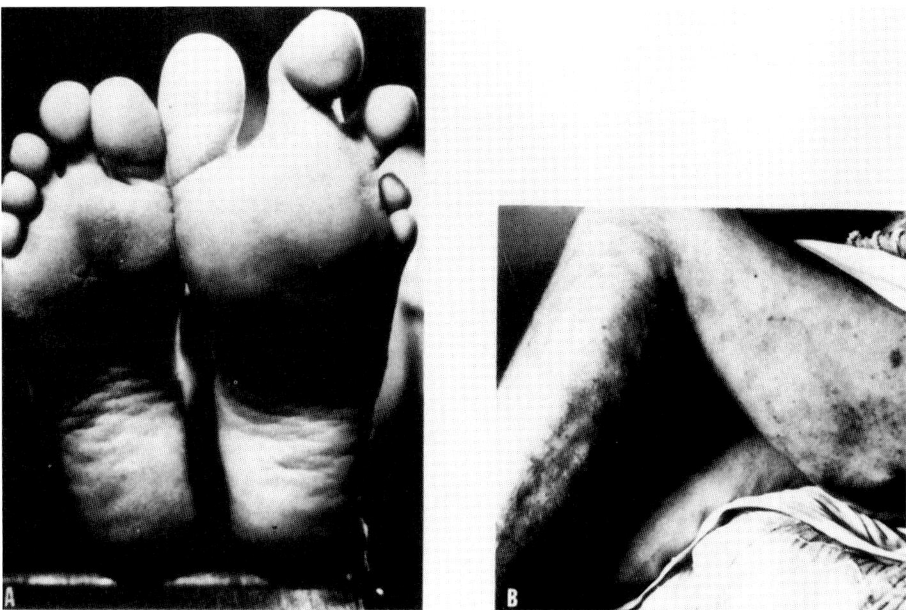

Figure 8.6. Inspection of the patient with an arteriovenous fistula may reveal an abnormally large and asymmetric extremity.

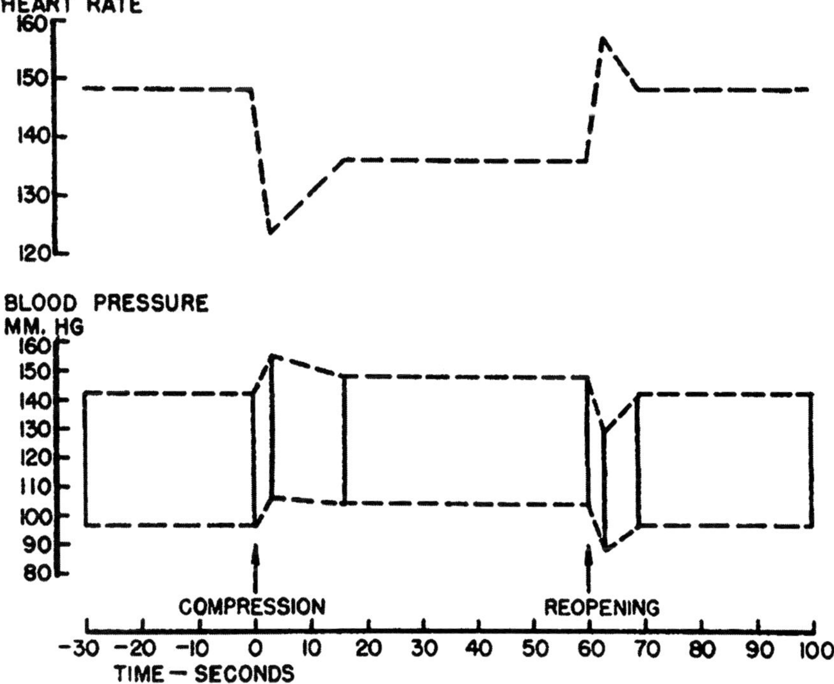

Figure 8.7. Schematic representation of the effects seen with compression of an arteriovenous fistula. The is a vagus-induced bradycardia and a decrease in venous return. These changes result in an initial bradycardia response and elevation of both the systolic and diastolic systemic arterial blood pressure. From Loo AV, Herringman EC. Circulatory changes in the dog produced by acute arteriovenous fistula. *Am J Physiol* 158:103–112, 1949. Reprinted with permission from author and publisher.

involvement manifested by congestive heart failure and restrictive cardiomyopathy, hepatic disease, and polyneuropathy.

DIAGNOSTIC CRITERIA

Patients with cardiovascular symptoms typically have widespread multiple myeloma. At this stage, the diagnosis is confirmed by the presence of marrow plasmacytosis of greater than 10% or a tumor nodule and a monoclonal protein or lytic bone lesion.[5]

DIFFERENTIAL DIAGNOSIS

Multiple myeloma should be differentiated from other causes of polyclonal plasmacytosis and bony lesions. The differential diagnosis of high-output cardiac states is noted above.

PATHOPHYSIOLOGY

Multiple Myeloma

Multiple myeloma is due to cancerous proliferation of heavy or light chain immunoglobin. Cardiovascular complications of multiple myeloma are common. Multiple myeloma is associated with systolic and diastolic dysfunction due to restrictive cardiomyopathy or constrictive pericarditis.[6,7] Secondary amyloidosis may be present. High-output congestive heart failure occurs in approximately 25% of patients with multiple myeloma.[8] This condition is probably due to coexisting anemia and extensive lytic bone lesions. Other factors implicated in producing the high-output cardiac state include increased splenic blood flow, positive chromotropic and inotropic humoral factors (interleukin-2 and -6, gamma interferon, tumor necrosis factor), and increased vascularity due to multiple small arteriovenous fistulas.[9,10]

High-Output Cardiac States

High-output congestive heart failure is due to volume overload. The direct runoff into a low-resistance system causes the high-output state in patients with large or small arteriovenous fistulas.[11] Some investigators have hypothesized that the increased cardiac output seen in patients with Paget's disease may be due to a cutaneous response to increased metabolic activity in the bones.[12] The volume overload causes ventricular dilation and remodeling due to an increase in the length, size, and assembly pattern of the sarcomeres and fibril slippage.[13,14]

NATURAL HISTORY OF THE DISEASE

Widespread bony resorption, severe anemia, and renal impairment are poor prognostic markers in patients with multiple myeloma. The mean survival of patients with these characteristics is approximately 2 years.[15]

CURRENT METHODS OF TREATMENT

Therapy of high-output congestive heart failure is directed at the underlying etiology. Successful use of chemotherapy may decrease the cardiac output in patients with multiple myeloma.[16] Transcatheter or surgical correction of large arteriovenous shunts has been successful.[17]

REFERENCES

1. Kosinski DJ, Roush K, Fraker TD Jr, et al: High cardiac output state in patients with multiple myeloma: Case report and review of the literature. *Clin Cardiol* 17:678–680, 1994.
2. Santana O, Vivas PH, Ramos A, et al: Multiple myeloma involving the pericardium associated with cardiac tamponade and constrictive pericarditis. *Am Heart J* 126:737–740, 1993.
3. McBride W, Jackman JD Jr, Gammon RS, et al: High-output cardiac failure in patients with multiple myeloma. *N Engl J Med* 319:1651–1653, 1988.
4. McAllister HA Jr, Seger J, Bossart M, et al: Restrictive cardiomyopathy with κ light chain deposits in myocardium as a complication of multiple myeloma: Histochemical and electron microscopic observations. *Arch Pathol Lab Med* 112:1151–1154, 1988.
5. Bergsagel DE: Plasma cell myeloma. In Hurst JW (ed): *Medicine for the Practicing Physician,* ed 3. Boston, Butterworth-Heinemann, 1992, pp 828–831.
6. Mitchell MA, Horneffer MD, Standiford TJ: Multiple myeloma complicated by restrictive cardiomyopathy and cardiac tamponade. *Chest* 103:946–947, 1993.
7. Goldberg E, Mori K: Multiple myeloma with isolated visceral (epicardial) involvement and cardiac tamponade. *Chest* 57:584–587, 1970.
8. McBride W, Jackman JD Jr, Grayburn P: Prevalence and clinical characteristics of a high cardiac output state in patients with multiple myeloma. *Am J Med* 89:21–24, 1990.
9. Leporrier M: High-output cardiac failure in multiple myeloma (letter). *N Engl L Med* 320:1419, 1989.
10. Lotze MT: High-output cardiac failure in multiple myeloma (letter). *N Engl L Med* 320:1419–1420, 1989.
11. Talley JD: Whose sign is it anyway: Nicoladoni's, Branham's, or Both? *Resident Staff Physician* 42:29–31, 1996.
12. Heistad DD, Abboud FM, Schmid PG, et al: Regulation of blood flow in Paget's disease of bone. *J Clin Invest* 55:69–74, 1975.
13. Linzbach AJ: Heart failure from the point of view of quantitative anatomy. *Am J Cardiol* 5:370–382, 1960.
14. Anversa P, Ricci R, Olivetti G: Quantitative structural analysis of the myocardium during physiologic growth and induced cardiac hypertrophy: A review. *J Am Coll Cardiol* 7:1140–1149, 1986.
15. MacLennan ICM, Chapman C, Dunn J, et al: Combined chemotherapy with ABCM versus melphalan for treatment of myelomatosis. *Lancet* 339:200–205, 1992.
16. Judson IR, Gore M, Tighe J, et al: Resolution of high-output cardiac failure following treatment of multiple myeloma (letter). *N Engl J Med* 321:1685–1686, 1988.
17. Sanchez FW, Chuang VP, Skolkin MD: Transcatheter treatment of myelomatous AV shunting causing high-output failure. *Cardiovasc Intervent Radiol* 9:219–221, 1986.

Cardiac Toxicity Due to Chemotherapy

J. David Talley, M.D.

PRESENTING MANIFESTATIONS

History

Obviously, the history is of critical importance in determining the cause of the cardiac toxicity. It is important to note that chemotherapy is used for diseases other than cancer. Cardiac toxicity due to chemotherapy is not necessarily related to the total dose of the medication. It may occur immediately after therapy or may be delayed for years. The major chemotherapeutic agents associated with cardiac toxicity are seen in Table 8.2.

Physical Examination

As noted in Table 8.2, myriad physical findings related to the cardiovascular system may be seen and are specific to the chemotherapeutic agent.

Laboratory Evaluation

The laboratory abnormalities are specific to the chemotherapeutic agent (Table 8.2).

DIAGNOSTIC CRITERIA

The diagnosis of cardiac toxicity due to chemotherapy depends on identifying the historical exposure to the responsible agent and the characteristic cardiovascular disease in the absence of other potentially related etiologies.

DIFFERENTIAL DIAGNOSIS

Many different chemotherapeutic agents are now used, either in combination or sequentially, in cancer treatment. Therefore, it may be difficult to pinpoint the agent responsible for the cardiovascular disease.

PATHOPHYSIOLOGY

Each chemotherapeutic agents has unique mechanisms of cardiovascular toxicity (Table 8.2).

NATURAL HISTORY

Doxorubicin myocardial toxicity with congestive heart failure is dose dependent. A total dose of less than 400 mg/m^2 is associated with a 2% occurrence of congestive heart failure. With a cumulative dose of more than 550 mg/m^2, the incidence approaches 10% (Figure 8.8). The development of congestive heart failure due to doxorubicin is associated with a mortality rate of approximately 50%.

Hemorrhage myocarditis due to cyclophosphamide toxicity occurs in 3% of patients. The mortality rate with this complication approaches 50%.

CURRENT TREATMENT

Treatment is usually supportive. Specific treatment regimens have been identified which can decrease the occurrence of the cardiovascular complications (Table 8.2).

TABLE 8.2. Cardiac Toxicity Due to Chemotherapy

Medication	Cardiac Toxicity	Pathophysiology	Diagnosis	Treatment	Ref
Amsacrine (AMSA)	Cardiomyopathy, arrhythmia, congestive heart failure			Avoid hypokalemia	1–3
Anthraquinones Mioxantrone Nonvantrone	Congestive heart failure		Reduced left ventricular ejection fraction		4–6
Anthracyclines Daunomycin Daunorubicin Doxorubicin	Acute or chronic myocardial toxicity, heart block, arrhythmia, pericarditis-myocarditis, myocardial infarction	Oxygen-free radical formation, damage to mitochondria and endoplasmic reticulum, myocyte death	Endomyocardial biopsy, resting and exercise left ventricular ejection fraction	Slow infusion of drug, ICRF-187, dose <450 mg/m^2, use of anthracycline analogue	7–12
Bleomycin	Pulmonary hypertension	Pulmonary fibrosis		Dose <450 mg/m^2	13
Cyclophosphamide	Congestive heart failure, pericardial effusion, pericarditis	Damage to microvascular bed, myocardial necrosis, lymphocytic myocarditis	Low ECG voltage, reduced left ventricular ejection fraction	dose <1.55 g/m^2	14–16
Esorubicin	Dilated cardiomyopathy				17
Estrogen	Increased cardiovascular death rate			Decrease dose to <1 mg/day	18–19
5-Fluorouracil	Myocardial ischemia, arrhythmia, sudden cardiac death, congestive heart failure	Corcnary vasospasm, coagulation abnormality		Coadministration of diltiazem, nifedipine	20–22 23
Granisetron	junctional bradycardia, junctional escape beats, atrioventricular block	stimu.atior. of the vagus nerve			24
Hyperthermia	Tachycardia, elevated cardiac output, hypotension	decreased systemic vascular resistance			25
Interleukin-2	Hyperdynamic state	Capillary leak			26
Taxol	Hypotension, arrhythmia, heart block	Cardiac toxicity of ethylated cater oil	Arrhythmia on ECG		27
Vinca alkaloids Vincristine Vindesine	Myocardial ischemia, infarction, orthostatic hypotension				28, 29

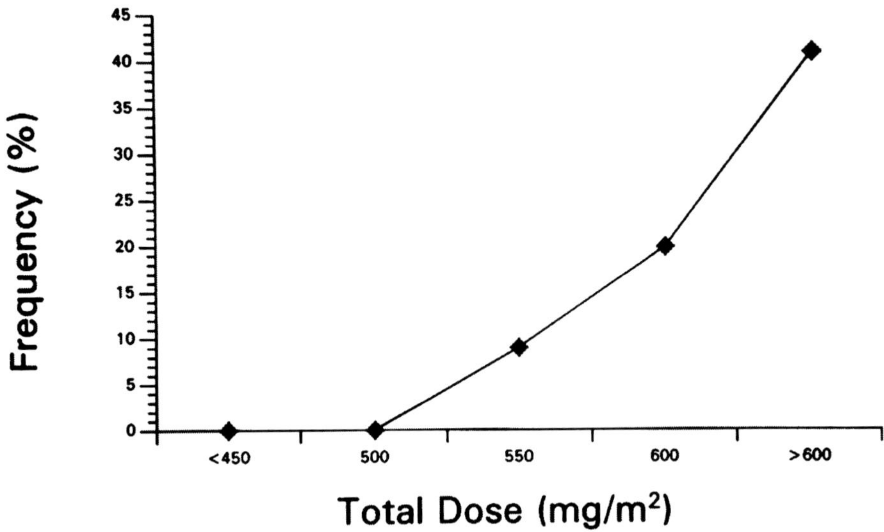

Figure 8.8.   The frequency of developing a dilated cardiomyopathy is directly correlated with the total lifetime dose of doxorubicin. It is unusual to develop a cardiomyopathy with a total dose less than 500 mg/m2, however, there is a progressive increase with higher doses. From Greene HL, Reich SD, Dalen JE. How to minimize doxorubicin toxicity. *J Cardiovasc Med* 7:306, 1982. Reprinted with permission from author and publisher.

REFERENCES

1. Lindpaintner K, Lindpaintner LS, Wentworth M et al: Acute myocardial necrosis during administration of amsacrine. *Cancer* 57:1284–1286, 1986.

2. Steinherz LJ, Steinherz PG, Mangiacasale D, et al: Cardiac abnormalities after AMSA administration. *Cancer Treat Rep* 66:483–488, 1982.

3. Weiss RB, Grillo-López AJ, Marsoni S, et al: Amsacrine-associated cardiotoxicity: An analysis of 82 cases. *J Clin Oncol* 4:919–928, 1986.

4. Coleman RE, Maisey MN, Knight RK, et al: Mitoxantrone in advanced breast cancer–A phase II study with special attention to cardiotoxicity. *Eur J Cancer Clin Oncol* 20:771–776, 1984.

5. Pratt CB, Vietti TJ, Etcubanas E, et al: Novantrone for childhood malignant solid tumors. A pediatric oncology group phase II study. *Invest New Drugs* 1986:4:43–48.

6. Landys K, Bergstrom S, Andersson T, et al: Mitoxantrone as a first line treatment of advanced breast cancer. *Invest New Drugs* 1985;3:133–137.

7. Speyer JL, Green MD, Kramer E, et al: Protective effect of the bispiperazinedione ICRF-187 against doxorubicin-induced cardiac toxicity in women with advanced breast cancer. *N Engl J Med* 319:745–752, 1988.

8. Porembka DT, Lowder JN, Orlowski JP, et al: Etiology and management of doxorubicin cardiotoxicity. *Crit Care Med* 17:569–572, 1989.

9. McKillop JH, Bristow MR, Goris ML, et al: Sensitivity and specificity of radionuclide ejection fraction in doxorubicin cardiotoxicity. *Am Heart J* 106:1048–1056, 1983.

10. Schwartz RG, McKenzie WB, Alexander J, et al: Congestive heart failure and left ventricular dysfunction complicating doxorubicin therapy: Seven-year experience using serial radionuclide angiography. *Am J Med* 82:1109–1118, 1987.

11. Bristow MR, Thompson PD, Martin RP, et al: Early anthracycline cardiotoxicity. *Am J Med* 65:823–832, 1978.

12. Steinherz LJ, Graham T, Hurwitz R, et al: Guidelines for cardiac monitoring of children during and after anthracycline therapy: Report of the Cardiology Committee of the Childrens Cancer Study Group. *Pediatrics* 89:942–949, 1992.

13. Yagoda A, Mukherji B, Young C, et al: Bleomycin, an antitumor antibiotic: Clinical experience in 274 patients. *Ann Intern Med* 77:861–870, 1972.

14. Baello EB, Ensberg ME, Ferguson DW, et al: Effect of high-dose cyclophosphamide and total-body irradiation on left ventricular function in adult patients with leukemia undergoing allogeneic bone marrow transplantation. *Cancer Treat Rep* 70:1187–1193, 1986.

15. Goldberg MA, Antin JH, Guinan EC, et al: Cyclophosphamide cardiotoxicity. An analysis of dosing as a risk factor. *Blood* 68:1114–1118, 1986.

16. Billingham ME: Pharmacotoxic myocardial disease: An endomyocardial study. In Sekiguchi M, Olsen EGJ, Goodwin JF (eds): *Myocarditis and Related Disorders.* Berlin, Springer-Verlag, 1985, pp 278–282.

17. Diehl LF, Banks A, Carter W, et al: Fatal esorubicin-induced cardiomyopathy: Report of a case and review of the literature. *Cancer Chemother Pharmacol* 21:347–350, 1988.

18. Henriksson P, Johansson S-E: Prediction of cardiovascular complication in patients with prostatic cancer treated with estrogen. *Am J Epidemiol* 125:970–978, 1987.

19. Henriksson P, Edhag O, Eriksson A, et al: Patients at high risk of cardiovascular complications in oestrogen treatment of prostatic cancer. *Br J Urol* 63:186–190, 1989.

20. Keefe DL, Roistacher N, Pierri MK: Clinical cardiotoxicity of 5-fluorouracil. *J Clin Pharm* 33:1060–1070, 1993.

21. Gradishar WJ, Vokes EE. 5-Fluorouracil cardiotoxicity: A critical review. *Ann Oncol* 1:409–414, 1990.

22. Kleiman NS, Lehane DE, Geyer CE Jr, et al: Prinzmetal's angina during 5-fluorouracil chemotherapy. *Am J Med* 82:566–568, 1987.

23. Baker WP, Dainer P, Lester WM, et al: Ischemic chest pain after 5-fluorouracil therapy for cancer. *Am J Cardiol* 57:497–498, 1986.

24. Watanabe H, Hasegawa A, Shinozaki T, et al: Possible cardiac side effects of granisetron, an antiemetic agent, in patients with bone and soft-tissue sarcomas receiving cytotoxic chemotherapy. *Cancer Chemother Pharmacol* 35:278–282, 1995.

25. Shime N, Lee M, Hatanaka T: Cardiovascular changes during continuous hyperthermic peritoneal perfusion. *Anesth Analg* 78:938–942, 1994.

26. Azar JJ, Theriault RL: Acute cardiomyopathy as a consequence of treatment with interleukin-2 and interferon-α in a patient with metastatic carcinoma of the breast. *Am J Clin Oncol* 14:530–533, 1991.

27. Biade O, Mengozzi G, Gherarducci G, et al: Evaluation of taxol cardiotoxicity in metastatic breast cancer. *Ann NY Acad Sci* 698:403–405, 1993.

28. Somers G, Abramow M, Wittek M, et al: Myocardial infarction: A complication of vincristine treatment? (Letter) *Lancet* 2:690, 1976.

29. DiBella NJ: Vincristine-induced orthostatic hypotension: A prospective clinical study. *Cancer Treat Rep* 64:359–360, 1980.

Radiation Therapy

Mark L. Mullens, M.D.
J. David Talley, M.D.

PRESENTING MANIFESTATIONS

History

Cardiovascular complications related to radiation therapy develop 5–9 months after the completion of x-ray therapy. However, they have been noted to occur 8–10 years in some

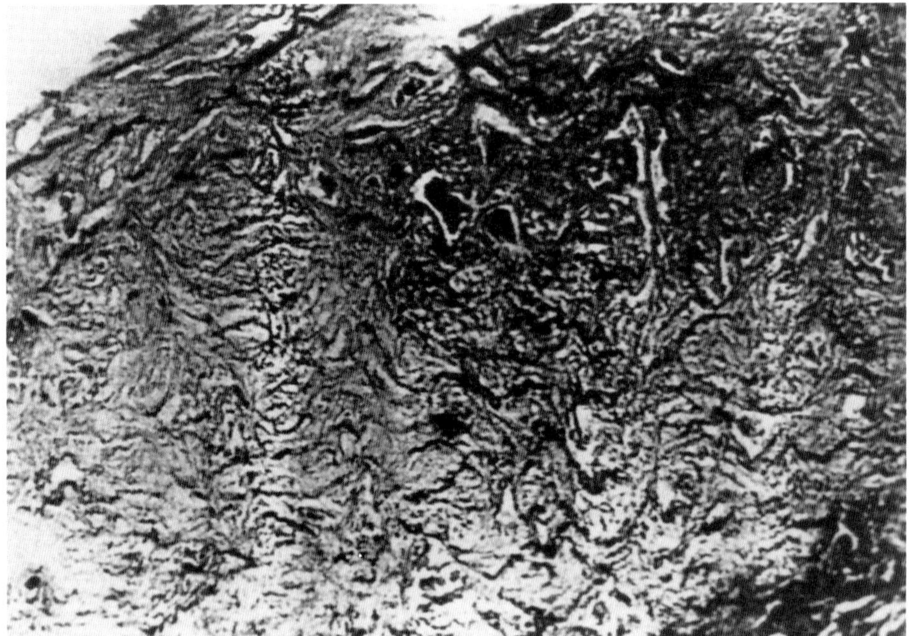

Figure 8.9.   Endothelial specimen (400x) obtained by directional coronary atherectomy from a patient with a severe stenosis of the mid-right coronary artery. Note the radiation-induced atypical cell proliferation and myxoid connective tissue matrix resulting in disruption of the internal elastic lamina. Permission obtained from author and publisher, Joseph A, Dunker D, Talley JD, et al. Directional coronary atherectomy for the diagnosis and treatment of radiation induced coronary artery stenosis. *J Interven Cardiol* 8:355–358, 1995. Reprinted with permission from author and publisher.

patients after completion of therapy. Patients who receive mantel radiation, especially in a dose greater than 1800 rads, are particularly likely to develop cardiovascular complications.

Physical Examination

Local skin changes (erythema and scaling due to radiation) may be apparent. Radiation-induced pericarditis has clinical features similar to those of other etiologies of pericarditis, with fever and pleuritic and pericardial pain. Endocardial radiation injury may result in new regurgitation murmurs.

Laboratory Evaluation

Echocardiography may show changes consistent with pericardial, myocardial, and endocardial damage. A transient decrease in myocardial function has been noted in some patients after radiation therapy for breast cancer.

DIAGNOSTIC CRITERIA

Cardiovascular complications (constrictive pericarditis or premature development of coronary artery disease) of radiation therapy should be considered in a patient who has had radiation therapy, especially if the complication occurs in the port where radiation was delivered. The histologic changes attributed to radiation-induced coronary artery disease include severe proliferation of the intima and adventitia, with an increase in the number of plasma cells without atherosclerosis (Figure 8.9).[1,2]

DIFFERENTIAL DIAGNOSIS

Other etiologies of pericardial, myocardial, and endocardial disease must be considered in patients in whom radiation-induced heart disease is considered.

PATHOPHYSIOLOGY

Radiation therapy was initially utilized to treat Hodgkin's lymphoma in the early 1900s. The heart was regarded as resistant to radiation until 1924, when Davis described myocardial and pericardial damage following radiation therapy.[3] Radiation-induced coronary artery disease was first reported in 1957.[4] Other reported complications attributed to radiation include pericarditis,[5] pericardial effusion,[6] restrictive cardiomyopathy,[7] valvular abnormalities,[8] and conduction abnormalities.[8]

Radiation-induced coronary artery disease is due to a combination of radiation injury to the vessel wall and hypercholesterolemia. Radiation results in loss of smooth muscle cells from the media, with proliferation in the subintima.[9] The additive role of hypercholesterolemia has been noted in both animals and humans. Amronim et al. reported that with radiation alone, rodent coronary arteries remained normal, yet with the addition of an atherogenic diet, coronary artery disease developed.[10] In an autopsy study of patients who received mediastinal irradiation, the cholesterol levels were higher than those of patients with significant coronary artery disease who had not had irradiation.[1] These findings imply that radiation transforms smooth muscle cells into a proliferative phase, and lipids promote vessel stenosis.

NATURAL HISTORY

The premature development of complications and the long-term effects of radiation suggest the progressive nature of the underlying cardiovascular abnormality.

CURRENT METHODS OF TREATMENT

Risk Factor Modification

Aggressive correction of all coronary artery disease risk factors, especially hyperlipidemia, is highly recommended. This is especially important, as radiation therapy is now used successfully in young patients with long-term survival.

Radiation Shielding

Advances in radiation therapy techniques, including shielding and multiple pinpoint ports of radiation delivery, have decreased the occurrence of radiation-induced heart disease. Previously, anterior mediastinal radiation was associated with a 10–15% incidence of complications. Improvements have decreased this risk to less than 5%, with no increase in the cancer relapse rate.[11]

Revascularization

Management of patients with radiation-induced coronary artery disease includes revascularization with coronary artery bypass graft surgery and percutaneous transluminal coronary angioplasty. Coronary artery bypass graft surgery is the therapy of choice for left main or osteal coronary lesions.[12] The use of the internal thoracic artery is favored; however, a disadvantage may be the development of sternal infection in irradiated tissue with little blood supply.[13] There are a few reports of percutaneous transluminal coronary angioplasty in these patients; limitations include failure to dilate the rigid lesion and enhanced recoil of the arterial wall.[14] Directional coronary atherectomy and intracoronary stenting may also be used to treat radiation-induced lesions by resisting elastic recoil of the vessel.[15]

REFERENCES

1. Brosius FC III, Waller BF, Roberts WE: Radiation heart disease: Analysis of 16 young (aged 15 to 33 years) necropsy patients who received over 3,500 rads to the heart. *Am J Med* 70:519–530, 1981.

2. Stewart JR, Cohn KE, Fajardo LF, et al: Radiation-induced heart disease. A study of twenty-five patients. *Radiology* 89:302–310, 1967.

3. Davis KS: Intrathoracic changes following X-ray treatment: A clinical and experimental study. *Radiology* 3:301–322, 1924.

4. Pearson HES: Coronary occlusion following thoracic radiotherapy: Two cases (letter). *Proc R Soc Med* 50:516–521, 1957.

5. Carmel R, Kaplan H: Mantle radiation in Hodgkin's disease: An analysis of technique, tumor eradication, and complications. *Cancer* 37:2813–2825, 1976.

6. Masland DS, Rotz CT Jr, Harris JH Jr: Postradiation pericarditis with chronic pericardial effusion. *Ann Intern Med* 69:97–102, 1968.

7. Fajardo LF, Stewart JR, Cohn KE: Morphology of radiation-induced heart disease. *Arch Pathol* 86:512–519, 1968.

8. Cohen SI, Bharati S, Glass J, et al: Radiotherapy as a cause of complete atrioventricular block in Hodgkin's disease: An electrophysiological-pathological correlation. *Arch Intern Med* 141:676–679, 1981.

9. McReynolds RA, Gold GL, Roberts WC: Coronary heart disease after mediastinal irradiation for Hodgkin's disease. *Am J Med* 60:39–45, 1976.

10. Amronim GD, Gildenhorn HL, Solomon RD, et al: The synergism of x-irradiation and cholesterol-fat feeding on the development of coronary artery lesions. *J Atherosclerosis Res* 4:325–334, 1964.

11. Green DM, Gingell RL, Pearce J, et al: The effect of mediastinal irradiation on cardiac function of patients treated during childhood and adolescence for Hodgkin's disease. *J Clin Oncol* 5:239–245, 1987.

12. Iqbal SM, Hanson EL, Gensini GG: Bypass graft for coronary artery stenosis following radiation therapy. *Chest* 71:664–666, 1977.

13. Grossi EA, Esposito R, Harris LJ, et al: Sternal wound infections and use of internal mammary artery grafts. *J Thorac Cardiovasc Surg* 102:342–347, 1991.

14. Sande LM, Casariego J, Llorian AR: Percutaneous transluminal coronary angioplasty for coronary stenosis following radiotherapy. *Int J Cardiol* 20:129–132, 1988.

15. Joseph A, Dunker D, Talley JD, et al: Directional coronary atherectomy for the diagnosis and treatment of radiation-induced coronary artery stenosis. *J Intervent Cardiol* 8:355–358, 1995.

— IX —

Cardiovascular Involvement with Diseases Related to Aging

David A. Lipschitz, M.D., Ph.D.
Section Editor

Effect of Age

David A Lipschitz, M.D., Ph.D.

PRESENTING MANIFESTATIONS

Well-described changes in the anatomy and function of the cardiovascular system occur with aging.[1] As with every other organ system, it is extremely difficult to distinguish the declines in heart function that accompany aging from those that occur because of coexisting age-dependent diseases. A major anatomic feature is an increase in arterial rigidity. Larger arteries such as the aorta increase in diameter and become elongated. Changes in arterial structure are due primarily to alterations in the composition of elastin and collagen that result in declines in elasticity. Increased vascular tone may contribute to the increased arterial rigidity that occurs with advancing age. Arterial rigidity leads to an increase in the velocity of the pulse wave, and pressure waves from peripheral sites are returned to the heart more rapidly in older compared with younger persons. It has been generally accepted that these changes lead to an increase in systolic blood pressure with advancing age. These increases have been reported in both longitudinal and cross-sectional studies. These observations are not universal and do not occur in isolated rural populations. This has led to the suspicion that age-related increases in blood pressure may well reflect pathology in an organ system rendered more susceptible due to age-related alterations in cardiac and vascular function.

PATHOPHYSIOLOGY

Pathologies are much more common in the hearts of older persons.[2] These include coronary artery disease, valvular lesions, and myocardial abnormalities. Lipofuscin deposition increases, the cellular content of the atrioventricular and sinus nodes is reduced, and the cardiac fat content is increased. The cause of these changes is not thought to be vascular insufficiency. Functionally, a reduction in the rate of diastolic filling has been reported with age. However, the atrial contribution to ventricular filling is increased, so that the net effect is no change in diastolic volume. When cardiac function is measured at rest, few differences are noted when older persons are compared to younger ones. Ejection fraction and stroke volume are not reduced, and no change in the resting heart rate is noted. Furthermore, no age-related alteration in cardiac output has been identified. Thus neither diastolic nor stroke volume is affected by aging.

The contraction time of the heart is prolonged with aging and the ability to respond to inotropic stimuli such as catecholamines is reduced.[3] Electrical currents are also slowed with aging. These effects may explain the age-related alterations in the cardiac response to exercise. Generally, aging is associated with a reduction in maximum exercise and maximum oxygen consumption. However, this may well be related to the age-related decline in muscle mass. If corrected for muscle mass and physical condition, the aerobic capacity of older persons is probably very similar to that of younger ones. In response to exercise, elderly persons have a significantly lower heart rate at high levels of exertion compared with younger persons. This decline in heart rate is accompanied by a much greater reduction in peak ventricular filling during maximum exercise. An analysis of the hemodynamics of exercise reveals that the reduced heart rate is accompanied by greater cardiac dilatation at the end of systole and diastole. The net effect is to maintain an adequate stroke volume.

While well-recognized differences between the cardiovascular systems of young and old persons can be demonstrated, the age effects by themselves are not sufficient to compromise cardiovascular function in any way. Nevertheless, the cardiovascular reserve capacity of the elderly is attenuated. This makes the presence of age-dependent cardiovascular disease more serious, and the morbidity and mortality of acute and chronic insults higher, and increases the susceptibility to cardiovascular toxicities of medications affecting the heart or vascular system.

REFERENCES

1. Lakatta EY, Goldsmith G: The cardiovascular system. In Hazzard WR, Bierman EL, Blass JP. et al: *Principles of Geriatric Medicine and Gerontology.* New York, McGraw-Hill, 1995, pp 493–508.
2. Wei JY, Gersh BJ: Heart disease in the elderly. *Curr Probl Cardiol* 12:7–65, 1987.
3. Lakatta EG: Altered autonomic modulation of cardiovascular function with adult aging: Perspectives from studies ranging from man to cell. In Stone HL, Weglicki WB, *Pathobiology of Cardiovascular Injury.* Boston, Nijhoff, 1985, p 441.

Isolated Systolic Systemic Arterial Hypertension

David A Lipschitz, M.D., Ph.D.

PRESENTING MANIFESTATIONS

Although very common in older persons, isolated systolic hypertension is silent. It is often detected as part of a routine medical evaluation or may be noted at the time of presentation with another illness that may or may not be related to the disease.[1]

TABLE 9.1.   Common Potentially Treatable Conditions Leading to Hypertension in Older Persons

Medications
  Steroids
  Antidepressants (tricyclics and monoamine oxidase inhibitors)
  Thyroid hormone replacement
  Beta-adrenergic agonists
  Nasal decongestants
Renovascular hypertension
  Consider if blood urea nitrogen and creatinine are elevated or if hypertension is difficult to control
Endocrine disorders
  Hyper- or hypothyroidism
  Primary or secondary Cushing's syndrome
  Primary hyperaldosteronism

DIAGNOSTIC CRITERIA

Isolated systolic hypertension is defined as a systolic blood pressure greater than 140 mm Hg with a diastolic blood pressure less than 90 mm Hg. The systolic level reflects a reduction from the previously observed value of 160 mm Hg that was thought to be the upper limit of normal in older persons.

DIFFERENTIAL DIAGNOSIS

Older persons are much more likely to have multiple comorbid conditions, some of which may contribute to hypertension. It is important to consider secondary causes of hypertension even if the systolic blood pressure alone is elevated. Although the list of conditions leading to hypertension in older persons is long, a smaller number of important conditions must always be considered. These are listed in Table 9.1. Medication usage and a simple evaluation of renal function and endocrine function should be a component of the initial workup. Renovascular hypertension should be considered in any older patient in whom hypertension control is difficult. Workup to exclude renal artery stenosis should be limited to those patients in whom active intervention (angioplasty or surgery) is feasible.

PATHOPHYSIOLOGY

The etiology of isolated systolic blood pressure is still not clear. Underlying increases in aortic rigidity and peripheral vascular resistance may be extremely important. It is thought that increased peripheral vascular resistance may result in reduced contractility of the heart. Isolated systolic hypertension has been shown to be associated with reduced intravascular volume. It is likely that these background age effects make the older person more susceptible to the generally recognized mechanisms leading to hypertension in younger persons. These include increased activity of the adrenergic system or reduced activity of substances that may assist in systolic blood pressure reduction, such as kallikreins, prostaglandins, and atrial natiuretic hormone.

NATURAL HISTORY OF THE DISEASE

Epidemiology data have clearly shown that increased morbidity and mortality accompany isolated systolic blood pressure in older persons. Multiple multicenter studies have shown a significant increase in cardiovascular and total morbidity and mortality with rises in either the systolic or diastolic blood pressure in older persons.[3] Recent evidence has shown that isolated systolic blood pressure is a much better predictor of cardiovascular complications than is elevated diastolic blood pressure. Isolated systolic blood pressure is associated with a 2- to 5-fold increase in the risk of death from cardiovascular disease and a 2.5-fold increase in the risk of stroke. Overall, the risk of mortality in patients with isolated systolic hypertension is about 50% higher than that of individuals with normal blood pressure. Most important is the fact that the risk of death from stroke and from fatal myocardial infarction decreases dramatically with treatment.[4]

CURRENT METHODS OF TREATMENT

Age per se is not a contraindication to treatment.[5] The benefit of therapy in subjects over the age of 80, however, is not yet proven. As a general rule, irrespective of age, therapy should be considered for functionally dependent ambulatory older persons with few comorbid conditions. Therapy should probably not be considered for frail, functionally dependent older persons with multiple medical problems.

For patients with isolated systolic hypertension, initial interventions should be nonpharmacologic. Prudent weight loss in overweight persons, sodium restriction, aerobic exercise, and avoidance of alcohol appear to be as beneficial, or more so, in older compared to younger persons. Blood pressure should be monitored closely. Any person who despite a controlled diet, exercise, and sodium restriction has a persistently elevated systolic blood pressure above 160 mm Hg should be treated pharmacologically. Thiazide diuretics (in the absence of diabetes, electrocardiographic evidence of ischemia, or left ventricular hypertrophy) or a water-soluble beta blocker are the medications of choice because of their low cost and proven efficacy. A water-soluble beta blocker such as atenolol is preferred to lipid-soluble agents because of their fewer central nervous system side effects (depression, memory loss). Therapy should commence with half of the usual recommended dose, and the dose should be increased cautiously. Disabling side effects such as vertigo and postural hypotension are a concern, and patients should be monitored for hypokalemia. When this is present, the use of potassium supplements or potassium-sparing agents must be considered. When serious side effects are present, therapy should either be discontinued or changed. Calcium channel blockers and ACE inhibitors are effective in the treatment of hypertension in the elderly. The use of these medications should be tailored to the particular clinical presentation and therapeutic response of the individual patient.

REFERENCES

1. Applegate WB: Hypertension in elderly patients. *Ann Intern Med* 110:901–915, 1989.

2. Soltis EE, et al: The vasculature in hypertension and aging. In Horan MJ, Steinberg GM, Dunbar JB, et al (ed). *Blood Pressure Regulation and Aging*. New York, NY Biomedical Information Corp., 1986.

3. The Systolic Hypertension in the Elderly Program (SHEP) Cooperative Research Group: Prevention of Stroke by Antihypertensive Drug Treatment in Older Patients with Isolated Systolic Hypertension: Final results of SHEP. *JAMA* 265:3255–3264, 1991.

4. MRC Working Party: Medical Research Council of trial treatment of hypertension in older adults: Principal results. *Br Med J* 304:405–412, 1992.

5. Applegate WB: Hypertension. In Hazzard WR, Bierman EL, Blass JP, et al: *Principles of Geriatric Medicine and Gerontology, ed. 3.* New York, McGraw-Hill, 1994, pp 541–554.

Orthostatic Hypotension

David A. Lipschitz, M.D., Ph.D.

PRESENTING MANIFESTATIONS

Physiologic reduction in blood pressure has been reported in some older persons. Its severity varies from day to day. It is believed to be benign based on the absence of symptoms and the lack of an identifiable pathology. It is diagnosed incidentally as part of a routine patient workup. Pathologic orthostatic hypotension presents with postural dizziness or syncope. When it is chronic, other features of autonomic dysfunction are often present. These include incontinence, impotence, and heat intolerance.

DIAGNOSTIC CRITERIA

Orthostatic hypotension is a common problem in older persons and is usually defined as a decline of 20 mm Hg or more in the systolic blood pressure upon standing. It is an extremely common condition, occurring in as many as 15–20% of ambulatory older persons.[1] Any decline in systolic blood pressure of 20 mm Hg is significant. Blood pressure in both arms should be taken in the recumbent, sitting, and standing positions.

DIFFERENTIAL DIAGNOSIS

In patients who present with vertigo, the condition must be distinguished from middle ear, cerebral, and cerebrovascular causes of dizziness. A careful history and blood pressure measurement are critical. Once the diagnosis has been made, it is critical to make every effort to identify the treatable causes. Dehydration and medication use are most important. Medications that can result in postural hypotension include antidepressants (tricyclics and monoamine oxidase inhibitors); phenothiazines and antipsychotic neuroleptics (haldol); antihypertensives including vasodilators, beta blockers, and calcium channel blockers; and dopamine. The list of medications that can lead to hypotension is so long that a careful analysis of all prescription and nonprescription medications is an essential part of the patient workup. Central nervous system lesions associated with postural hypotension include vertebrobasilar insufficiency, brainstem lesions, Parkinson's disease, and the Shy-Drager syndrome. The last disorder presents with dementia, orthostatic hypotension, and cerebellar and extrapyramidal syndrome. Secondary causes of autonomic dysfunction that can lead to orthostatic hypotension include diabetes, alcohol abuse, and paraneoplastic syndromes. In a small fraction of older patients, symptomatic orthostatic hypotension is not associated with any other underlying pathology. By exclusion, this idiopathic condition is referred to as *pure autonomic failure.*

PATHOPHYSIOLOGY

As indicated above, modest reductions in systolic blood pressure may be noted in otherwise healthy older persons. When this is symptomatic, the mechanism in older persons is usually secondary to an underlying problem leading to fluid depletion or affecting autonomic control of vascular tone. Patients with pure autonomic failure have reduced basal concentrations of norepinephrine and no increase in the level of the hormone upon standing.

NATURAL HISTORY OF THE DISEASE

If orthostatic hypotension is present as a component of a primary treatable condition, significant improvement may be noted. If not, this condition is often very disabling to older persons.

CURRENT METHODS OF TREATMENT

A major goal of treatment is to identify and correct disorders that may be the cause or may contribute to postural hypotension. Analyzing medication use and avoiding drugs that can contribute to the problem is important. Many older persons develop hypotension in association with meals. This may require timing the use of antihypertensive drugs to minimize their impact on postprandial reduction in systolic blood pressure with posture changes. The patient should also be trained to be aware of the risks of blood pressure drops with sudden changes in posture. After lying flat, the patient should sit at the side of the bed for an appropriate period of time before standing and should have support available when standing. The most successful pharmacologic agent is fludrocortisone acetate, a synthetic mineralocorticoid that increases plasma volume and, at high doses, sensitizes adrenergic receptors to circulating norepinephrine. Therapy should commence with a low dose (0.1 mg) and should be increased slowly until peripheral edema develops. Other medications that may have a place in therapy include indomethazine, the alpha-2 agonist, clonidine and the beta-adrenergic agonist pindolol.

REFERENCE

1. Johnson RH: Orthostatic hypotension in elderly patients. In: Evans JG, Williams TF, *Oxford Textbook of Geriatric Medicine.* Oxford, England, Oxford Medical Publications, 1994, pp 526–537.

Congestive Heart Failure

David A Lipschitz, M.D., Ph.D.

PRESENTING MANIFESTATIONS

Although the clinical presentation of heart failure may be similar to that in younger persons, including breathlessness, ankle edema, and right upper quadrant pain, unusual clinical features are more common in older persons. Heart failure can present with somnolence, confusion, anorexia, and weight loss. Not infrequently, breathlessness is not present and the diagnosis may be especially difficult in demented patients. Patients who have primarily diastolic dysfunction tend to present more acutely and have less evidence of right heart failure than those with systolic dysfunction, in whom the presentation may be more insidious.

DIAGNOSTIC CRITERIA

The lack of a classical history makes it critical for the physician to have a high index of suspicion of heart failure in older persons presenting with fatigue, weakness, somnolence, or delirium. The clinical findings may also be subtle. However, the diagnostic features on examination, x-ray, and electrocardiogram are similar in older compared to younger persons. It is essential that a noninvasive evaluation of ventricular function be performed. A normal or near-normal ejection fraction suggests diastolic dysfunction.

DIFFERENTIAL DIAGNOSIS

Pulmonary disorders with breathlessness may be mistaken for heart failure. Ankle edema due to venous insufficiency may be mistaken for heart failure in older persons. In some patients, no cause for ankle edema can be found.

PATHOPHYSIOLOGY

Age-related alterations in peripheral vascular resistance and changes in myocardial function may make older persons more prone to develop cardiac decompensation.[1] Thyroid disorders, inappropriate medication use, electrolyte abnormalities, infections, hypoxia, and anemia are frequent contributory factors to heart failure in older persons. Isolated systolic or systolic/diastolic hypertension is found in a large majority of older persons with heart failure. Other common underlying conditions that can lead to heart failure in older persons include coronary artery disease, ischemic cardiomyopathy, and valvular heart disease. Diastolic dysfunction is a more common cause of heart failure in older persons than is systolic dysfunction.[2] The former disorder is characterized by elevated left-sided diastolic pressure at rest and during exercise. In contrast to patients with systolic dysfunction, the ejection fraction in patients with diastolic dysfunction is either normal or only slightly reduced. Coronary artery disease and hypertension are common underlying etiologies of diastolic dysfunction in the elderly, whereas cardiomyopathy is a more common cause of systolic dysfunction.

NATURAL HISTORY OF THE DISEASE

It does not follow that older persons with congestive heart failure carry a poor prognosis. Patients respond well to therapy, and the prognosis can be excellent if an underlying correctable condition (inappropriate medication use, electrolyte abnormality, arrhythmia) is present.

CURRENT METHODS OF TREATMENT

Initial approaches should be directed at correcting coexisting conditions that have either aggravated or caused heart failure. These include electrolyte abnormalities, thyrotoxicosis or myxedema, hypertension, inappropriate medication use or toxicities, anemia, and hypoxia. In some circumstances, surgical correction may be required for patients with valvular heart disease. For patients with systolic dysfunction, treatment with diuretics, digoxin, and vasodilators such as an ACE inhibitor is indicated. For patients with diastolic dysfunction, calcium channel blockers or beta blockers are indicated. Digoxin should be avoided if possible. Since older persons are more dependent on atrial filling than younger persons, pharmacologic or electrical cardioversion of arrhythmias should be attempted.

REFERENCES

1. Wei JY: Age and the cardiovascular system. *N Engl J Med* 327:1735–1739, 1992
2. Kannel WB: Epidemiological aspects of heart failure. *Cardiol Clin* 7:1–9, 1989.

— X —

Cardiovascular Involvement with Neuromuscular Diseases

Sami I. Harik, M.D.
Section Editor

Stroke

Stacy A. Rudnicki, M.D.
Sami I. Harik, M.D.

INTRODUCTION

The brain is a fastidious organ that requires a large, uninterrupted supply of oxygen and glucose. Even under resting conditions, it does not accept any appreciable debt when it comes to the delivery of oxygen and glucose. The brain requires about 15% of the cardiac output and uses about 20% of the body's oxygen consumption. Because oxygen and glucose are carried to the brain by the blood pumped by the heart, it is not surprising that malfunction of the heart has immediate repercussions on central nervous system function. Every clinician is painfully aware of the drastic consequences for nervous system function when cardiac output decreases or stops or when a blood clot from the heart lodges within the arterial supply to the central nervous system. The neurologic complications of cardiac disease have been the subject of several reviews and monographs and will not be discussed further in this chapter. This chapter will focus on the cardiac complications of relatively common neuromuscular diseases.

Two major threads connect the neuromuscular system to the heart. The first is the autonomic nervous system, which innervates the heart and modulates its function. The second stems from the similarities between cardiac and skeletal muscles. It is thus expected that the cardiac muscle is affected by the numerous diseases that afflict voluntary muscles, such as the muscular dystrophies and mitochondrial myopathies.

STROKE

It is widely recognized that emboli emanating from the heart are an important, and often underestimated, cause of strokes. It is also well documented that strokes are associated with electrocardiographic (ECG) abnormalities and cardiac arrhythmias.[1–4] Although the majority of patients with stroke are reported to have nonspecific ECG abnormality, it is rather unusual for these abnormalities to be associated with serious trouble.[4] Hemorrhagic strokes are more likely to cause cardiac abnormalities than are ischemic strokes, and strokes in the posterior fossa are associated with a higher prevalence of cardiac abnormalities than those affecting the forebrain. On the other hand, it is well recognized that subarachnoid hemorrhage from intracranial aneurysms or malformations is associated with the so-called neurogenic pulmonary edema, which can be fatal. Neurogenic pulmonary edema is thought to be mediated by the

199

autonomic nervous system via the noradrenergic sympathetic components, and is believed to result from the leakage of plasma proteins from the pulmonary circulation into the alveoli and the lung interstitium.[5] Neurogenic pulmonary edema is thought to result from an acute rise in the hydrostatic pressure in the lung capillaries and from increased pulmonary endothelial permeability, both due to increased sympathetic activity and/or increased adrenalin and noradrenalin in the circulation. However, there is no conclusive evidence that heart failure plays an important role. Neurogenic pulmonary edema does not occur in subarachnoid hemorrhage alone; it is also found in other neurologic catastrophes.

Like strokes and subarachnoid hemorrhage, major traumatic brain injury induces cardiac arrhythmias and ECG abnormalities, probably via the same mechanisms.

REFERENCES

1. Davis TP, Alexander J, Lesch M: Electrocardiographic changes associated with acute cerebrovascular disease: a clinical review. *Prog Cardiovasc Dis* 36:245–260, 1993.
2. Diamant J, Grob D: Electrocardiographic changes and myocardial damage in patients with acute cerebrovascular accidents. *Stroke* 8:448–455, 1977.
3. Goldstein DS: The electrocardiogram in stroke: relationship to pathophysiological type and comparison with prior tracings. *Stroke* 10:253–259, 1979.
4. Oppenheimer SM, Hachinski VC: The cardiac consequences of stroke. *Neuro. Clin* 10:167–176, 1992.
5. Malik A: Mechanisms of neurogenic pulmonary edema. *Circ Res* 57:1–18, 1985.

Epilepsy

Stacy A. Rudnicki, M.D.
Sami I. Harik, M.D.

Cardiac arrhythmias and ECG changes frequently accompany seizures, usually those of the generalized motor type. Sudden death presumably from cardiac arrythmias, is a rare complication of seizures. Cardiac problems in seizures are markedly increased in subjects with *status epilepticus*, which is defined as repetitive, generalized major motor seizures, with the patient remaining unconscious between seizures.[1] In some series, the mortality of untreated or unresponsive status epilepticus can be higher than 50%, particularly in older patients. The cause of death is often cardiac and is attributed to ischemic heart disease given the marked increases in cardiac output and in systemic arterial pressure during seizures. In animal models of status epilepticus, there is severe hypertension and pulmonary edema which are thought to be mediated via increased sympathetic activity. Transection of the cervical spinal cord in these animals promptly prevents the hypertension and cardiopulmonary abnormalities of experimental status epilepticus. The systemic hypoxemia that accompanies major motor seizures, along with the increased workload on the heart from the increased cardiac output and the increased systemic resistance, contribute to the cardiac manifestations of generalized epileptic seizures that can result in death.

REFERENCES

1. Aminoff MJ, Simon RP: Status epilepticus: causes, clinical features, and consequences in 98 patients. *Am J Med* 69:657–666, 1980.

Myotonic Dystrophy

Stacy A. Rudnicki, M.D.
Sami I. Harik, M.D.

PRESENTING MANIFESTATIONS

The most common muscular dystrophy of adults is myotonic dystrophy, inherited in an autosomal dominant fashion.[1] First described in the late eighteenth and early nineteenth centuries, it is also known in the older literature as *Steinert's disease* and *dystrophia myotonica*. *Myotonia* refers to failure of muscle relaxation after contraction, frequently causing the patient to complain of muscle cramp with use. For example, when shaking a person's hand, the patient will have difficulty releasing the grip. Patients may also complain of weakness, and this is the most common reason to seek medical attention. Symptoms can begin at any age, but the most common age of symptom onset is in the teens or early adulthood.[2] In 10–15% of patients, symptoms are present at birth; when this is the case, the condition is referred to as *congenital myotonic dystrophy*. There is marked hypotonia; respiratory distress is common and is associated with significant morbidity and mortality in the affected neonate. The neonate can have ineffectual sucking as well as dysphagia, requiring tube feedings. Myotonia is conspicuously absent during infancy, frequently not appearing clinically until 5 years of age and universally evident by age 10. If the child survives, motor milestones are delayed but with time the child's strength improves. In such cases, the affected parent is invariably the mother; occasionally, she may not realize that she has the disease until she bears an affected child.[3,4]

While there may be a paucity of symptoms, findings on physical exam can be numerous, including facial weakness, ptosis, and distal weakness of the extremities. Weakness of the tongue, jaw, and pharyngeal muscles leads to slurred speech, and difficulty in chewing and swallowing. Because of this distribution of weakness, patients frequently have a very distinctive facies: facial muscles appear slack, the jaw hangs open, and temporal wasting causes a hollowed-out appearance of the cheeks. Frontal balding is often found in both sexes at an early age. While patients may show a restricted range of eye movements on formal testing, complaints of diplopia are rare. In contrast to most myopathies, proximal muscles are spared until late in the disease. Myotonia can be elicited by asking the patient to make a fist or close the eyes tightly for several seconds. Attempts to reopen the hand or eyelids require much effort and take several seconds. Percussion myotonia can be detected by tapping over the thenar eminence with a reflex hammer; the thumb rises as if it is abducting and will not relax for a few seconds.

Myotonic dystrophy, however, is not solely a disease of skeletal muscles. Besides the heart (see below), a number of nonnervous system problems are seen. Patients can have respiratory problems related to weakness of respiratory muscles, and because of aspiration. Hypersomnia is seen and is believed to be related to abnormalities of central nervous system respiratory drive. Endocrinologic problems include reduced fertility or infertility, peripheral resistance to insulin, and frontal balding. Eye manifestations include cataracts at a young age and pigmentary retinal abnormalities. Patients frequently have mild mental retardation, particularly those with congenital myotonic dystrophy. There is no decline of cognitive function over time.[3]

CARDIAC DISEASE

Heart involvement is common in myotonic dystrophy, although frequently asymptomatic. Abnormal ECGs were reported in 202 of 236 patients.[5] Conduction defects are found most frequently, with arrhythmias (atrial more than ventricular) also being a problem. ECGs can show atrioventricular (AV) block, intraventricular conduction delays, bundle branch blocks, and hemiblocks. Other ECG abnormalities include abnormal Q waves, ST-T wave changes, right and left axis deviation, and right and left ventricular hypertrophy. The conduction disturbances tend to worsen with time, though they can appear suddenly in a patient previously not known to have heart problems.[6] There is a tendency for the heart problems to correlate in severity with the neurologic status of the patient, but some patients can have major heart problems with mild neurologic disease. Electrophysiologic studies reveal that the His-Purkinje system is the most strongly affected area, though all areas of the conducting system can be involved.[7] Ventricular late potentials, believed to be possibly predictive of a predisposition to reentrant arrhythmias, have been found in 75% of patients with myotonic dystrophy versus 5% of controls. These patients were asymptomatic and had no evidence for conduction block on routine ECG.[8] Some patients will require a permanent pacemaker. Sudden death in a myotonic patient may be due to either heart block or, less commonly, ventricular arrhythmia. Cardiac disease is more frequently encountered in some families than in others. Whether there is an increased incidence of mitral valve prolapse in patients with myotonic dystrophy remains controversial. Coronary artery disease is not prevalent in these patients. Ventricular dysfunction is found rarely, and heart failure is not commonly encountered. Hypotension was reported, although it is typically asymptomatic.[6] Because of the unpredictable nature of the cardiac disease in myotonic dystrophy, it is recommended that patients have yearly ECGs. If symptoms such as syncope, near-syncope, or palpitations arise, then 24-hr Holder monitoring is appropriate.[9]

DIAGNOSIS

In a patient suspected of having myotonic dystrophy, the family history is of prime importance. Blood work can show a mild elevation of serum creatine phosphokinase (CPK). Electromyogram (EMG) and nerve conduction studies (NCS) are useful in establishing the diagnosis. The NCS are normal, but the EMG almost invariably shows myotonic discharges with needle movement, percussion of the muscle, or after voluntary contraction. The exception occurs in the young child, who may not develop EMG myotonia until the age of 3.[10] In a patient with a positive family history, appropriate findings on neurologic exam, and EMG evidence of myotonia, no further workup is needed. In patients in whom the diagnosis is still unclear, a muscle biopsy may be helpful. Findings include internal nuclei, type 1 fiber atrophy, and ringbinden.[11] However, muscle biopsy is not necessarily diagnostic. Genetic testing is now available for myotonic dystrophy. A CTG (cytosine, thymine, guanine) repeat in increased number is found on chromosome 19q in patients with myotonic dystrophy. A normal gene has 5 to 35 repeats, while patients with the disease have at least 50 repeats. There is a direct correlation between the number of repeats and the severity of the disease. Diagnostic methods can now identify and quantify the repeat. There is a tendency for the repeat to increase with generations, explaining the anticipation phenomenon (i.e., offspring tend to have more severe disease at an earlier age than their affected parent).[12]

DIFFERENTIAL DIAGNOSIS

When a patient presents with weakness and a family history of muscle disease, the pattern of inheritance can help exclude Duchenne dystrophy and Becker dystrophy, both of which are X-linked recessive disorders. These diseases also lack myotonia, ptosis, and facial weakness and tend to cause more proximal than distal weakness. Fascioscapulohumeral dystrophy, as its name implies, causes facial and shoulder weakness. Although it is inherited as an autosomal dominant trait, there is again no myotonia and no involvement of tissues other than skeletal muscles. Oculopharyngeal dystrophy is not associated with extremity weakness and usually occurs in middle to late life.

Other disorders associated with myotonia that enter into the differential diagnosis include myotonia congenita, hyperkalemic periodic paralysis, and paramyotonia congenita. Myotonia congenita can be either autosomal dominant (Thomsen's disease) or autosomal recessive (Becker's disease). In general, these are nonprogressive disorders associated with painless myotonia that improves with exercise. Hyperkalemic periodic paralysis is an autosomal dominant condition characterized by transient episodes of weakness associated with hyperkalemia. Patients with paramyotonia congenita have spells of weakness and myotonia precipitated most commonly by exposure to cold, and exercise tends to exacerbate the myotonia. EMG can frequently distinguish between these myotonic disorders.[10]

PATHOPHYSIOLOGY

The gene for myotonic dystrophy has been identified. This gene codes for an abnormal protein kinase that is believed to alter phosphorylation of muscle ion channels, leading to membrane instability. This alteration in phosphorylation (and, as a result, changes in ion channel function) is not believed to be limited to skeletal muscle. It may also be present in the heart, brain, pancreas, and so on, explaining other manifestations of the disease.[13]

NATURAL HISTORY OF THE DISEASE

Myotonic dystrophy is a progressive disorder with no known treatment. The weakness worsens over time, but there is great variability in the degree of disability among patients, even those within the same family. In severe cases, patients become wheelchair bound. Myotonia usually becomes less of a problem as the weakness worsens. Studies on mortality are somewhat scanty, but most report a shortened life span, with a mean age at death of approximately 50 years. Respiratory failure is a leading cause of death, followed by heart disease and pneumonia.[14] In congenital myotonic dystrophy, there is a 25% mortality by 18 months of age.[15] The most common cause of death in congenital myotonic dystrophy, regardless of age, is respiratory failure, followed by cardiac failure.[15]

CURRENT METHODS OF TREATMENT

Symptomatic improvement of the myotonia can be achieved in some patients with medication; benefits have been reported with dilantin, quinine, procainamide, tocainamide, and mexilitene. Cardiac disease may prevent the use of at least some of these drugs. These drugs have no impact on the weakness or other symptoms.[2]

REFERENCES

1. Brooke MH: *A Clinician's View of Neuromuscular Disease, 2nd ed.* Baltimore, Williams & Wilkins, 1986, p194.
2. Harper PS: *Myotonic Dystrophy, 2nd ed.* London, WB Saunders, 1989, p13.
3. Harper PS: Congenital myotonic dystrophy in Britain. 1. Clinical aspects. *Arch Dis Child* 50: 505–513, 1975.
4. Harper PS: Congenital myotonic dystrophy in Britain. 2. Genetic Basis. *Arch Dis Child* 50: 514–521, 1975.

5. Church SC: The heart in myotonia atrophica. *Arch Intern Med* 119:176–181, 1967.

6. Fragola PV, Luzi M, Calo L, et al: Cardiac involvement in myotonic dystrophy. *Am J Cardiol* 74:1070–1072, 1994.

7. Motta J, Guilleminault C, Billingham M, et al: Cardiac abnormalities in myotonic dystrophy: electrophysiologic and histopathologic studies. *Am J Med* 67:467–473, 1979.

8. Milner MR, Hawley RJ, Jachim M, et al: Ventricular late potentials in myotonic dystrophy. *Ann Intern Med* 115:607–613, 1991.

9. Anonymous: The heart in myotonic dystrophy. *Lancet* 339:528–529, 1992. Editorial.

10. Streib E: AAEE minimonograph #27: Differential diagnosis of myotonic disorders. *Muscle Nerve* 10:603–615, 1987.

11. Dubowitz V: *Muscle Biopsy.* Philadelphia, PA, WB Saunders, 1985, pp380–395.

12. Shelbourne P, Davies J, Buston J, et al: Direct diagnosis of myotonic dystrophy with a disease-specific DNA marker. *N Engl J Med* 328:471–475, 1993.

13. Ptacek LJ, Johnson KJ, Griggs RC: Genetics and physiology of the myotonic muscle disorders. *N Engl J Med* 328:482–489, 1993.

14. Moriuchi T, Kagawa N, Mukoyama M, et al: Autopsy analyses of the muscular dystrophies. *Tokushima J Exp Med* 40(1-2):83–93, 1993.

15. Reardon W, Newcombe R, Fenton I, et al: The natural history of congenital myotonic dystrophy: Mortality and long term clinical aspects. *Arch Dis Child* 68:177–181, 1993.

Duchenne's Muscular Dystrophy

Stacy A. Rudnicki, M.D.
Sami I. Harik, M.D.

PRESENTING MANIFESTATIONS

Duchenne's muscular dystrophy (DMD) is an X-linked recessive disorder with an incidence of 1 per 3500 male births. Children usually appear normal at birth, but most will have delayed motor milestones. Language skills can also lag behind the norm. Rarely, a child will appear normal until the age of 3 or even 6 years, but typically, weakness is apparent by the age of 3 years, with a waddling gait, the start of a lumbar lordosis; some of the boys are toe walkers. Frequently, the child is never able to jump and lags behind peers in running. On examination, there is proximal muscle weakness of the arms and legs, with a positive Gower's sign (when rising from the floor, the child will push himself up by placing his hands on his thighs and pushing his buttocks up first). The calf muscles are large; this pseudohypertrophy is due to fat replacement. Weakness above the neck is quite rare; only mild facial weakness is seen late in the disease. There is hypotonia and hyporeflexia, with the exception of preserved ankle jerks.[1]

The heart is almost always involved in DMD (see below). Smooth muscles in the gastrointestinal tract are abnormal, leading to gastrointestinal problems. Intelligence testing usually yields results that are about 1 standard deviation below the mean. This deficit is nonprogressive. Laboratory testing will reveal a serum CPK of 50–100 times normal; occasionally it is much higher. A high serum CPK is present from birth and can be used as a screening tool, although it is not specific for DMD. The CPK continues to rise until the ages of 3–6 years and then declines as muscle fibers are lost and replaced with fat.[2]

CARDIAC DISEASE

Up to 90% of patients with DMD will have an abnormal ECG. Common findings include tall R waves in the right precordial leads and narrow Q waves in the limb and left precordial leads.[3] Sinus nodal dysfunction, atrial and ventricular arrhythmias, and AV block have been described. Ventricular arrhythmias become more frequent with age and increasing neurologic dysfunction, with one study showing a frequency of 38% at study onset, rising to 75% 5 years later. Sudden death is seen occasionally in DMD and is believed to be related to ventricular arrhythmias. Patients who have the R-on-T phenomenon during monitoring are at particularly high risk for sudden death.[4] Cardiomyopathy develops with time, being universally found by the age of 18. Preclinical cardiomyopathy is found in 25% of patients under the age of 6. In those over 18, three-fourths have a dilated cardiomyopathy and one-quarter have a hypertrophic myopathy.[5]

DIAGNOSIS

When a high serum CPK level is found in a young boy with proximal muscle weakness, an EMG/NCS is often requested. In DMD, the EMG shows fibrillation potentials and positive sharp waves at rest. Motor unit potentials are polyphasic, short in duration, and small in amplitude, with an enhanced interference pattern. While this picture is consistent with DMD, it is not unique to this disease.[6] Muscle biopsy, if adequately done, is usually diagnostic. The muscle to be biopsied should be carefully chosen; if the muscle is very weak, it has probably been replaced by fat and no muscle fibers will be seen. Routine stains show variability in fiber size, with an increase in type I fibers and a decrease in type II b fibers. There is also muscle fiber necrosis with regeneration. Fat replaces necrotic/fibrotic muscle. A definitive diagnosis is established by immunostaining for dystrophin, which is absent or reduced to <5% in DMD (see "Pathophysiology").[7]

DIFFERENTIAL DIAGNOSIS

The disease that is considered most commonly in the differential diagnosis of DMD is Becker's muscular dystrophy (BMD), another X-linked recessive disease. However, the age of onset is earlier in DMD and the progression is more rapid, with death at an earlier age. There are instances when the differentiation can be made only by staining the muscle for dystrophin; in BMD it is diminished compared to controls but is present to some extent.

PATHOPHYSIOLOGY

The gene for muscular dystrophy is located on chromosome Xp21 and codes for dystrophin, a protein which is an essential component of the muscle fiber cytoskeleton, contributing to its membrane integrity. In patients with DMD dystrophin is absent, and this is believed to cause leakiness of the membrane. This results in calcium influx into muscle fibers, which ultimately leads to their death. Many different mutations can occur at the dystrophin gene, resulting in either DMD or BMD. In DMD, about 55% of mutations are deletion mutations, 40% are point mutations, and 5% are duplications.[8] It is believed that BMD patients have preserved the translational reading frame, so that some dystrophin is synthesized, although it is abnormal in quantity or structure. In patients with DMD, the gene is altered in such a way that translation can no longer occur and dystrophin is essentially absent.[1] This gene is expressed in the heart muscle, and absence of dystrophin in the heart leads to fibrosis, particularly in the basolateral free wall of the left ventricle. This area is very vascular, as well as being capable of generating significant force. Abnormalities in this region result in decreased ventricular function.[9] There is also evidence that dystrophin plays an important role in the function of Purkinje cells, and its absence in DMD likely contributes to the conduction problems.[10]

NATURAL HISTORY OF THE DISEASE

Extremity weakness continues to progress as the child grows older, although there is occasionally a seeming improvement in strength during the growth spurt around age 5 or 6. Most children are wheelchair bound by the age of 13, though the range is 6–14 years. Prolonged bed rest can accelerate the weakness, so attempts should be made to avoid surgery while the child is still ambulatory. Large joint contractures worsen over time. Once the patient is in a wheelchair, scoliosis may become problematic, further worsening an already poor respiratory status. When ambulation is lost, forced vital capacity decreases to 50–60% of normal and continues to decline at the rate of about 5% per year.[1] Death is usually the result of respiratory failure, with congestive heart failure and sudden death being less common. The mean age of death is 19 years. In patients who are artificially ventilated ventricular failure is the leading cause of death.[11]

CURRENT METHODS OF TREATMENT

There is no known treatment for DMD. Prednisone therapy was shown to slow the progression of weakness, and in some patients it may transiently improve strength when first begun.[12,13] However, it does not affect the life span, though it does delay progression to a wheelchair. The best time to begin prednisone therapy is not yet entirely clear, but many physicians begin using it when strength obviously starts to deteriorate, frequently between the ages of 6 and 8 years. Once the patient is wheelchair bound, it is tapered and discontinued. It is not entirely clear how it works; most believe it slows the rate of muscle breakdown. Since azathioprine was tried without benefit, it is less likely that the mode of action is through immunosuppression.[14] There is no evidence to suggest that steroids have a beneficial effect on the cardiac involvement in DMD.

REFERENCES

1. Rosenberg RM, Prusine SB, Di Mauro S, et al: *The Molecular and Genetic Basis of Neurological Disease.* Boston, Raven Press, 1993, pp613–615.
2. Miller RG, Hoffman EP: Molecular diagnosis and modern management of Duchenne muscular dystrophy. *Neurol Clin* 12:699–725, 1994.
3. Perloff JK, Roberts WC, de Leon AC, Jr et al: The distinctive electrocardiogram of Duchenne's progressive muscular dystrophy. An electrocardiographic-pathologic correlative study. *Am J Med* 42(2):179–188, 1967.
4. Yanagisawa A, Miyagawa M, Yotsukura M, et al: The prevalence and prognostic significance of arrhythmias in Duchenne type muscular dystrophy. *Am Heart J* 124:1244–1250, 1992.
5. Nigro G, Comi LI, Politano L, et al: The incidence and evolution of cardiomyopathy in Duchenne muscular dystrophy. *Int J Cardiol* 26:271–277, 1990.
6. Kimura J: *Electrodiagnosis in Diseases of Nerve and Muscle: Principles and Practice.* Philadelphia, Churchill Livingstone, 1984, pp528–529.

7. Hoffman EP, Fischbeck KH, Brown RH, et al: Characterization of dystrophin in muscle biopsy specimens from patients with Duchenne's or Becker's muscular dystrophy. *N Engl J Med* 318: 1363–1368, 1988.

8. Fong PY, Turner PR, Denetclaw WF, et al: Increased activity of calcium leak channels in myotubes of Duchenne human and mdx mouse origin. *Science* 250(4981):673–676, 1990.

9. Cziner DG, Levin RI: The cardiomyopathy of Duchenne's muscular dystrophy and the function of dystrophin. *Med Hypotheses* 40(3):169–173, 1993.

10. Bies RD, Friedman D, Roberts R, et al: Expression and localization of dystrophin in human cardiac Purkinje fibers. *Circulation* 86:147–153, 1992.

11. Moriuchi T, Kagawa N, Mukoyama M, et al: Autopsy analyses of the muscular dystrophies. *Tokushima J Exp Med* 40:83–93, 1993.

12. Fenichel GM, Florence JM, Pestronk A, et al: Long-term benefit from prednisone therapy in Duchenne muscular dystrophy. *Neurology* 41:1874–1877, 1991.

13. Griggs RC, Moxley RT III, Mendell JR, et al: Prednisone in Duchenne dystrophy. A randomized, controlled trial defining the time course and dose response. Clinical investigation of Duchenne dystrophy group. *Arch Neurol* 48:383–388, 1991.

14. Griggs RC, Moxley RT III, Mendell JR: Duchenne dystrophy: randomized, controlled trial of prednisone (18 months) and azathioprine (12 months). *Neurology* 43:520–527, 1993.

Becker's Muscular Dystrophy

Stacy A. Rudnicki, M.D.
Sami I. Harik, M.D.

PRESENTING MANIFESTATIONS

Becker's muscular dystrophy (BMD) is an X-linked recessive disease which has a more benign course than DMD. It is less common than DMD, with an incidence of 3–6/100,000 male births. Onset of symptoms is usually between the ages of 5 and 15 years, almost always by the age of 25 years. Early symptoms are related to gait, with difficulty running or climbing stairs. On exam, the patient will initially have proximal muscle weakness in the legs and a tendency to be a toe walker because of shortened Achilles tendons. As in DMD, pseudohypertrophy of the calf muscles is common. Upper extremity weakness develops 2–10 years after the onset of leg weakness. Tendon reflexes are diminished early in the course of the disease and are lost as the disease progresses. Mental retardation is occasionally seen, and there are fewer problems with contractures and scoliosis. Patients will have an increased CPK in the range seen in DMD. It falls with increasing age and will be 1–10 times normal by the age of 20.[1]

CARDIAC DISEASE

Most patients with BMD have no symptoms of cardiac disease, but many have abnormalities on testing. In one study of 31 patients, 68% had an abnormal ECG and 62% had an abnormal echocardiogram. ECG abnormalities included Q waves in lateral and inferior leads and tall R waves (as seen in DMD), nonspecific ST-T wave changes, and bundle branch blocks. Right ventricular dysfunction was found in 52%, primarily in younger patients, while 39% showed left ventricular dysfunction, typically in the older patients. Left ventricular dysfunction occurred in isolation in 10% and was associated with right heart dysfunction in 29%. A decreased left ventricular ejection fraction was found in 29%, usually in the older patients. Ventricular arrhythmias were found in 4 of the 31 patients. No correlation was found between degree of neuromuscular weakness, amount of dystrophin, and cardiac status. There was a suggestion that families with deletions between exons 48 and 49 had an increased incidence of cardiac disease.[2] Another study, however, failed to show such a relationship. Nor did this study find right ventricular problems. Instead, it found that 67% of the patients had decreased left ventricular function and another 31% had left ventricular dilatation. ECG changes were similar in type and incidence in the two studies.[3] Rapidly progressive heart failure, seen in DMD, is rare in BMD. However, Donofrio reported on a 17-year-old boy who developed severe congestive heart failure over 1 month. His weakness was mild, and a successful heart transplant was performed but the patient died of lymphoma 3 years later.[4] The disparity between the extent of heart disease and the severity of skeletal muscle weakness has led to heart transplants in patients with BMD.[5]

DIAGNOSIS

As with other muscle diseases, the EMG shows fibrillations and positive sharp waves at rest, with motor units which are small, polyphasic, and of brief duration, with an enhanced interference pattern. Occasionally, myotonic discharges are seen.[6] Findings on routine muscle biopsy are similar to those in DMD, with fiber splitting, internal nuclei, variation of fiber size, degenerating fibers, and fibrosis. However, immunostaining for dystrophin shows that it is present albeit in decreased amounts.[7]

DIFFERENTIAL DIAGNOSIS

DMD may be confused with BMD but can be distinguished on clinical grounds in many cases and definitively with dystrophin immunostaining of muscle biopsy specimens. Spinal muscular atrophy may be inherited on an X-linked recessive basis and can cause weakness in childhood and adolescence. Since this is a neurogenic rather than a myogenic disorder, it can be distinguished on EMG; while CPK can be mildly elevated, it should not be as markedly abnormal as it is in BMD. Limb girdle dystrophy is likely more than one disease entity; and the inheritance pattern is usually autosomal dominant.

PATHOPHYSIOLOGY

Decreased dystrophin in skeletal and heart muscles is believed to underlie the neuromuscular and cardiac problems. Symptoms are slower to appear and progress compared to those of DMD because some dystrophin is present. It is believed that some mutations allow the dystrophin to be made to at least some degree (resulting in BMD), while in DMD the mutation is in a more strategic location of the gene to totally disrupt the ability to make dystrophin. Patchy staining for dystrophin in a heart muscle biopsy specimen was reported in a patient with BMD.[8]

NATURAL HISTORY OF THE DISEASE

Patients with BMD have a relentlessly progressive course, but at a slower tempo than DMD. On average, the ability to walk is lost by age 27, with a wide range of (12–63 years). Mean life expectancy is 42 years, with a range of 23–63 years. Death is attributed to respiratory failure, with or without pneumonia; cardiac failure is the second most common cause of death.[9]

CURRENT METHODS OF THERAPY

To date there are no therapies reported to be of benefit.

REFERENCES

1. Bradley WG, Jones MZ, Mussini JM: Becker-type muscular dystrophy. *Muscle Nerve* 1:111–132, 1978.
2. Melacini P, Fanin M, Danieli GA, et al: Cardiac involvement in Becker muscular dystrophy. *J Am Coll Cardiol* 22:1927–1934, 1993.
3. Steare SE, Dubowitz V, Benatar A: Subclinical cardiomyopathy in Becker muscular dystrophy. *Br Heart J* 68(3):304–308, 1992.
4. Donofrio PD, Challa VR, Hackshaw BT, et al: Cardiac transplantation in a patient with muscular dystrophy and cardiomyopathy. *Arch Neurol* 46(6):705–707, 1989.
5. Orlov YS, Brodsky MA, Allen BJ, et al: Cardiac manifestations and their management in Becker's muscular dystrophy. *Am Heart J* 128(1):193–196, 1994.
6. Griggs RC, Moxley RT III, Mendell JR: Duchenne dystrophy: Randomized, controlled trial of prednisone (18 months) and azathioprine (12 months). *Neurology* 43:520–527, 1993.
7. Miller RG, Hoffman EP: Molecular diagnosis and modern management of Duchenne muscular dystrophy. *Neurol Clin* 12:699–724, 1994.
8. Anan R, Higuichi I, Ichinari K, et al: Myocardial patchy staining of dystrophin in Becker's muscular dystrophy associated with cardiomyopathy. *Am Heart J* 123:1088–1089, 1992.
9. Walton J: *Disorders of Voluntary Muscle.* Edinburgh, Churchill Livingstone, 1988, p539.

Guillain-Barré Syndrome

Stacy A. Rudnicki, M.D.
Sami I. Harik, M.D.

PRESENTING MANIFESTATIONS

Rapidly progressive weakness, with or without sensory symptoms, is the hallmark of Guillain-Barré syndrome (GBS). Although the disease is traditionally described as ascending weakness, symptoms can also progress in other fashions. Symptom severity can range widely, from slight difficulty with walking and trouble with fine motor skills of the hands to quadriplegia. Sensory symptoms are usually vague and transient. Cranial nerve–innervated muscles can be affected; when they are, patients complain of facial weakness, double vision, slurring of speech, and difficulty in chewing and swallowing. Patients may report shortness of breath if the respiratory musculature is impaired, and respiratory failure can occur precipitously.[1]

On exam, patients will have fairly symmetric weakness associated with areflexia. Early on, reflexes may still be present but they will be lost with time. Despite sensory complaints, not all patients will have sensory findings on exam. When they do, it is more distal than proximal, and tends to involve proprioception and vibration more than pain and temperature. Patients may or may not have facial, jaw, tongue, and neck weakness. Vital capacity should be checked to assess respiratory function.[2]

About two-thirds of patients will have an antecedent viral illness, surgery or vaccinations a few weeks before the onset of neurologic symptoms. Serologic confirmation of *Campylobacter* enteritis can be found in some patients. Certain underlying medical illnesses seem to predispose to the development of GBS, including Hodgkin's disease, lymphoma, sarcoid, collagen vascular disease, and human immunodefiency virus (HIV) (see below).

Two variants of GBS warrant special mention. The Fisher variant is characterized by the triad of ophthalmoplegia, areflexia, and ataxia.[3] Another variant is manifested by pandysautonomia alone.[4]

CARDIAC MANIFESTATIONS

Most of the cardiac manifestations are related to dysautonomia; one study found autonomic dysfunction in 67% of patients studied.[5] Both hypertension and hypotension are found, although the former is more common. Hypertension can be extreme and severe but is usually short-lived. It is believed to be related to abnormalities of the afferent nerves from baroreceptors. Hypotension is frequently orthostatic, and is associated with quadriplegia, ventilatory support, and involvement of the 9th and 10th cranial nerves. A partial sympathectomy is believed to be responsible. Sinus tachycardia is the most common evidence of dysautonomia, with some authors reporting its occurrence in up to 80% of patients with GBS. The likely etiology is decreased vagal innervation. Vagal spells, manifested by bradycardia, sinus arrest, asystole, and atrioventricular block are seen in fewer than 10% of patients and tend to be precipitated by vagal stimulation such as tracheal suctioning or Valsalva-type maneuvers. Other arrhythmias include premature ventricular contractions, paroxysmal atrial tachycardia, premature atrial contraction, atrial fibrillation, ventricular tachycardia, and ventricular fibrillation. The rare patient requires a pacemaker.[2,6] Patients can have extreme sensitivity to vasoactive drugs, and life-threatening arrhythmias have been reported with the use of suxemethonium.[7,8] A study of 100 patients with GBS found serious arrhythmias, most often in patients with systolic hypertension and a reduced RR interval. Only ventilated patients developed serious cardiac arrhythmias; in this group, wide fluctuations in pulse or blood pressure, or tracheal suctioning preceded the arrhythmia.[9]

In addition to rhythm disturbances, other ECG changes were reported in 50–80% of GBS patients. The most common changes are flattened and/or inverted T waves in lateral leads and ST segment depression. Left axis deviation, widened QRS interval, bundle branch block, various degrees of heart block, and tall, peaked T waves have rarely been found.[2]

DIAGNOSIS

When GBS is being considered, NCS are very useful in establishing the diagnosis. Evidence of demyelination includes prolonged distal latencies, slowed conduction velocities, conduction block, temporal dispersion, and prolonged F waves and H reflexes. The latter two findings are seen earliest and may be the only abnormalities when the patient is studied early. Changes are seen on both sensory and motor studies.[10] A spinal tap will show increased cerebrospinal fluid (CSF) protein, with no cells and a normal glucose level; however, it may take 7 days from symptom onset to protein elevation. White cells are occasionally found; when present, they raise the possibility that the patient is HIV positive. Occasionally, patients will develop GBS when they seroconvert, so the diagnosis may be unknown at the time of presentation.[1] Progressive motor weakness in more than one limb and areflexia are important features for the diagnosis. Supporting the diagnosis are relative symmetry, sensory signs and symptoms, cranial nerve involvement, autonomic dysfunction, absence of fever, and recovery. Sphincter dysfunction is unusual; if present, it is transient. Pupillary abnormalities are rare.[11]

DIFFERENTIAL DIAGNOSIS

Certain toxins can cause a rapidly progressive neuropathy, including *n*-hexane (found in glue), lead, and arsenic. A history of exposure and confirmation by determining the lead and arsenic levels are helpful. Also, the neuropathy of *n*-hexane and lead is axonal rather than demyelinating. Porphyria too can cause a rapidly progressive axonal neuropathy; the patient usually has a past history of abdominal pains and psychiatric manifestations. Frequently, the patient was recently given a drug such as an anticonvulsant, which can precipitate the neuropathy in porphyria. This diagnosis can be confirmed by finding delta-aminolevulinic acid and porphobilinogen in the urine. Weakness in diptheria usually develops more slowly than that seen in GBS. These patients will have a gray membrane on the back of the throat; frequently, initial symptoms are visual blurring and dysphagia. Rarely, polio, botulism, tick paralysis, and organophosphate poisoning are confused with GBS, but the spinal tap, history, and NCS will sort out these diagnoses.[2]

PATHOPHYSIOLOGY

GBS is believed to be an immune-mediated disease in which the nerve is damaged through both humoral and cell-mediated processes. Antibodies have been identified that react with the nerve, but damage to the nerve and the myelin sheath is also believed to be mediated by cytokines and through complement activation. There is focal segmental demyelination, with perivascular and endoneural infiltration of lymphocytes and macrophages; the latter is believed to be a primarily cell-mediated response. In regard to changes in the heart, most autopsies reveal no changes in the myocardium. Some have reported findings suggestive of myocarditis, with focal areas of perivascular lymphocytic infiltration particularly near the conduction system and cardiac ganglion.[12] One case showed extensive destruction of the dorsal root ganglia and infiltration of the necrotic myocardium with inflammatory cells. The myocarditis was, however, believed to be viral in nature and not a direct result of the DBS.[13]

NATURAL HISTORY OF THE DISEASE

The disease can progress for up to 4 weeks, but 50% stop progressing by 2 weeks and 80% by 3 weeks. The biggest fear is respiratory failure requiring intubation. Frequent measurements of simple respiratory functions and prophylactic intubation of patients when these measurements fall is recommended.[14] Autonomic instability (see above) can also be a major cause of morbidity and mortality. In addition, patients can develop secondary infections (pneumonia, urinary tract infections) and deep venous thrombosis because of inactivity. In patients with evidence of autonomic instability, rapidly progressive weakness, or significant respiratory decline, monitoring in an intensive care unit (ICU) setting is appropriate. Mortality ranges from 3% to 8%, with the causes of death being aspiration pneumonia, pulmonary embolus, infection, and autonomic dysfunction. After the patient has stabilized, there is usually a plateau period of a few weeks before gradual improvement begins. Approximately 10% of patients have a biphasic course with a period of worsening during recovery. Two percent of patients have recurrence after recovery, which may follow the initial episode by many years.

Only 15% of patients return to a neurologically normal state; 65% are left with minor weakness. Significant neurologic deficits with major disability are seen in 5–10%.[2] The single strongest predictor of a poor outcome is a low compound muscle action potential amplitude on NCS (<20% of normal).[15] Advanced age, need for respiratory support, and rapidly progressive disease correlated with poor outcomes in one study but not in others.[16,17]

TREATMENT OF THE DISEASE

For many years, GBS was treated with steroids; anecdotal reports were the basis for their use, but a controlled study showed no benefit.[18] In the past decade plasma exchange was reported to be of benefit. Specifically, plasma exchange decreases the time needed to walk unassisted, decreases the need for and duration of ventilatory support, shortens the length of time in the ICU and decreases the period of acute care hospitalization. Four to six plasma exchanges are performed, usually every-other-day. The greatest benefit is achieved if the patient has had symptoms for fewer than 2 weeks, but it can still be considerable when therapy is started later.[19,20] Contraindications include recent myocardial infarction, angina, sepsis, and significant dysautonomia. Plasma exchange removes a number of circulating factors believed to play a role in the pathogenesis of the disease, including antibodies, cytokines, and complement. It may also favor immune suppressor systems. Intravenous immunoglobulins (IVIg) was shown to be as effective as plasma exchange in one study, although the plasma exchange group in this particular study did not do as well as in previously reported exchange groups.[21] The benefits of IVIg include its ready availability and the ease with which it could be administered. Preliminary data, however, suggest that it may increase the chance of exacerbating symptoms from 1 day to 5 weeks after treatment.[22,23] IVIg has multiple possible mechanisms of action: formation of anti-idiotypic antibodies, blockage of Fc receptors, down regulation of cytokines and B cells, and induction of T-suppressor cells.[24]

REFERENCES

1. Ropper AH: The Guillain-Barré syndrome. *N Engl J Med* 326:1130–1136, 1992.
2. Ropper A, Wijdicks EF, Truax BT: *Guillain Barré Syndrome,* Philadelphia, FA Davis, 1991, pp73–101.
3. Fisher M: An unusual acute idiopathic polyneuritis (syndrome of ophthalmoplegia, ataxia, and areflexia). *N Engl J Med* 255:57–65, 1956.
4. Young RR, Asbury AK, Corbett JL, et al: Pure pan-dysautonomia with recovery: description and discussion of diagnostic criteria. *Brain* 98:613–636, 1975.
5. Singh NK, Jaiswal AK, Misra S, et al: Assessment of autonomic dysfunction in Guillain-Barré syndrome and its prognostic implications. *Acta Neurol Scand* 75:101–105, 1987.
6. Zochodne DW: Autonomic involvement in Guillain-Barré syndrome: a review. *Muscle Nerve* 17:1145–1155, 1994.
7. Lichtenfield P: Autonomic dysfunction in the Guillain-Barré syndrome. *Am J Med* 50:772–780, 1971.
8. Fergusson RJ, Wright DJ, Willey RF, et al: Suxamethonium is dangerous in polyneuropathy. *Br Med J* 282:298–299, 1981.
9. Winer JB, Hughes RA: Identification of patients at risk of arrhythmia in the Guillain-Barré syndrome. *Q J Med* 68(257):735–739, 1988.
10. Ropper AH, Wijdicks EF, Shahani BT: Electrodiagnostic abnormalities in 113 consecutive patients with Guillain-Barré syndrome. *Arch Neurol* 47:881–887, 1990.
11. Asbury AK, Aranson BG, Korp HR: Criteria for the diagnosis of Guillain-Barré syndrome. *Ann Neurol* 3:565–567, 1978.

12. Hartung HP, Pollard JD, Harvey GK, et al: Immunopathogenesis and treatment of the Guillain-Barré syndrome—Part I. *Muscle Nerve* 18:137–153, 1995.

13. Hodson AK, Hurwitz BJ, Abrecht R: Dysautonomia in Guillain-Barré syndrome with dorsal root ganglioneuropathy, Wallerian degeneration and fatal myocarditis. *Ann Neurol* 15:88–95, 1984.

14. Chevrolet JC, Deleamont P: Repeated vital capacity measurements as predictive parameters for mechanical ventilation need and weaning success in the Guillain-Barré syndrome. *Am Rev Respir Dis* 144:814–818, 1991.

15. Cornblath DR, Mellits ED, Griffin JW, et al: Motor conduction studies in Guillain-Barré syndrome: description and prognostic value. *Ann Neurol* 23:354–359, 1988.

16. McKhann GM, Griffin JW, Cornblath DR, et al: Plasmapheresis and Guillain-Barré syndrome: analysis of prognostic factors and the effect of plasmapheresis. *Ann Neurol* 23:347–353, 1988.

17. Eisen A, Humphreys P: The Guillain-Barré syndrome: a clinical and electrodiagnostic study of 25 cases. *Arch Neurol* 30:438–443, 1974.

18. Hughes RA, Newsom-Davis J, Perkin GD, et al: Controlled trial of prednisolone in acute polyneuropathy. *Lancet* 2:750–753, 1978.

19. Anonymous: Efficiency of plasma exchange in Guillain-Barré syndrome: role of replacement fluids. French Cooperative Group on Plasma Exchange in Guillain-Barré syndrome. *Ann Neurol* 22:753–761, 1987.

20. The Guillain-Barré Study Group: Plasmapheresis and acute Guillain-Barré syndrome. *Neurology* 35:1096–1104, 1985.

21. van der Meche FG, Schmitz PI: A randomized trial comparing intravenous immune globulin and plasma exchange in Guillain-Barré syndrome. Dutch Guillain-Barré Study Group. *N Engl J Med* 326:1123–1129, 1992.

22. Castro LH, Ropper AH: Human immune globulin infusion in Guillain-Barré syndrome: worsening during and after treatment. *Neurology* 43:1034–1036, 1993.

23. Irani DN, Cornblath DR, Chaudhry V, et al: Relapse in Guillain-Barré syndrome after treatment with human immune globulin. *Neurology* 43:872–875, 1993.

24. Hartung HP, Pollard JD, Harvey GK, et al: Immunopathogenesis and treatment of the Guillain-Barré syndrome—Part II. *Muscle Nerve* 18(2):154–164, 1995.

Friedreich's Ataxia

Stacy A. Rudnicki, M.D.
Sami I. Harik, M.D.

PRESENTING MANIFESTATIONS

Friedreich's ataxia (FA) is a type of spinocerebellar degeneration (SPCD). SPCDs are inherited progressive disorders with a variable age of symptom onset. There is primary involvement of the cerebellum, the large primary afferent neurons, and later, and to a lesser extent, the motor neurons.[1] FA is the most common of the early-onset ataxias, with a prevalence of 1–2/100,000. It is inherited as an autosomal recessive disease. Symptom onset ranges from 18 months to 27 years but typically occurs between the ages of 8 to 15 years. The first symptoms are usually gait related, with progressive limb and trunk ataxia as well as dysarthria. Weakness follows the ataxia by several years. Exam shows ataxia, usual leg weakness, absent tendon reflexes in the lower extremities, and positive Babinski responses. Usually, there is evidence of a sensory neuropathy, with distal loss of vibration and proprioception and occasional pain. Skeletal abnormalities include scoliosis, pes cavus, and equinovarus feet. Sensorineural deafness is demonstrated in 10%. Type I diabetes mellitus is found in 10% of patients, and another 10–20% have impaired glucose tolerance.[2,3]

CARDIAC MANIFESTATIONS

ECG abnormalities are found frequently, with one study reporting them in 92% of patients with FA. The abnormalities found included ST-T wave changes in 79%, right axis deviation in 40%, short PR interval in 24%, abnormal Q wave in 14%, and left ventricular hypertrophy (LVH) in 16%. Arrhythmias include supraventricular tachycardia, atrial fibrillation, atrial flutter, and rare ventricular tachycardia. There is some controversy surrounding the cardiomyopathy associated with FA. In most patients it is concentric left ventricular hypertrophy, occurring in 11–71% of the patients studied. While generally concentric and not associated with decreased output, the hypertrophy is occasionally asymmetric and can cause aortic outflow obstruction. In rare patients, global cardiac hypokinesia with a dilated cardiomyopathy and decreased cardiac output occurs. There is debate as to whether this process is separate from the LVH, with a different pathogenesis, or whether it is the end result of LVH and replacement of the heart muscle by fibrosis. This dilated cardiomyopathy has been referred to as a *dystrophic heart.*[4–8] No correlation was found between the degree of neurologic impairment and the severity of myocardial disease. Small coronary arteries with intimal proliferation have been reported, but the influence of diabetes mellitus (found in increased frequency in FA) on this finding remains undetermined.[9] A detailed study of autonomic function in 15 patients with FA failed to show evidence of sympathetic or parasympathetic dysfunction.[10]

DIAGNOSIS

Computed cranial tomography can occasionally show mild cerebellar atrophy, but magnetic resonance imaging is better at demonstrating not only the cerebellar atrophy but also the atrophy of the medulla and spinal cord.[11] The gene locus in FA was mapped to 9q 22-CEN.[12] Since FA is autosomal recessive, a positive family history may be lacking. Primary criteria include ataxia, dysarthria, absent tendon reflexes, weakness, and proprioceptive and vibratory loss in the lower extremities. The NCS will demonstrate a sensory axonal neuropathy with absent or very small sensory nerve action potentials. Motor NCS and EMG are usually normal; any abnormality is mild.[11]

DIFFERENTIAL DIAGNOSIS

Other ataxias can be distinguished from FA by the age of symptom onset; multisystem atrophies are usually late-onset disorders. There is an early-onset cerebellar ataxia with retained tendon reflexes and no cardiac, skeletal, or eye findings which is also inherited in an autosomal recessive fashion. Cerebellar ataxia with hypogonadism is also autosomal recessive, but abnormal sexual development is obvious by puberty; there is no associated heart disease. There is also cerebellar ataxia with myoclonus and ataxia associated with hearing loss. Behr's syndrome is characterized by ataxia with optic atrophy, spasticity, and mental retardation. Marinesco-Sjögren syndrome features ataxia with cataracts, mental retardation, and hypogonadism.[13]

PATHOPHYSIOLOGY

The etiology of FA remains a mystery. An abnormality in pyruvate metabolism was postulated but is not universally accepted.[13] In the nervous system, there is degeneration of the dorsal columns, pyramidal tracts, and spinocerebellar tracts, as well as loss of cells in the dorsal root ganglia and cerebellar Purkinje cells. There is also loss of large, myelinated axons. The heart shows symmetric myocytic hypertrophy and focal interstitial fibrosis, together with a myocytopathy with bizarre-shaped myocytes.[11]

PROGNOSIS

The rate of progression is variable, but there is almost universal loss of the ability to walk, with 90% of patients wheelchair bound by the age of 45 years. On average, the ability to walk is lost 15 years after the onset of symptoms. This is often the result of profound ataxia rather than weakness. The median age of death is 35 years and is unrelated to the age of symptom onset. There is a wide range in the time of death, from the 30s to the 70s. For unclear reasons, women have a much better survival than men, with 20-year survival after symptom onset of 100% for women and only 63% for men. Death is usually secondary to a cardiomyopathy, with either congestive heart failure or an arrhythmia being the terminal event. Scoliosis is progressive and causes respiratory compromise.[2] A small group of families (5–10%) have prolonged survival and slower disease progression.[14]

CURRENT METHODS OF TREATMENT

A number of agents have been tried in FA, but none showed sustained benefit. Medications tried include amantadine, choline, physostigmine, 5-hydroxytryptophan, and thyrotropin-releasing factor.[13,15]

REFERENCES

1. Dyck PJ: Neuronal atrophy and degeneration predominantly affecting peripheral sensory and autonomic neurons. In Dyck PJ, Thomas PK, Lambert EH, Bunge R: *Peripheral Neuropathy*, Philadelphia, WB Saunders, 1984, pp1589–1591.
2. Harding AE: Friedreich's ataxia: a clinical and genetic study of 90 families with analysis of early diagnostic criteria and intrafamilial clustering of clinical features. *Brain* 104:589–620, 1981.
3. Werdelin L: Hereditary ataxias. Occurrence and clinical features. *Acta Neurol Scand Suppl* 106:1–124, 1986.
4. Child JS, Perloff JK, Bach PM, et al: Cardiac involvement in Friedreich's ataxia: a clinical study of 75 patients. *J Am Coll Cardiol* 7:1370–1378, 1986.
5. Therriault L, Lamoureux G, Cote M, et al: The cardiomyopathy in Friedreich's ataxia: isotopic ventriculography and myocardial imaging with Thallium-201. *Can J Neurol Sci* 11:588–591, 1984.
6. Steinsapir K, Lewis W: Dilated cardiomyopathy associated with Friedreich's ataxia. *Arch Pathol Lab Med* 109:454–456, 1985.
7. Zimmermann M, Gabathuler J, Adamec R, et al: Unusual manifestations of heart involvement in Friedreich's ataxia. *Am Heart J* 111:184–187, 1986.
8. Hawley RJ, Gottdiener JS: Five-year follow-up of Friedreich's ataxia cardiomyopathy. *Arch Intern Med* 146:483–488, 1986.
9. James TN, Cobbs BW, Coghlan HC, et al: Coronary disease, cardioneuropathy, and conduction system abnormalities in the cardiomyopathy of Friedreich's ataxia. *Br Heart J* 57:446–457, 1987.

10. Ingall TJ, McLeod JG: Autonomic function in Friedreich's ataxia. *J Neurol Neurosurg Psychiatry* 54:162–164, 1991.

11. Calne DB: *Neurodegenerative Diseases,* Philadelphia, WB Saunders, 1994, pp792–794.

12. Chamberlain S, Shaw J, Rowland A, et al: Mapping of mutation causing Friedreich's ataxia to human chromosome 9. *Nature* 334:248–250, 1988.

13. Conner KE, Rosenberg RN: The hereditary ataxias. In Rosenberg RN, Prusiner SB, Di Mauro S, et al: *The Molecular and Genetic Basis of Neurologic Disease.* Boston, Raven Press, 1993, p697–736.

14. Evans RW, Baskin DS, Yatsu FM: *Prognosis of Neurological Disorders,* New York, Oxford University Press, 1992, pp479–481.

15. Filla A, De Michele G, Orefice G, et al: A double-blind cross-over trial of amantadine hydrochloride in Friedreich's ataxia. *Can J Neurol Sci* 20(1):52–55, 1993.

Polymyositis and Dermatomyositis

Stacy A. Rudnicki, M.D.
Sami I. Harik, M.D.

PRESENTING MANIFESTATIONS

Polymyositis (PM) and dermatomyosits (DM) are inflammatory myopathies. Symptoms progress over weeks to months, with proximal muscle weakness as the most common and major initial symptom. Pain in the form of myalgias and muscle tenderness is another common complaint. Patients can have weakness of pharyngeal and neck muscles, but the face and eye muscles are usually spared. Although patients can have weakness affecting the muscles of respiration as the disease progresses, this is rarely observed at presentation.[1] DM is a disease of childhood and adulthood, with women being affected 1.4–2.0 times as often as men.[1,2] PM develops after the second decade of life and has a similar female preponderance in most studies. In both disorders, the exam reveals proximal muscle weakness affecting the legs more often than the arms, and weakness of neck flexors more than extensors. Myotatic reflexes are normal to diminished, and sensation is normal.[3] The rash in DM can occur before or at the onset of weakness. The rash can include a heliotropic hue to the upper eyelids, a malar rash across the cheeks, an erythematous rash over the extensor surfaces of the joints, or dilated capillaries around the fingernail beds.[4]

Both DM and PM can occur in association with other mixed connective tissue diseases, scleroderma, rheumatoid arthritis, Sjögren's syndrome, and systemic sclerosis.[3] There has been some controversy over the association of malignancy with PM and DM. A large study of 788 patients with DM or PM in Sweden followed these patients for 5 to 25 years and found an increased incidence of cancer in both groups, but higher in DM. A higher mortality rate from cancer was found only in DM. The risks of cancer and of death from cancer were higher in women than in men with PM.[5]

Pulmonary problems can occur in DM and PM and have several etiologies. Some patients develop weakness of the respiratory muscles. Others develop interstitial lung disease, and an occasional patient will develop a drug-induced pneumonitis from treatment with methotrexate.[4]

CARDIAC MANIFESTATIONS

The frequency of cardiac disease in patients with PM and DM depends on how long the patient has had the disease and on how intensively the cardiac status is investigated. Early on, approximately 20% will have some cardiac problems, but later in the disease under heavy scrutiny, the number can approach 75%.[3] Studies have reported abnormal ECGs in 32–52% of patients with PM and DM. Changes are numerous and include nonspecific ST-T wave changes, left or right ventricular hypertrophy, left or right bundle branch block, and first-degree heart block.[1,6,7] Other studies have emphasized the finding of ventricular, atrial, and sinus arrhythmias.[8] There was no correlation between the ECG changes and the severity of the muscle disease; only rarely did ECG changes improve with treatment.[6] In a study of 13 patients, 9 had pulmonary hypertension but none had significant valvular disease or decreased left ventricular function on echocardiogram.[9] Another echocardiographic study of 21 patients with PM found mitral valve prolapse in 65% and increased systolic left ventricular function compared to controls. Rarely, an echocardiogram shows pericarditis. Coronary artery disease also occurs, though the frequency is uncertain since relatively few patients undergo cardiac catheterization. An autopsy series of 16 patients showed abnormalities in the coronary arteries in 5; 3 patients had vasculitis, 1 had intimal proliferation, and 1 had medial sclerosis.[10] Myocardial disease has been reported in as many as 70% of patients with PM. This encompasses a broad spectrum of pathology ranging from mild diffuse or focal infiltrates of inflammatory cells to severe inflammation with necrosis and fibrosis.[8] Fibrosis of the conduction system is believed to lead to the arrhythmias. Patients with more severe skeletal muscle disease do not have a higher incidence of myocarditis.[10] There is some controversy concerning the significance of an elevated MB fraction of the CPK. It is frequently found in patients with PM or DM, and while some believe that more than a 3% fraction correlates with cardiac disease, this conclusion is not universally accepted.[3,11] There is a consensus that cardiac disease is frequently asymptomatic but, when present, is associated with increased mortality.[3] Cardiac symptoms include congestive heart failure, angina, and syncope.[1]

DIAGNOSIS

Criteria for the diagnosis of PM and DM were proposed by Bohan et al. in 1975 and include proximal, symmetric muscle weakness developing over weeks to months; muscle biopsy evidence of necrosis, degeneration, and regeneration with an interstitial mononuclear infiltrate; increased CPK; and an abnormal EMG. For a definitive diagnosis, all four features need to be present; a probable diagnosis requires three. If only two features are present, the diagnosis is possible. For DM, a rash also needs to be present.[12] The EMG/NCS findings typically include a normal NCS; rarely, motor amplitudes are reduced. On EMG, there is abnormal rest activity including positive sharp waves, fibrillations, and complex, repetitive discharges. Motor unit potentials are small, polyphasic, and of brief duration, with an enhanced interference pattern. Occasionally, myotonia is found. The EMG can be normal in up to 11% of patients, but the yield is improved by sampling multiple muscles, particularly the paraspinal muscles.[13] Because inflammation can be patchy, a muscle biopsy may be normal; if suspicion is high, a second biopsy may be warranted.

DIFFERENTIAL DIAGNOSIS

The hereditary myopathies, primarily limb girdle dystrophy, are occasionally confused with PM, but they progress over years instead of months and do not show inflammation on biopsy.

The more difficult disorder to distinguish from PM is inclusion body myositis (IBM), another inflammatory myopathy. In contrast to PM, however, it is not responsive to steroids. IBM is more common in men than in women, with a ratio of 3:1. Onset is usually more insidious than in PM, with progression over years instead of months. The age of onset is usually after 50. Pain is usually absent, and the CPK is typically normal or only mildly elevated. In some patients, weakness is more distal than proximal. Muscle biopsy shows endomysial inflammation and vacuoles which, on electron microscopy, contain membranous whorls. While one study suggested that the rate of cardiac disease in this group of patients was similar to that in PM and DM, it included hypertension; without this inclusion, the incidence of cardiac disease would have been lower.[4,14]

Patients who are HIV positive can develop PM, although in some of these patients the myopathy is actually secondary to zidovudine therapy, which can cause a mitochondrial myopathy.[15] HIV antigens have not been isolated in muscle fibers in seropositive patients with PM, so the myopathy is not believed to be related to direct invasion by the virus.[16] Other disorders which can be distinguished from PM by muscle biopsy include sarcoid myopathy, eosinophilic PM, and eosinophilic fasciitis.[17]

PATHOPHYSIOLOGY

PM and DM are believed to be auotimmune-mediated diseases, in part because of their association with other immune disorders and their response to immunosuppression. In patients with PM, muscle biopsy shows predominantly cell populations of CD8+ T cells and macrophages which surround and invade muscle fibers expressing major histocompatibility complex I antigens. What triggers the antigen expression is unknown, but some believe that a viral disease is the underlying cause.[16]

NATURAL HISTORY OF THE DISEASE

The natural history of untreated disease is difficult to ascertain because today all patients are treated with some form of immunosuppression. A retrospective study from 1968 comparing patients treated with prednisone versus those not treated showed that 35 of 122 patients not treated died (29%); of those treated with steroids, an identical percentage (45 of 157) also died. Causes of death included heart disease, secondary infections seen in the chronically disabled, and malignancy. Of the 122 patients in the series who were not treated with prednisone, 48 went into remission (39%), 13 improved (11%), 12 did not improve (10%), and 14 became weaker (11%). One problem with this and other early studies was the failure to establish clear criteria for the diagnosis of PM or DM.[2]

CURRENT METHODS OF TREATMENT

Immunosuppression is the mainstay of treatment for PM and DM. Interestingly, a prospective placebo-controlled trial was never done to establish its efficacy. Instead, retrospective studies of prednisone were used to support its use. The study from the Mayo Clinic divided patients into low-dose (<50 mg/day) and high-dose groups.[2] It found that 75 of 119 patients treated with high-dose prednisone achieved remission or improved, while 12 of 38 patients treated with low-dose prednisone and 61 of 122 receiving no prednisone went into remission or improved. Only one patient on low-dose treatment went into remission. The study also found a reduced death rate in those treated with high-dose compared to no prednisone (28 of 119 in the high-dose group died compared to 35 of 122 in the no-prednisone group). In addition, remission was achieved faster in those taking high-dose prednisone than in those untreated.

The study concluded that prednisone in high doses was effective in treating PM and that low-dose prednisone not recommended.[2]

A study of 118 patients with PM and DM showed the greatest chance of improving with prednisone therapy if it was instituted in the first 3 years of the disease. Approximately 20% of patients have active disease for more than 10 years, but two-thirds of the patients who survive are not functionally disabled. Mortality was essentially identical to that of the other study, at 28%.[1]

Many other forms of immunosuppression have been tried in patients with DM and PM. Azathioprine (imuran) is frequently added to prednisone if the latter is not sufficiently effective, or it can be used in conjunction with prednisone as an initial therapy.[3,17] One study failed to show improvement when comparing azathioprine (imuran) and prednisone to prednisone alone, but patients were followed for only 3 month, which is not sufficient time for azathioprine (imuran) to exert its effects.[18] Both leukopheresis and plasma exchange failed to show benefit in steroid-resistant PM in a placebo-controlled trial.[19] Several small studies have shown IVIg to be of benefit in patients with DM and PM who failed to respond adequately to steroids alone; some patients treated with IVIg subsequently decreased or tapered their steroids completely.[20–22] Cyclosporin A was reported to be of benefit in an anecdotal report.[23] Lastly, total body irradiation has shown benefit in an occasional patient.[24]

REFERENCES

1. De Vere R, Bradley WG: Polymyositis: its presentation, morbidity and mortality. *Brain* 98:637–666, 1975.

2. Winkelmann RK, Mulder DW, Lambert EH, et al: Course of dermatomyositis-polymyositis: comparison of untreated and cortisone-treated patients. *Mayo Clin Proc* 43:545–556, 1968.

3. Dalakas MC: *Polymyositis and Dermatomyositis,* Boston, Butterworth, 1988.

4. Dalakas MC: Polymyositis, dermatomyositis and inclusion-body myositis. *N Engl J Med* 325(21): 1487–1498, 1991.

5. Sigurgeirsson B, Lindelof B, Edhag O, et al: Risk of cancer in patients with dermatomyositis or polymyositis. A population based study. *N Engl J Med* 326:363–367, 1992.

6. Stern R, Godbold JH, Chess Q, et al: ECG abnormalities in polymyositis. *Arch Intern Med* 144:2185–2189, 1984.

7. Gottdiener JS, Sherber HS, Hawley RJ, et al: Cardiac manifestations in polymyositis. *Am J Cardiol* 41:1141–1149, 1978.

8. Byrnes TJ, Baethge BA, Wolf RE: Noninvasive cardiovascular studies in patients with inflammatory myopathy. *Angiology* 42(10):843–848, 1991.

9. Askari AD: Cardiac abnormalities. *Clin Rheum Dis* 10:131–149, 1984.

10. Haupt HM, Hutchins GM: The heart and cardiac conduction system in polymyositis-dermatomyositis: a clinicopathologic study of 16 autopsied patients. *Am J Cardiol* 50:998–1006, 1982.

11. Strongwater SL, Annesley T, Schnitzer TJ: Myocardial involvement in polymyositis. *J Rheumatol* 10:459–463, 1983.

12. Bohan A, Peter JB: Polymyositis and dermatomyositis. *N Engl J Med* 292:344–347, 1975.

13. Robinson LR: AAEM case report #22: polymyositis. *Muscle Nerve* 14:310–315, 1991.

14. Lotz BP, Engel AG, Nishino H, et al: Inclusion body myositis. Observations in 40 patients. *Brain* 112:727–747, 1989.

15. Dalakas MC, Leon-Monzon ME, Bernardini I, et al: Zidovudine-induced mitochondrial myopathy is associated with muscle carnitine deficiency and lipid storage. *Ann Neurol* 35:482–487, 1994.

16. Illa I, Nath A, Dalakas M: Immunocytochemical and virological characteristics of HIV-associated inflammatory myopathies: similarities with seronegative polymyositis. *Ann Neurol* 29:474–481, 1991.

17. Walton J: The idiopathic inflammatory myopathies and their treatment. *J Neurol Neurosurg Psychiatry* 54:285–287, 1991.

18. Bunch TW, Worthington JW, Comps J, et al: Azathioprine with prednisone for polymyositis. *Ann Intern Med* 92:365–369, 1980.

19. Miller FW, Leitman SF, Cronin ME, et al: Controlled trial of plasma exchange and leukopheresis in polymyositis and dermatomyositis. *N Engl J Med* 326:1380–1384, 1992.

20. Dalakas MC, Illa I, Dambrosia JM, et al: A controlled trial of high-dose intravenous immune globulin infusions as treatment for dermatomyositis. *N Engl J Med* 329:1993–2000, 1993.

21. Cherin P, Herson S, Wechsler B, et al: Efficacy of intravenous gammaglobulin therapy in chronic refractory polymyositis and dermatomyositis: an open study with 20 adult patients. *Am J Med* 91:162–168, 1991.

22. Lang BA, Laxer RM, Murphy G, et al: Treatment of dermatomyositis with intravenous gammaglobulin. *Am J Med* 91:169–172, 1991.

23. Lueck CJ, Trend P, Swash M: Cyclosporin in the management of polymyositis and dermatomyositis. *J Neurol Neurosurg Psychiatry* 54:1007–1008, 1991.

24. Kelly JJ, Madoc-Jones H, Adelman LS, et al: Response to total body irradiation in dermatomyositis. *Muscle Nerve* 11:120–123, 1988.

Mitochondrial Myopathies

Stacy A. Rudnicki, M.D.
Sami I. Harik, M.D.

CLINICAL MANIFESTATIONS

The mitochondrial myopathies are heterogeneous in their clinical manifestations and biochemical abnormalities resulting in different attempts at classification. Petty et al., suggested three groups: (1) chronic progressive external ophthalmoplegia (CPEO) with limb weakness, with or without fatigability; (2) limb weakness alone; and (3) primary central nervous system involvement, including ataxia, dementia, deafness, seizures, and movement disorders.[1] Another classification system used clinically "distinct" syndromes. Kearns-Sayre syndrome (KSS) includes the triad of CPEO, pigmentary retinopathy, and heart block. Mitochondrial encephalomyopathy, lactic acidosis, and stroke-like episodes syndrome (MELAS) lacks *eye* involvement and ataxia.[2] Myoclonic epilepsy and ragged red fibers (MERRF) includes myoclonus, ataxia, weakness, hearing loss, seizures, and dementia, but again, eye findings are lacking.[3] Others have suggested a classification based on the specific defects in mitochondrial metabolism. The problem with all of these classification systems is that there is considerable overlap between the groups described clinically, and there is no correlation between the clinical picture and the biochemical defect.[1,4]

The largest clinical study of patients with mitochondrial myopathy was reported by Petty and included 66 patients. Though there was considerable overlap in clinical features, patients were divided into those with CPEO and limb weakness (55%), limb weakness alone (18%), and primary central nervous system involvement (27%). Pigmentary retinopathy was found in 36% of all patients and included patients in all three groups. The age of onset was quite variable, ranging from infancy to 68 years, but with most patients (61%) developing symptoms prior to age 20.[1] Others reported an age of onset as late as 75 years.[5] Males and females are equally affected. The most common symptoms at disease onset, in order of descending frequency, were ptosis, fatigue, and proximal more than distal limb weakness. On exam, most patients had preserved tendon reflexes, while 14 had hyporeflexia and only 1 had brisk reflexes. However, a Babinski sign was found in 16 patients. Eleven patients had mild distal sensory loss, and five had marked sensory abnormalities. Thirteen patients were demented.[1]

CARDIAC MANIFESTATIONS

In general, the cardiac manifestations fall into two categories: conduction defects and cardiomyopathy. Conduction defects include first-degree heart block, intraventricular conduction delays, right bundle branch block, and complete heart block. Nonspecific ST-T wave changes are also seen. There is no correlation between the severity of neurologic disease and the presence or absence of cardiac disease.[1] Several authors pointed out the significance of a bifascicular block in patients with KSS. In contrast to ischemic heart disease, when bifascicular block is found in KSS, it is a harbinger of complete heart block. Therefore, it is recommended that affected patients have electrophysiologic testing, as they may require a pacemaker.[6,7]

Patients with mitochondrial myopathies infrequently develop a rapidly progressive cardiomyopathy; some of these patients have had successful heart transplants. It is proposed that congestive heart failure may occur more frequently as patients receive pacemakers and live to an older age.[8,9] Hypertrophic cardiopathy has also been found in patients with MELAS and, less often, in MERRF, but in general, their central nervous system disease is a greater problem. There have also been rare reports of mitochondrial disease limited to the heart muscle. Histocytoid cardiopathy of infancy causes death typically in the first year of life from heart failure and is associated with complex II deficiency. It has also been noted that within the same family there can be patients with a myopathy alone, while others have both a myopathy and a cardiopathy.[10]

DIAGNOSIS

The hallmark of mitochondrial myopathy is the muscle biopsy finding of ragged red fibers on Gomori trichrome stain. These fibers are related to the accumulation of abnormal mitochondria, typically in subsarcolemmal locations.[11] Although most patients have a normal CPK, occasionally it may be mildly elevated. EMG/NCS findings are variable, ranging from myopathic or neuropathic to normal results. The electroencephalogram can be normal, or can show epileptiform activity or nonspecific slowing. About half of the patients have a normal cranial computed tomography scan; and cerebral and/or cerebellar atrophy are the most common abnormalities. White matter changes, stroke, and basal ganglia and white matter calcifications were reported. Laboratory abnormalities include increased CSF protein, low serum and folic acid, and increased lactic acid.[1,12]

PATHOPHYSIOLOGY

The percentage of patients with affected family members ranges from 18 to 33%.[1,13] Though occasionally autosomal modes of inheritance have been reported, the families usually seem to have non-Mendelian inheritance patterns. The ratio of maternal to paternal transmission is a striking 9:1.[13] This pattern of maternal inheritance led to the suggestion that mitochondrial disease, at least in some patients, was related to a problem with the mitochondrial DNA (mtDNA). Besides maternal inheritance of mtDNA, several other features are noteworthy. When a mutation occurs in the mtDNA, the result is a mix of normal and mutant mtDNA (referred to as *heteroplasmy*). This may lead to some cells having mostly normal mtDNA and to other cells having very abnormal mtDNA. Tissues which depend heavily on oxidative metabolism, such as skeletal and cardiac muscles and brain, are more sensitive to abnormal mtDNA. While defects in nuclear DNA (nDNA) also play a role in mitochondrial disease, mtDNA genes are 10–17 times more likely to have mutations than are nDNA genes.[14]

MtDNA codes for 13 of 67 subunits of the mitochondrial respiratory chain and oxidative phosphorylation systems. In patients with mitochondrial myopathy diagnosed by ragged red fibers on muscle biopsy, 40% had deletions of mtDNA. While similar clinical presentations could be found with different mitochondrial abnormalities, one constant finding was that patients with mtDNA deletions had CPEO.[15] There is no correlation between the amount of abnormal mtDNA and the clinical or biochemical severity of the disease.[16] Defects in mitochondrial metabolism include deficiencies of complexes I, III, IV, and V. Again, no correlation exists between the clinical features and the biochemical defect.[1]

At autopsy, the heart shows fatty infiltration and fibrosis in both a patchy and a diffuse distribution. These changes are frequently found in the His-Purkinje system. Abnormal mitochondria are found throughout the heart.[7,9,17]

PROGNOSIS

In Perry's study, patients had their disease for a mean period of 20 years. Of 66 patients, 9 were severely disabled and 42 were still working. The prognosis was worst in the patients with central nervous system disease, with only 2 of 18 able to work after a mean disease duration of 17 years. The patients with CPEO and extremity weakness had the best prognosis. Those with extremity weakness alone had a mixed prognosis; some fared well, while others had significant disability.[1]

CURRENT METHODS OF TREATMENT

Coenzyme Q10 plays a role in electron transport, and vitamins K_3 and C are believed to improve oxidative phosphorylation. Riboflavin, thiamine, and niacin are cofactors in the electron transport chain. Therefore, these substances were given to patients with mitochondrial myopathy. No improvement, either clinically or by measures of oxidative metabolism (as demonstrated by the amount of lactate in urine and blood, by exercise tolerance, and by spectroscopy), was observed. Some patients with mitochondrial myopathy have been found to have carnitine insufficiency. In an uncontrolled trial, these patients were given l-carnitine and a number of them showed improvement in muscle weakness and cardiomyopathy, though the way improvement was measured was not well defined.[18]

REFERENCES

1. Petty RK, Harding AE, Morgan-Hughes JA: The clinical features of mitochondrial myopathy. *Brain* 109:915–938, 1986.
2. Pavlakis SG, Phillips PC, Di Mauro S, et al: Mitochondrial myopathy, encephalopathy, lactic acidosis, and stroke-like episodes: a distinctive clinical syndrome. *Ann Neurol* 16:481–488, 1984.
3. Fukuhara N, Tokiguichi S, Shirakawa K, et al: Myoclonus epilepsy associated with ragged-red fibers (mitochondrial abnormalities): disease entity or syndrome? Light- and electron-microscopic studies of two cases and review of literature. *J Neurol Sci* 47:117–133, 1980.
4. Morgan-Hughes JA, Cooper JM, Holt IJ, et al: Mitochondrial myopathies: clinical defects. *Biochem Soc Trans* 18:523–526, 1990.
5. Johnston W, Karpati G, Carpenter S, et al: Late-onset mitochondrial myopathy. *Ann Neurol* 37:16–23, 1995.
6. Kenny D, Wetherbee J: Kearns-Sayre syndrome in the elderly: mitochondrial myopathy with advanced heart block. *Am Heart J* 120:440–443, 1990.
7. Gallastegui J, Hariman RJ, Handler B, et al: Cardiac involvement in the Kearns-Sayre syndrome. *Am J Cardiol* 60:385–388, 1987.
8. Channer KS, Channer JL, Campbell MJ, et al: Cardiomyopathy in the Kearns-Sayre syndrome. *Br Heart J* 59:486–490, 1988.

9. Hubner G, Gokel JM, Pongratz D, et al: Fatal mitochondrial cardiomyopathy in Kearns-Sayre syndrome. *Virchows Arch A Pathol Anat Histopathol* 408:611–621, 1986.

10. Servidei S, Bertini E, Di Mauro S: Hereditary metabolic cardiomyopathies. *Adv Pediatr* 41:1–33, 1994.

11. Schapira AH, Di Mauro S: *Mitochondrial Disorders in Neurology.* Cambridge, Butterworth, 1994, pp76–77.

12. Matthews PM, Ford B, Dandurand RJ, et al: Coenzyme Q_{10} with multiple vitamins is generally ineffective in treatment of mitochondrial disease. *Neurology* 43:884–890, 1993.

13. Harding AE, Petty RK, Morgan-Hughes JA: Mitochondrial myopathy: a genetic study of 71 cases. *J Med Genet* 25:528–535, 1988.

14. Brown MD, Wallace DC: Molecular basis of mitochondrial DNA disease. *J Bioenerg Biomembr* 26:273–289, 1994.

15. Holt IJ, Harding AE, Cooper JM, et al: Mitochondrial myopathies: clinical and biochemical features of 30 patients with major deletions of muscle mitochondrial DNA. *Ann Neurol* 26:699–708, 1989.

16. Harding AE, Holt IJ, Cooper JM, et al: Mitochondrial myopathies: genetic defects. *Biochem Soc Trans* 18:519–522, 1990.

17. Bussieres LM, Pflugfelder PW, Guiraudon C, et al: Exercise responses after cardiac transplantation in mitochondrial myopathy. *Am J Cardiol* 71:1003–1006, 1993.

18. Campos Y, Huertas R, Lorenzo G, et al: Plasma carnitine insufficiency and effectiveness of L-carnitine therapy in patients with mitochondrial myopathy. *Muscle Nerve* 16:150–153, 1993.

Cardiovascular Involvement With Special Conditions

Jon P. Lindemann, M.D.
Section Editor

Pregnancy

Mark L. Mullens, M.D.
J. David Talley, M.D.

PRESENTING MANIFESTATIONS

History

Chest discomfort is common during pregnancy. While the most common etiology is gastro-esophageal reflux, other possibilities include myocardial ischemia and pulmonary infarction. The treatment of choice for angina pectoris is beta-adrengeric blocking medication. Nitrates and calcium channel blockers are generally avoided. Low-dose aspirin should be withheld until the 13th week of gestation, but then it can be continued until delivery, with minimal potential for complications.

Palpitations and arrhythmias are also common during pregnancy. Since nearly all antiarrhythmic medications have potentially harmful side effects, an exact diagnosis should be made. Initial treatment of symptomatic but not life-threatening arrhythmias begins with avoidance of excessive fatigue, caffeine, alcohol, and the use of vagal maneuvers.[1]

Physical Examination

The first heart sound may be loud and widely split due to early closure of the mitral valve. The second heart sound is usually normal, but there may be decreased respiratory variation late in pregnancy. A third heart sound is heard in 85% of normal pregnant patients, and a fourth heart sound is infrequent. A murmur louder than grade 2 (on a scale from 1 to 6) is abnormal. A systolic ejection murmur is heard in more than 90% patients, usually at the left sternal border, but may occur throughout the pericardium. Rarely, a soft diastolic murmur of increased tricuspid valve flow is noted. The intensity of the systolic ejection murmur auscultated over the breasts (the mammary soufflé) may be diminished with pressure applied at the point of auscultation. This murmur has been attributed to flow in the mammary and/or intercostal arteries. Continuous murmurs over the breasts are referred to as a *venous hum* and are due to increased venous blood flow.

Laboratory Evaluation

Submaximal stress echocardiography is safe for risk stratification in the evaluation of chest discomfort, but maximal stress testing may cause fetal bradycardia. Radionuclide imaging is

224

TABLE 11.1. Hemodynamic Changes During Pregnancy

Cardiovascular Index	Change
Total peripheral vascular resistance	Decreased
Pulmonary vascular resistance	Decreased
Heart rate	Increased
Stroke volume	Increased
Cardiac output	Increased
Blood volume	Increased
Systemic arterial blood pressure	Decreased

Modified from Sullivan JM, Ramanathan KB. Management of medical problems in pregnancy—severe cardiac disease. *N Engl J Med* 313:304–309, 1985. Reprinted with permission of author and publisher.

contraindicated due to fetal radiation exposure. Cardiac catheterization with abdominal shielding is done only if the results crucially influence the treatment choices.

PATHOPHYSIOLOGY

Hemodynamics

The normal pregnancy involves widespread physiologic changes affecting the cardiovascular system (Table 11.1). After fertilization, the effects of continued progesterone production accompanied by high estrogen levels result in decreased peripheral vascular resistance accompanied by a positive ionotropic effect on the heart.[2] Renin, angiotensin, and aldosterone production promote increased plasma volume secondary to sodium and water retention. Total body water rises throughout pregnancy by 6 to 8 L, a 50% increase in volume compared to the nonpregnant condition. A relative increase in the plasma volume per erythrocyte mass results in the normal hemotocrit in pregnancy ranging from 33% to 35% (11–12 g/dL hemoglobin).

The heart rate, stroke volume, and cardiac output increase in pregnancy. Heart rate increases by 10–20 beats per minute, beginning at the onset of pregnancy and leveling off during the 32nd week. Stroke volume begins to increase at 8 weeks and peaks at 20 weeks. Thus, cardiac output rises during pregnancy as a function of heart rate and stroke volume.

At the time of delivery, cardiac output, already increased above normal, may increase another 34%. This is due to the continued increase in heart rate and stroke volume and to the return of 500 mL of blood to the circulation when the placenta is delivered. After delivery, cardiac output remains high for 2 days, with a return to normal levels over the following 10 to 14 days.

Valvular Disease

Aortic Stenosis

Severe aortic stenosis in pregnancy requires close attention to fluid status, since volume overload may result in pulmonary edema and hypovolemia may cause serious ischemic complications. Pulmonary edema will usually respond to bed rest, digitalis, oxygen, and diuresis. Hypovolemia, if not rapidly corrected, is associated with maternal mortality of nearly 40% and fetal mortality of 30%. When medical treatment fails, valvuloplasty, commissurotomy, or valve replacement may be considered.[3,4]

Aortic Regurgitation

Aortic regurgitation in pregnancy usually responds to traditional measures such as salt restriction, digitalis, and diuretics. Afterload reduction with hydralazine may be used. Endocarditis prophylaxis may be given at the time of delivery.

Mitral Stenosis

The increased plasma volume and heart rate increase left atrial pressure and predispose the patient to pulmonary edema and atrial fibrillation. Cardiac output may drop due to the rapid ventricular response or to overly aggressive diuresis. Digoxin is commonly used to control the ventricular response. Cardioversion may be attempted to restore sinus rhythm. It is generally well tolerated; however, external fetal monitoring is recommended due to the theoretical possibility of induction of fetal asystole with cardioversion. Subcutaneous heparin administration under close supervision may prevent thromboembolic complications. At the time of delivery, pulmonary artery pressure and the capillary wedge pressure should be monitored.[5] Labor should take place in the lateral recumbent position to avoid compression of the inferior vena cava. Anesthetic agents which reduce venous return due to peripheral vasodilatation may avoid postpartum pulmonary edema. Antibiotic prophylaxis for endocarditis is recommended for mitral stenosis, and rheumatic fever prophylaxis is indicated for patients with a history of rheumatic fever. When medical treatment for mitral stenosis fails, mitral valve balloon valvuloplasty, mitral valve commissurotomy, and mitral valve replacement can be used.[6]

Mitral Valve Prolapse

Mitral valve prolapse and mitral regurgitation are generally well tolerated in pregnancy. Endocarditis prophylaxis is recommended for mitral valve prolapse accompanied by mitral regurgitation.

Pulmonary and Tricuspid Valve Disease

The initial management of pulmonary stenosis involves reduction of activity. Pulmonary valve balloon angioplasty may be considered for medially refractory right heart failure. Endocarditis prophylaxis is recommended for patients with pulmonary stenosis. Tricuspid regurgitation is well tolerated in pregnancy.[7]

Congenital Heart Disease

Eisenmenger's Syndrome

Uncorrected cyanotic congenital heart disease is a contraindication to pregnancy due to excessive maternal and fetal risk. If pregnancy occurs, it should be terminated. Cyanotic congenital heart disease, when corrected prior to surgery, has an outcome comparable to that of other forms of congenital heart disease.[8]

Tetralogy of Fallot

This congenital defect (overriding aorta from both the right and left ventricles, pulmonary outflow tract stenosis, ventricular septal defect, and right ventricular hypertrophy) places the patient and fetus at increased risk. Commonly, an increase in the right-to-left shunt necessitates interruption of the pregnancy. Surgical correction of tetralogy of Fallot prior to pregnancy decreases complications.

Patent Ductus Arteriosus

An isolated patent ductus arteriosus, without pulmonary hypertension, is well tolerated in pregnancy. When clinical deterioration occurs, the patient responds to bed rest, digitalis, and diuretics. For the rare patient who does not respond to medical therapy, catheter-based or surgical intervention may be attempted.

Ventricular Septal Defect

The risk of complications related to a ventricular septal defect during pregnancy depends upon the size and direction of the shunt. Small left-to-right shunts are well tolerated. Complications include congestive heart failure, arrhythmias, right ventricular failure, and emboli. The decrease in systemic vascular resistance seen with pregnancy may reverse a left-to-right shunt, causing progressive hypoxemia. Vasopressors and volume replacement may control this shunt.

Atrial Septal Defect

The completely repaired atrial septal defect represents no increased risk of complications to the mother or fetus. Large atrial septal defects are well tolerated in pregnancy. If pulmonary hypertension is present, maternal and fetal risks are increased and termination of the pregnancy should be considered.

Coarctation of the Aorta

This condition may be complicated by congestive heart failure and endocarditis. Complications unique to coarctation of the aorta are the risks of aortic dissection and rupture of an intracranial aneurysm. These risks are further increased by pregnancy, and the maternal mortality rate is approximately 5%.

Hypertrophic Obstructive Cardiomyopathy

Due to the volume expansion that occurs during pregnancy, this abnormality is generally well tolerated. Maternal morbidity includes fatigue, chest pain, congestive heart failure, palpitations, and syncope. The patient should have ambulatory monitoring performed for detection of symptomatic ventricular arrhythmias. The initial treatment of these rhythm disturbances is a beta-blocking agent. The risks of amiodarone use in pregnancy are not known, so it should be used as a last resort. The role of dual-chamber pacing and the use of an automatic implantable cardioverter-defibrillator are being investigated. Hemodynamic monitoring for excessive fluid shifts should be done at the time of delivery.[9]

Marfan's Syndrome

There is nearly a 50% mortality rate during pregnancy in patients who have Marfan's syndrome and an enlarged aortic root. Serial echocardiograms should be performed to detect progressive aortic root enlargement; physical activity should be avoided and beta-blocker therapy begun. Delivery by cesarean section is recommended in patients with Marfan's syndrome to prevent any potentially deleterious effect of the Valsalva maneuver during labor.[10,11]

Peripartum Cardiomyopathy

Peripartum cardiomyopathy is defined as a dilated cardiomyopathy which occurs during the last month of pregnancy or within 5 months of delivery in the absence of another identifiable cause.[12] Approximately one-half of the patients who develop congestive heart failure due to peripartum cardiomyopathy recovery over the next 6 months; the other half develop chronic congestive heart failure. Those patients who recover from peripartum cardiomyopathy have a normal life expectancy in the absence of repeated pregnancy. If they become pregnant again, the risk of death associated with the second pregnancy is 10%. Patients who develop chronic congestive heart failure have a 50% mortality rate with repeat pregnancy.[13]

Treatment of peripartum cardiomyopathy during pregnancy includes conventional ther apy for congestive heart failure with oxygen, digoxin, diuretics, and afterload reduction with hydrazine and nitrates. Heparin may be used to prevent thromboembolic complications.

Coronary Artery Disease

Coronary artery disease is rare in women of childbearing age. The risk factor most highly correlated with the risk of myocardial infarction in pregnancy is cigarette smoking. Myocardial infarction in the peripartum period may be due to atherosclerosis, coronary spasm or dissection, and in situ thrombosis. Cardiac catheterization in pregnant patients with a myocardial infarction shows abnormal coronary artery morphology in only 30% of the patients. Overall mortality rates with peripartum myocardial infarction are nearly 30%, and the mortality from myocardial infarction in the third trimester is 40%. Patients less than 35 years of age with peripartum myocardial infarction have a 50% mortality rate.[14]

REFERENCES

1. Cox JL, Gardner MJ: Treatment of cardiac arrhythmias during pregnancy. *Prog Cardiovasc Dis* 36:137–178, 1993.
2. Metcalfe J, Ueland K: Maternal cardiovascular adjustments to pregnancy. *Prog Cardiovasc Dis* 41;363–374, 1975.
3. Arias F, Pineda J: Aortic stenosis and pregnancy. *J Reprod Med* 20:229–232, 1978.
4. Angel JL, Chapman C, Knuppel RA, et al: Percutaneous balloon aortic valvuloplasty in pregnancy. *Obstet Gynecol* 72:438–440, 1988.
5. Clark SL, Phelan JP, Greenspoon J, et al: Labor and delivery in the presence of mitral stenosis: Central hemodynamic observations. *Am J Obstet Gyncol* 152:984–988, 1985.
6. Esteves CA, Ramos AIO, Braga SLN, et al: Effectiveness of percutaneous balloon mitral valvotomy during pregnancy. *Am J Cardiol* 68:930–934, 1991.
7. Donnelly JE, Brown JM, Radford DJ: Pregnancy outcome and Ebstein's anomaly. *Br Heart J* 66:368–371, 1991.
8. Jeyamalar R, Sivanesaratnam V, Kuppuvelumani P: Eisenmenger syndrome in pregnancy. *Br Heart J* 3:275–277, 1992.
9. Shah DM, Sunderji SG: Hypertrophic cardiomyopathy and pregnancy: Report of a maternal mortality and review of literature. *Obstet Gynecol* 40:444–448, 1985.
10. Pyeritz RE: Maternal and fetal complications of pregnancy in the Marfan syndrome. *Am J Med* 71:784–790, 1981.
11. Mor-Yosef S, Younis J, Granat M, et al: Marfan's syndrome in pregnancy. *Obstet Gynecol Surv* 43:382–385, 1988.
12. Homans DC: Peripartum cardiomyopathy. *N Engl J Med* 312:1432–1437, 1985.
13. O'Connell JB, Costanzo-Nordin MR, Subramanian R, et al: Peripartum cardiomyopathy: Clinical, hemodynamic, histologic and prognostic characteristics. *J Am Coll Cardiol* 8:52–56, 1986.
14. Frenkel Y, Etchin A, Barkai G, et al: Myocardial infarction during pregnancy: A case report. *Cardiology* 78:363–368, 1991.

Exercise

Jon P. Lindemann, M.D.

This section considers the interaction between exercise and preexisting heart disease. Space limitations preclude consideration of the role of stress testing in the evaluation of heart disease and the value of exercise-based training programs in the rehabilitation of patients with heart disease.

TABLE 11.2. Mechanisms of Exercise-Induced Symptoms and Related Conditions

Symptom	Causes	Conditions
Chest discomfort	Myocardial ischemia	Coronary disease, left ventricular outflow obstruction
Dyspnea	Pulmonary congestion	Mitral disease, left ventricular dysfunction (increased left ventricular end-diastolic pressure
	Arterial oxygen desaturation	Congenital heart disease with shunt
Palpitations	Tachycardia, bradycardia, extrasystoles	Any
Cyanosis	Right-to-left shunt	Congenital heart disease with shunt
Syncope	Fixed cardiac output with peripheral vasodilatation	Valvular stenosis
	Ventricular tachycardia/ fibrillation	Any

PRESENTING MANIFESTATIONS

History

The hallmark of impaired cardiac function is a reduction in the ability of the heart to increase its performance in response to a variety of demands. Patients notice a progressive decrease in their ability to exert themselves to the same extent (level of activity or duration) compared to their activity level at the onset of their disease. Symptoms that predictably occur at the same level of exercise are highly suggestive of cardiac disease. Symptoms that may limit activity include chest discomfort, dyspnea, palpitations, cyanosis, syncope, and presyncope (Table 11.2). Which symptom occurs in response to exercise is determined largely by the nature of the underlying disease. Thus, ischemic heart disease frequently results in exertional chest pain, whereas conditions impairing left ventricular function result predominantly in dyspnea. Ischemia may also result in impaired left ventricular function, giving rise to dyspnea as well. Exercise may precipitate cardiac dysrhythmia (usually tachyarrhythmias) which would not have occurred in the absence of cardiac disease. In conditions associated with an inability to increase the cardiac output, peripheral vasodilatation may result in syncope, presyncope, or undue fatigue.

Extensively trained athletes, particularly if endurance trained, develop functional and anatomic changes in the heart—the so-called athlete's heart. These findings mimic chronic volume overloading with chamber dilation and eccentric hypertrophy.

Physical Examination

Physical examination at rest may be normal or may reveal findings consistent with the underlying cardiac disease. A transient third or fourth heart sound may be heard in patients with exercise-induced systolic or diastolic function, respectively. Basilar crackles due to pulmonary congestion may occur in such cases. Exercise-induced cyanosis may occur in patients with congenital heart disease and right-to-left intracardiac shunts. Inappropriate acceleration of the heart rate may be observed in patients with atrial fibrillation or flutter with inadequate pharmacologic control of the ventricular response.

Laboratory Evaluation

Exercise testing may be useful in determining the degree of functional impairment, as well as providing an indication of heart rate and blood pressure products with which objective evidence of decompensation develops.

DIAGNOSTIC CRITERIA

Criteria for establishing cardiac disease that is evident only in response to exercise generally derive from demonstration of the underlying cardiac disorder. Intolerance to exercise may be due to anatomic disorders such as coronary artery disease or congenital heart disease or to functional disorders such as dysrhythmias. Further, diagnostic testing employing invasive or noninvasive assessments of cardiac structure or function at rest and in response to stress may be required to establish the presence of disease. Diagnosis of the athlete's heart requires demonstration of chamber dilation and eccentric hypertrophy combined with excellent exercise tolerance in an individual with a history of endurance training.

DIFFERENTIAL DIAGNOSIS

The differential diagnosis of cardiac disease producing exercise intolerance includes those conditions that impair the end result of cardiac function, namely, tissue nutrition and oxygenation. Conditions impairing oxygenation include pulmonary diseases, anemia, and hemoglobinopathies. Disorders that increase the generalized metabolic demand, such as hyperthyroidism and chronic infection, may also impair exercise tolerance.

PATHOPHYSIOLOGY

Exercise may be broadly categorized into two groups: isometric and isotonic. Isotonic exercise is characterized by rhythmic, repetitive changes in muscle length against light loads developing little force. Isometric exercise is characterized by the rather sudden development of a large force with little muscle movement. Examples of isotonic exercise include walking, running, and swimming. Examples of isometric exercise include heavy weight lifting and wrestling.

Physical exercise or the anticipation of physical exercise results in an increase in cardiac output. The increase in cardiac output is mediated in part by alterations in autonomic tone, preload, afterload, heart rate, and the Frank-Starling mechanism. Normally, cardiac output can be increased four- to fivefold by these mechanisms (Figure 11.1).

Alterations in autonomic tone, including increased sympathetic tone and reduced vagal tone, increase heart rate and myocardial contractility. Peripheral vasoconstriction occurs in both arterial and venous beds, except in exercising musculature, where local factors including adenosine and endothelial-derived relaxing factor produce local vasodilatation. The constriction of venous capacitance vessels maintains or increases venous return to the heart. The effects of sympathetic venoconstriction are more marked with exercise in the upright position, where blood pooling in the lower extremities reduces end-diastolic volume and stroke volume at rest. Increased venous return (preload) during upright exercise may increase end-diastolic and stroke volumes significantly. By contrast, in supine exercise, there is little change in end-diastolic and stroke volumes, with the change in cardiac output coming largely from the increase in heart rate.

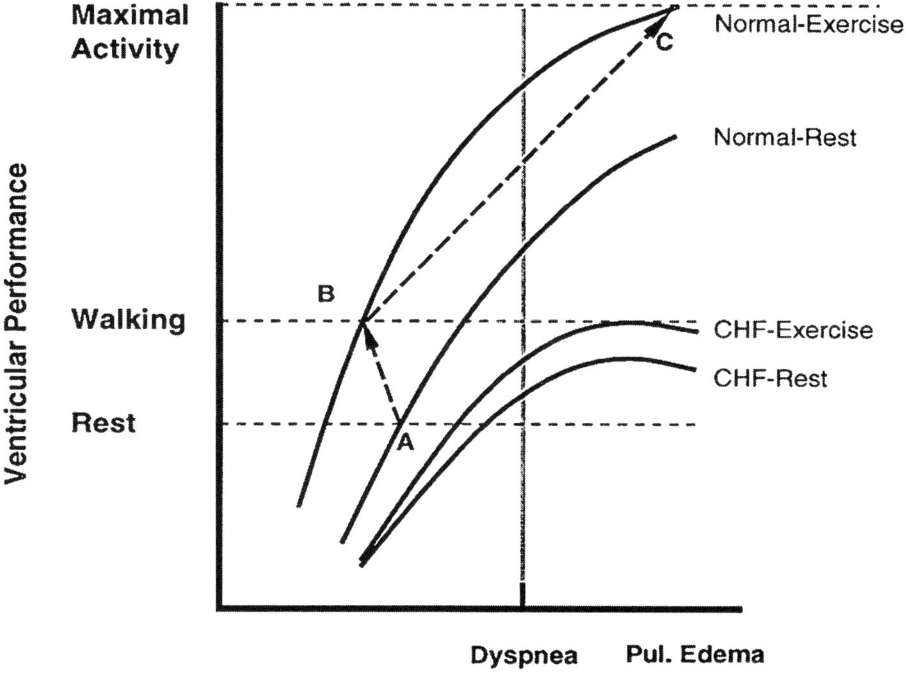

Figure 11.1. Schematic depicting the relationship between end-diastolic volume, contractility, and symptoms in response to exercise. In response to mild isometric exercise, sympathetic tone increases, resulting in a shift of the Frank-Starling curve upward and to the left (A→B). Continued exercise with accompanying increases in preload increases ventricular performance essentially by moving along the same curve (B→C). Patients with depressed left ventricular function (congestive heart failure) have a depressed contractility curve at rest. The initial shift induced by sympathetic tone is blunted, with the increase in ventricular performance coming largely from an increase in end-diastolic volume (and pressure). The increased end-diastolic pressure results in increased left atrial pressure and pulmonary venous pressure, leading to dyspnea. Dyspnea is experienced at much lower levels of activity than in normal individuals.

Patients with valvular heart disease or end-stage cardiomyopathies have a limited ability to increase their cardiac output. In these conditions, peripheral vasodilatation in response to isometric exercise may result in significant reductions in blood pressure, leading to presyncope or syncope. Syncope may also arise from the development of ventricular tachycardia or ventricular fibrillation.

NATURAL HISTORY OF THE DISEASE

The natural history of exercise intolerance in patients with cardiac disease is related to the underlying disease. Patients must exert themselves in order to have exertional symptoms. As the disease progresses, less exertion is required to produce symptoms, to the point where many patients voluntarily and often unknowingly limit their exertion.

Although once thought to be abnormal, the structural alterations in athlete's heart now appear to be benign and to reverse rapidly on cessation of training.

CURRENT METHODS OF TREATMENT

Treatment is generally directed at the underlying disorder. Evidence now exists that conditioning programs may improve exercise tolerance in patients with left ventricular dysfunction or frank heart failure (for a review, see Ref. 1). For example, Levy et al. showed that endurance exercise training improved the diastolic dysfunction observed in elderly patients.[2] In patients with chronic congestive heart failure, improvement of the easily fatigability may derive in part from reversal of the biochemical changes that occur in skeletal muscle.[3] Continued investigation in this area should provide important insight into better nonpharmacologic methods to improve exercise tolerance in patients with cardiac disease.

REFERENCES

1. McKelvie RS, Teo KK, McCartney N, et al. Effects of exercise training in patients with congestive heart failure: A critical review. *J Am Col Cardiol* 23:789–796, 1995.
2. Levy WC, Cerqueira MD, Abrass IB, et al. Endurance exercise training augments diastolic filling at rest and during exercise in healthy young and older men. *Circulation* 88:116–126, 1993.
3. Adamopoulous S, Coats AJ, Brunotte F, et al. Physical training improves skeletal muscle metabolism in patients with chronic heart failure. *J Am Coll Cardiol* 21:1101–1106, 1993.

Electrical Shock and Lightning

Jon P. Lindemann, M.D.

PRESENTING MANIFESTATIONS

History

The history is important in determining the type of electrical shock received, the likelihood that the heart is involved, and the magnitude of current exposure the heart might have received. Moreover, the history suggests the likelihood of nonelectrical injury to the victim as a consequence of other trauma secondary to the shock. For recent reviews of electrical injuries see references 1–4.

The type of electrical shock is suggested by the environment of the patient when the shock was received. *Alternating current (AC)* injuries occur in response to contact with electrical sources in household or utility locations. Shocks from residential or office electrical equipment are most frequently 110 V. By contrast, higher-consumption appliances such as electric dryers or stoves or heavy electrical equipment are generally associated with sources of 220 V or more. Both of these levels are considered to be low-voltage AC contacts. Household electrocutions most frequently result from improperly grounded electrical circuits and/or appliances or from using electrical devices near water or plumbing. High-voltage AC shocks (>1000 V) are generally limited to electrical utility or construction workers exposed to high-voltage utility or transmission lines. Similarly, nonoccupational exposure may occur with accidental exposure to downed utility lines.

Sources of *direct current* (*DC*) shocks include batteries, railway systems, automobile electrical systems, and high-voltage power supplies in electronic equipment, particularly that used in conjunction with cathode ray tubes. Examples of the latter include televisions and computer monitors. External defibrillators in medical facilities constitute a risk for DC injury as well. Lightning is a special case of DC electrocution.

The type of current (AC or DC) also may be suggested by reviewing the history of the patient's physical response to the exposure. AC exposure from grasping a source frequently renders the patient unable to let go of the source due to tetanic stimulation of skeletal muscle by the 60-Hz AC. By contrast patients receiving a DC shock are frequently thrust back from the source. This difference is also important in determining the duration of exposure to the current source and the degree of injury resulting therefrom.

Apart from the type of exposure, several additional factors should be determined. These include the involvement of water in the exposure (e.g., bathtubs, other plumbing fixtures, or swimming pools) and the location of the victim at the time of the exposure. The involvement of water is important because wet skin has considerably lower resistance than does dry skin. The location of the patient at the time of injury is also important because of the possibility of additional trauma secondary to the shock. Since the majority of serious high-voltage electrical injuries involve utility and construction workers, falls from ladders, utility poles, and trees are common and may result in additional injury to the cardiovascular system.

In spite of the immense currents and voltages involved, approximately 70% of individuals struck by lightning survive. Lightning strikes occur in association with thunderstorms. Thus, the greatest likelihood of a lightning strike coincides with peak periods of thunderstorm activity when individuals are outdoors.

Three types of lightning strikes have been described: direct strike, side strike, and ground strike. Direct strikes most often have distinct entry and exit sites, and are associated with extensive burns and barotrauma. Side strikes occur when the lightning strike current "jumps" from an object such as a tree to the victim standing next to it. Most victims are solitary, but when groups are involved, several individuals may be shocked as a result of the same strike. Ground strikes occur when the current passes from the ground into the subject. Of the three types of lightning strikes, side strikes are more likely to occur when the individual is standing next to a tall object, whereas direct strikes are more likely to occur when the individual is standing in the open.

Physical Examination

The most immediate life-threatening consequence of electrical shock is cardiopulmonary arrest. The absence of pulses in victims of AC electrocution is generally due to ventricular fibrillation, whereas in DC shock victims frequently manifest asystole.

Classically, external signs of damage in response to electrical injury do not estimate the potential existence of internal injury.[1-4] However, identification of entrance and exit points is important in estimating the path of current travel. Although the pathway cannot be precisely delineated, identification of these points can predict the potential for myocardial involvement. The risk of myocardial exposure is greatest with transthoracic pathways resulting from upper to lower extremity, upper to upper extremity, and head to lower extremity exposures. Typically, entrance and exit wounds are small third-degree burns which result from the heat generated by current entering the skin. The heat generated is determined by the magnitude of the current and is inversely related to the area of contact. Entrance wounds may be absent if the victim was submerged at the time of exposure, with large amounts of current entering the body through a broad area. Such exposures are frequently fatal.

Survivors of lightning strikes present with a variety of cutaneous manifestations according to the type of strike. Because the majority of the current of the strike "flashes over" the surface of the victim, entrance and exit wounds are uncommon. Because lightning strikes occur during thunderstorms, individuals struck are frequently wet because of being in the rain. As a result, much of the current flows over the skin of the individual. "Feathering" burns are fern-like patterns over the skin and are evident within several hours of the strike. These are not actually burns but result from electrons passing over the surface of the skin. Additionally, the current may heat the water contained in wet clothing to steam, destroying the victim's clothing by a blast effect. Burns may include punctate entrance and exit burns, linear burns which occur in the axilla and groin, and thermal burns resulting from ignition of clothing. As with other electrical injuries, the location of nonthermal burns in lightning strike victims may suggest the potential for cardiovascular exposure. Neurologic signs observed following lightning strike include confusion, amnesia, loss of consciousness, and paralysis. Prolonged apnea may follow lightning strikes and persist well beyond resolution of ventricular fibrillation or asystole. Ruptured tympanic membranes occur frequently, presumably due to associated barotrauma. This finding may be useful in differentiating electrical injuries due to lightning strikes from contact with downed utility lines.

Laboratory Evaluation

Electrocardiographic abnormalities are frequently observed in victims of electrical injury. As indicated previously, ventricular fibrillation or ventricular standstill may be observed in patients with cardiopulmonary arrest. Virtually all forms of tachy- and bradyarrhythmias, as well as atrioventricular and intraventricular blocks including bundle branch blocks, have been described. Most are transient and observed only during the first 1–2 days after the shock. Additional abnormalities include transient, nonspecific ST- and T-wave abnormalities. These electrocardiographic changes may be observed in the absence of significant contractile abnormalities and may not occur in cases of significant structural damage. Prolongation of the QT interval without obvious myocardial damage has also been reported. Victims of lightning strikes have been reported to display deep, symmetric T-wave inversion in the anterior precordial leads mimicking ischemia or infarction, as well as broad-based anterior T-wave inversion mimicking an acute central nervous system event. This T-wave inversion may arise from autonomic instability rather than from myocardial injury or intracranial hemorrhage. Victims of direct strikes resulting in transthoracic involvement frequently demonstrate ST-segment elevation consistent with epicardial injury. In one large series of lightning victims, ST-segment elevation was seen only in victims of direct strikes, whereas nonspecific ST- and T-wave abnormalities were frequently seen in victims of side and ground strikes.[5]

In addition to electrocardiographic changes, elevation of serum creatine kinase (CK) activities (both total and the MB-isoenzyme) may occur, suggesting the presence of myocardia injury and necrosis. Early elevations in total or MB-CK activity may reflect damage of skeletal rather than cardiac muscle; late elevations in CK and particularly CK-MB may reflect myocardial damage.

Noninvasive imaging modalities such as echocardiography are useful in the evaluation and management of patients who have survived cardiac arrest from electrical injury.[6] Such patients may demonstrate global or regional wall motion abnormalities including hypokinesis and akinesis. In one large series of lightning strike victims, these echocardiographic abnormalities seem to be limited to victims of direct lightning strikes.[5] Similar findings have been observed in high-voltage DC shock victims.[6] Myocardial prefusion imaging may reveal perfusion defects, but the myocardial necrosis observed in autopsy series appears not to be related to thrombotic occlusion of epicardial coronary arteries. Neither diagnostic modality can differentiate between acute and preexisting abnormalities, an important consideration in older victims who are at increased risk for preexisting cardiac disease.

DIAGNOSTIC CRITERIA

The diagnosis of electric shock–induced cardiac disease requires the presence of structural or functional cardiac abnormalities in the absence of diseases known to produce similar abnormalities. Thus a history of electrical shock is essential to establish the diagnosis.

DIFFERENTIAL DIAGNOSIS

The differential diagnosis of electrical injury to the heart includes preexisting cardiac abnormalities or cardiac injury due to trauma secondary to the electrical exposure. In younger victims, the likelihood of coincident disease, i.e., coronary heart disease or systemic arterial hypertension, is relatively less than in older ones. Thus cardiac abnormalities noted on either physical examination or laboratory testing are most likely related to the acute electrical injury or related trauma. In older patients, the initial electrocardiographic findings of ST elevation and/or symmetric T-wave inversion may be difficult to distinguish from those due to acute myocardial infarction, pericarditis, or acute intracerebral hemorrhage. Other etiologies of cardiac dysfunction or injury occurring in electrical shock victims but not related to direct cardiac electrical exposure include trauma and prolonged ischemia.

PATHOPHYSIOLOGY

Major mechanisms of electrical injury to the heart include the direct effect of electrical stimulation and heat arising from passage of current through the tissues. Lightning strikes also may produce cardiac injury by barotrauma. Lethal arrhythmias may be induced with relatively small currents, whereas large current exposures may be sustained with an excellent chance of survival. The heart, like the nervous system, is highly vulnerable to electrical stimulation. As little as 100 mA of current across the myocardium is sufficient to cause ventricular fibrillation.

The magnitude of current delivered to the body is determined by Ohm's law:

$$E = IR$$

where E is voltage, I is current, and R is resistance. Since the current of a source is frequently unknown, the magnitude of the current is estimated from the voltage, which is linearly related to the current. This relationship also points out the danger of water with electrical exposure. Wetting the skin reduces its electrical resistance nearly 1000-fold, reducing the current requirements for ventricular fibrillation a similar degree (Table 11.3).

Current flow through the body generally occurs through the tissues with the lowest electrical resistance. These include the nervous system and blood. Thus the likelihood of significant transcardiac current flow is increased by contacts directed from the head or arm to the foot or leg and from arm to arm. Moreover, these two systems are most susceptible to direct

TABLE 11.3. Effect of Water on Voltage Requirements for Ventricular Fibrillation

Factor	Wet Skin	Dry Skin
Average resistance (ohms/cm^2)	30,000	1,200
Current required for ventricular fibrillation (mA)	100	100
Voltage required for ventricular fibrillation	3,000	120

Modified from Cooper MA: Electrical lightning injuries. *Emerg Med Clin North Am* 2:489–501, 1984. Reprinted with permission from author and publisher.

electrical injury; central nervous system dysfunction (apnea/paralysis) and cardiac arrhythmia can lead to death with little structural damage.

Most of the structural damage related to electrical injury is caused by heat generation. The amount of thermal energy imparted to a tissue is defined by Joule's law:

$$\text{Heat} = K(I)RT$$

where I and R are current and resistance, respectively. T is the duration of contact and K is a constant. Although cardiac muscle has relatively low electrical resistance, significant damage my be observed. In one autopsy series of four patients, diffuse myocardial necrosis was observed in patients dying of either low- or high-voltage AC electrocution.[7] Whether this damage was due to direct heating or mediated by ischemia, neuronal catecholamine release, or small vessel occlusion could not be established.

Barotrauma, produced by the shock wave generated by the superheated column of air surrounding the lightning bolt, may also produce myocardial damage. Such injury may result in a myocardial contusion or global hypokinesis much like stunned myocardium.[5] In this study, only patients with direct strikes demonstrated echocardiographic abnormalities.

NATURAL HISTORY

The major causes of morbidity and mortality from electrical cardiac injury are determined by the magnitude and duration of current exposure. Arrhythmia and respiratory arrest are the most common causes of death in electrocution.[2] Most electrocution victims who are promptly resuscitated have an excellent chance of survival. In the series of lightning victims reported by Lichtenberg et al.,[5] 18/19 survived, with the single death being a direct strike victim. The survivors of direct strikes, all of whom demonstrated severe systolic dysfunction on the initial study returned to normal systolic function.[5] There are no reports of recurrent arrhythmia on long-term follow-up.

CURRENT METHODS OF TREATMENT

The immediate mortality of electrical injury is due to cardiopulmonary arrest. Initial management demands *safely* removing the victim from the current source, followed by prompt cardiopulmonary resuscitation. Resuscitation should even be initiated and sustained for victims who appear to be dead. Such victims may remain apneic due to brain stem depression even when ventricular fibrillation or asystole has resolved spontaneously. Sustained or symptomatic arrhythmias are treated as they would be in any patient with acute myocardial injury. Invasive hemodynamic monitoring and aggressive management of hypertension or hypotension are indicated. Echocardiography is indicated to assess the degrees of cardiac dysfunction and injury in patients who require cardiopulmonary resuscitation, or who manifest significant abnormalities or arrhythmia on the presenting electrocardiograms. Regardless of the type or degree of electrical injury, patients who manifest tachy- or bradyarrhythmia during the initial 4–6 hr after the strike should be monitored electrocardiographically for at least 24 hr.

REFERENCES

1. Cooper MA. Electrical and lightning injuries. *Emerg Med Clin North Am* 2:489–501, 1984.
2. Browne BJ, Gaasch WR. Electrical injuries and lightning. *Emerg Med Clin North Am* 10:211–228, 1992.

3. Fontanarossa PB. Electrical shock and lightning strike. *Ann Emerg Med* 22:378–387, 1993.
4. Carlton SC. Cardiac problems associated with electrical injury. *Cardiol Clin* 13:263–266, 1995.
5. Lichtenberg R, Dries D, Ward K, et al. Cardiovascular effects of lightning strikes. *J Am Coll Cardiol* 21:531–536, 1993.
6. Homma S, Gillam LD, Weyman AE. Echocardiographic observations in survivors of acute electrical injury. *Chest* 97:103–105, 1990.
7. James TN, Riddick L, Embry JH. Cardiac abnormalities demonstrated postmortem in four cases of accidental electrocution and their potential significance relative to nonfatal electrical injuries of the heart. *Am Heart J* 120:143–157, 1990.

Index

A

Acromegaly, 31–34
  diagnostic criteria, 32
  differential diagnosis, 32
  macroglossia, *33*
  natural history, 33, *33*
  pathophysiology, 32
  presenting manifestations, 31–32
    history, 31
    laboratory abnormalities, 32
    physical examination, 31
  treatment, 33–34
    cardiovascular symptoms, 34
    growth hormone, excessive secretion of, 33–34
      pharmacotherapy, 33
      radiation, 33
      surgery, 34
Adrenal insufficiency, 17–19
  diagnostic criteria, 17
  differential diagnosis, 18
  hyperpigmentation, *18*
  natural history, 18
  pathophysiology, 18
  presenting manifestations, 17
    history, 17
    laboratory evaluation, 17
    physical examination, 17, *18*
  treatment, 19
Aging, cardiac involvement in diseases, 191–98
  congestive heart failure, 197–98
    diagnostic criteria, 197
    differential diagnosis, 197
    natural history, 198
    pathophysiology, 197
    presenting manifestations, 197
    treatment, 198
  orthostatic hypotension, 195–96
    diagnostic criteria, 195
    differential diagnosis, 195–96
    natural history, 196
    pathophysiology, 196
    presenting manifestations, 195
    treatment, 196
  pathophysiology, 191–92
  presenting manifestations, 191
  systolic hypertension, isolated, 192–95, 193t
    diagnostic criteria, 193
    differential diagnosis, 193, 193t
    natural history, 194
    pathophysiology, 193
    presenting manifestations, 192
    treatment, 194
Alcoholic heart disease, 55–60
  consumption, death rates, correlation, *58*
  diagnostic criteria, 55–56, *56*
  differential diagnosis, 56
  natural history, 59
  pathophysiology, 57–59, *58*
  presenting manifestations, 55
    history, 55
    laboratory evaluation, 55
    physical examination, 55
  treatment, 59
  ventricular ejection fraction, decline in, alcohol con-
    sumption and, *56*

Amyloidosis, 165–68
  differential diagnosis, 166
  natural history, 167
  pathophysiology, 166–67
  presenting manifestations, 165, *166*
    diagnostic criteria, 165–66
    history, 165
    laboratory evaluation, 165, *166*
    physical examination, 165
  treatment, 167
    cardiovascular manifestations of, 167
Ankylosing spondylitis, 42–45, *44*
  diagnostic criteria, 43
  differential diagnosis, 43, *44*
  natural history, 45
  pathophysiology, 43–44
  presenting manifestations, 42–43
    history, 42–43
    laboratory evaluation, 43
    physical examination, 43
  treatment, 45
Aortic regurgitation, pregnancy and, 225
Aortic stenosis, pregnancy and, 225
Arrhythmias, 74
Arthritis, rheumatoid, 48–51
  diagnostic criteria, 48
  differential diagnosis, 49
  natural history, 50
  pathophysiology, 49
  presenting manifestations, 48
    history, 48
    laboratory evaluation, 48
    physical examination, 48
  treatment, 50
Ataxia, Friedreich's, 213–16
  cardiac manifestations, 214
  diagnosis, 214
  differential diagnosis, 214
  pathophysiology, 215
  presenting manifestations, 213–14
  prognosis, 215
  treatment, 215
Atrial septal defect, pregnancy and, 227

B

Becker's muscular dystrophy, 207–09
  cardiac disease, 207–08
  diagnosis, 208
  differential diagnosis, 208
  natural history, 208–09
  pathophysiology, 208
  presenting manifestations, 207
  treatment, 209

C

CAD, *see* Coronary artery disease
Calcium homeostasis, disorders of, 107–13
  diagnostic criteria, 108
  differential diagnosis, 108–09, *109*
  natural history, 109
  pathophysiology, 109
  presenting manifestations, 108
    history, 108

Calcium homeostasis (*contd.*)
    laboratory evaluation, 108
    physical examination, 108
    treatment, 109–10
Carcinoid syndrome, 168–73, *170*
  carcinoid plaques, *172*
  diagnostic criteria, 171
  differential diagnosis, 171, 171t
  natural history, 172
  pathophysiology, 171–72, *172*
  presenting manifestations, 168–71, *169*
    history, 168–69
    laboratory evaluation, *170,* 170–71
    physical examination, 169, *169*
  treatment, 172–73
    cardiovascular symptoms, 173
    chemotherapy, 172
    excess vasoactive substances, 172
Cardiac malignancies, 74
Cardiac toxicity, from chemotherapy, 183–87, *186*
  diagnostic criteria, 184
  differential diagnosis, 184
  natural history, 184, *186*
  pathophysiology, 184, 185t
  presenting manifestations, 183–84, 185t
    history, 183–84, 185t
    laboratory evaluation, 184, 185t
    physical examination, 184, 185t
  treatment, 184, 185t
Cardiomyopathy, 72–73
  alcohol-induced, 55–60
    consumption, death rates, correlation, *58*
    diagnostic criteria, 55–56, *56*
    differential diagnosis, 56
    natural history, 59
    pathophysiology, 57–59, *58*
    presenting manifestations, 55
      history, 55
      laboratory evaluation, 55
      physical examination, 55
    treatment, 59
    ventricular ejection fraction, decline, lifetime dose of
      alcohol consumed, *56*
  diabetic, 2
  etiology, 72–73
  hypertrophic obstructive, pregnancy and, 227
  peripartum, 227
  presentation, 72
  treatment, 73
Chemotherapy, cardiac toxicity from, 183–87, *186*
  diagnostic criteria, 184
  differential diagnosis, 184
  natural history, 184, *186*
  pathophysiology, 184, 185t
  presenting manifestations, 183–84, 185t
    history, 183, 185t
    laboratory evaluation, 184, 185t
    physical examination, 184, 185t
  treatment, 184, 185t
Chronic obstructive pulmonary disease, 139–43
  diagnostic criteria, 139
  differential diagnosis, 139
  natural history, 141
  pathophysiology, 140–41
  presenting manifestations, 139
  treatment, 141–42
Cigarette smoking, disease from, 60–62
  diagnostic criteria, 60–61
  differential diagnosis, 61
  natural history, 61–62
  pathophysiology, 61
  presenting manifestations, 60
    history, 60

    laboratory evaluation, 60
    physical examination, 60
  treatment, 62
Cirrhosis, autonomic dysfunction in, 132
Coarctation of aorta, pregnancy and, 227
Cocaine-related cardiac disorders, 62–66
  cardiotoxic effects, mechanisms, *64*
  diagnostic criteria, 63
  differential diagnosis, 63
  natural history, 65
  pathophysiology, 63–65, *64*
  presenting manifestations, 62–63
    history, 62–63
    laboratory evaluation, 63
    physical examination, 63
  treatment, 65
Congestive heart failure, 197–98
  diagnostic criteria, 197
  differential diagnosis, 197
  natural history, 198
  pathophysiology, 197
  presenting manifestations, 197
  treatment, 198
Connective tissue disease, 35–54
  alcoholic heart disease, 55–60
  ankylosing spondylitis, 42–45, *44*
    diagnostic criteria, 43
    differential diagnosis, 43, *44*
    natural history, 45
    pathophysiology, 43–44
    presenting manifestations, 42–43
      history, 42–43
      laboratory evaluation, 43
      physical examination, 43
    treatment, 45
  Marfan's syndrome, 51–54
    aortic root, echocardiography, *53*
    diagnostic criteria, 52, 52t
    differential diagnosis, 52
    natural history, 53–54
    pathophysiology, 53
    presenting manifestations, 51–52, 52t, *53*
    treatment, 54
  Reiter's syndrome, 46–47
    diagnostic criteria, 46
    differential diagnosis, 47
    natural history, 47
    pathophysiology, 47
    presenting manifestations, 46
      history, 46
      laboratory evaluation, 46
      physical examination, 46
    treatment, 47
  rheumatoid arthritis, 48–51
    diagnostic criteria, 48
    differential diagnosis, 49
    natural history, 50
    pathophysiology, 49
    presenting manifestations, 48
      history, 48
      laboratory evaluation, 48
      physical examination, 48
    treatment, 50
  systemic lupus erythematosus, 35–39
    classification of, criteria for, 36t
    diagnostic criteria, 36, 36t
    differential diagnosis, 36
    mitral valve leaflet, rupture, with vegetations, *38*
    natural history, 36–38
      antiphospholipid antibody syndrome, 37
      conduction defects, 38
      coronary artery disease, 37
      myocarditis, 36–37

pericarditis, 36
  valvular disease, 37, *38*
pathophysiology, 36
presenting manifestations, 35
  history, 35
  laboratory evaluation, 35
  physical examination, 35
treatment, 38–39
systemic sclerosis, 39–42
  diagnostic criteria, 40
  differential diagnosis, 40
  natural history, 41
  pathophysiology, 40
  presenting manifestations, 39–40
    history, 39–40
    laboratory evaluation, 40
    physical examination, 40
  treatment, 41–42
Coronary artery disease (CAD), pregnancy and, 227–28
Cushing's syndrome, 22–25
  diagnostic criteria, 22
  differential diagnosis, 23
  natural history, 24
  pathophysiology, 23–24
  presenting manifestations, 22
    history, 22
    laboratory evaluation, 22
    physical examination, 22, *23*
  treatment, 24
  truncal obesity, *23*
Cystic fibrosis, 143–46
  diagnostic criteria, 144
  differential diagnosis, 144
  natural history, 145
  pathophysiology, 144–45
  presenting manifestations, 143
  treatment, 145–46

D

Dermatomyositis, 216–20
  cardiac manifestations, 217
  diagnosis, 217
  differential diagnosis, 217
  natural history, 218
  pathophysiology, 218
  presenting manifestations, 216
  treatment, 218–19
Diabetes mellitus, 1–4
  diagnostic criteria, 2
  differential diagnosis, 2
  history, 1
  laboratory evaluation, 1–2
  natural history, 3
  pathophysiology, 2
    atherosclerosis, 2
    diabetic cardiomyopathy, 2
    systemic arterial hypertension, 2
  physical examination, 1
  presenting manifestations, 1–2
  treatment, 3
    atherosclerosis, 3
    diabetic cardiomyopathy, 3
    systemic arterial hypertension, 3
Drugs, excessive use of, diseases related, 55–68
  alcoholic heart disease, 55–60
    consumption, correlation, *58*
    diagnostic criteria, 55–56, *56*
    differential diagnosis, 56
    natural history, 59
    pathophysiology, 57–59, *58*
    presenting manifestations, 55
      history, 55
      laboratory evaluation, 55

      physical examination, 55
    treatment, 59
    ventricular ejection fraction, decline in, *56*
  cigarette smoking, 60–62
    diagnostic criteria, 60–61
    differential diagnosis, 61
    natural history, 61–62
    pathophysiology, 61
    presenting manifestations, 60
      history, 60
      laboratory evaluation, 60
      physical examination, 60
    treatment, 62
  cocaine-related cardiac disorders, 62–66
    cardiotoxic effects, mechanisms, *64*
    diagnostic criteria, 63
    differential diagnosis, 63
    natural history, 65
    pathophysiology, 63–65, *64*
    presenting manifestations, 62–63
      history, 62–63
      laboratory evaluation, 63
      physical examination, 63
    treatment, 65
  miscellaneous drugs/prescription medications, 66–68
    cardiovascular side effects, drugs with, 67t
    diagnostic criteria, 67
    differential diagnosis, 67
    history, 66
    laboratory evaluation, 66
    natural history, 68
    pathophysiology, 67, *67*
    physical examination, 66
    presenting manifestations, 66
    treatment, 68
Duchenne's muscular dystrophy, 204–07
  cardiac disease, 205
  diagnosis, 205
  differential diagnosis, 205
  natural history, 206
  pathophysiology, 205–06
  presenting manifestations, 204
  treatment, 206

E

Eisenmenger's syndrome, pregnancy and, 226
Electrical shock, 232–37
  diagnostic criteria, 235
  differential diagnosis, 235
  natural history, 236
  pathophysiology, 235–36
  presenting manifestations, 232–34
    history, 232–33
    laboratory evaluation, 234
    physical examination, 233–34
  treatment, 236
  ventricular fibrillation, effect of water, 235t
calcium homeostasis, disorders of, 107–13
  hyperkalemia, 100–04
    diagnostic criteria, 101, *102*
    differential diagnosis, 102, *103*
    ECG findings in, *101*
    natural history, 102
    pathophysiology, 102
    presenting manifestations, 101
      history, 101
      laboratory evaluation, 101
      physical examination, 101
    treatment, 103–04
  hypokalemia, 104–06
    diagnostic criteria, 104
    differential diagnosis, 104, *105*
    natural history, 106

Electrical shock (*contd.*)
   pathophysiology, 105
   presenting manifestations, 104
    history, 104
    laboratory evaluation, 104
    physical examination, 104
   treatment, 106
  potassium balance, disorders of, 100–07
Embolism, pulmonary, 158–62, *159, 160*
  diagnostic criteria, 60, *159–60*
  differential diagnosis, 160
  natural history, 161
  pathophysiology, 160–61
  presenting manifestations, 158
   history, 158
   laboratory evaluation, 158, *159*
   physical examination, 158
  treatment, 161
Endocarditis, 73–74
  presentation, 73–74
  treatment, 74
Endocrine system, 1–34
  acromegaly, 31–34
   diagnostic criteria, 32
   differential diagnosis, 32
   macroglossia, *33*
   natural history, 33, *33*
   pathophysiology, 32
   presenting manifestations, 31–32
    history, 31
    laboratory abnormalities, 32
    physical examination, 31
   treatment, 33–34
    cardiovascular symptoms, 34
    growth hormone, excessive secretion of, 33–34
     pharmacotherapy, 33
     radiation, 33
     surgery, 34
  adrenal insufficiency, 17–19
   diagnostic criteria, 17
   differential diagnosis, 18
   hyperpigmentation, *18*
   natural history, 18
   pathophysiology, 18
   presenting manifestations, 17
    history, 17
    laboratory evaluation, 17
    physical examination, 17, *18*
   treatment, 19
  Cushing's syndrome, 22–25
   diagnostic criteria, 22
   differential diagnosis, 23
   natural history, 24
   pathophysiology, 23–24
   presenting manifestations, 22
    history, 22
    laboratory evaluation, 22
    physical examination, 22, *23*
   treatment, 24
   truncal obesity, *23*
  diabetes mellitus, 1–4
   diagnostic criteria, 2
   differential diagnosis, 2
   history, 1
   laboratory evaluation, 1–2
   natural history, 3
   pathophysiology, 2
    atherosclerosis, 2
    diabetic cardiomyopathy, 2
    systemic arterial hypertension, 2
   physical examination, 1

   presenting manifestations, 1–2
   treatment, 3
    atherosclerosis, 3
    diabetic cardiomyopathy, 3
    systemic arterial hypertension, 3
  glucocorticoid excess, *see* Cushing's syndrome
  hyperaldosteronism, 19–21
   diagnostic criteria, 20
   differential diagnosis, 20
   natural history, 21
   pathophysiology, 20
   presenting manifestations, 19–20
    history, 19
    laboratory evaluation, 20
    physical examination, 20
   treatment, 21
    cardiovascular symptoms, management
     of, 21
    excessive aldosterone secretion, management
     of, 21
     pharmacotherapy, 21
     surgery, 21
  hyperthyroidism, 10–17
   diagnostic criteria, *12,* 12–13
   differential diagnosis, 13
   natural history, 14
   pathophysiology, 13–14
   presenting manifestations, 10–11
    assessment, thyroid function, thyroid stimulating
     hormone assay, *12*
    history, 10–11
    laboratory evaluation, 11
    physical examination, 11, *11*
   treatment, 14–16
  hypothyroidism, 4–10
   diagnostic criteria, 6
   differential diagnosis, 7–8
   natural history, 8–9
   pathophysiology, 8
   presenting manifestations, 4–6
    facial appearance, *5*
    history, 4–5
    laboratory evaluation, 6
    physical examination, 5, *5*
    puffiness, *5*
   treatment, 9
  obesity, 25–27
   causes of, 26t
   diagnostic criteria, 25
   differential diagnosis, 25, 26t
   natural history, 26
   pathophysiology, 25–26
   presenting manifestations, 25
    history, 25
    laboratory evaluation, 25
    physical examination, 25
   treatment, 26–27
    behavioral modification, 26
    pharmacotherapy, 26
    surgical therapy, 27
  pheochromocytoma, 27–31
   diagnostic criteria, 29
   differential diagnosis, 29, 29t
   methods of treatment, 30
   natural history, 30
   pathophysiology, 29–30
   presenting manifestations, 27–28
    history, 27–28, 28t
    laboratory evaluation, 28
    physical examination, 28
   symptoms, 28t

End-stage liver disease, conditions affecting cardiovascular system, 132–33
Epilepsy, 200
Exercise, cardiovascular disease and, 228–32, 229t, *231*
  diagnostic criteria, 230
  differential diagnosis, 230
  natural history, 231
  pathophysiology, 230–31, *231*
  presenting manifestations, 229–30
    history, 229, 229t
    laboratory evaluation, 230
    physical examination, 229
  treatment, 232

F

Fibrosis, cystic, 143–46
  diagnostic criteria, 144
  differential diagnosis, 144
  natural history, 145
  pathophysiology, 144–45
  presenting manifestations, 143
  treatment, 145–46
Friedreich's ataxia, 213–16
  cardiac manifestations, 214
  diagnosis, 214
  differential diagnosis, 214
  pathophysiology, 215
  presenting manifestations, 213–14
  prognosis, 215
  treatment, 215

G

Gastrointestinal system, disease related to, 119–38
  liver disease, cardiac involvement in, 126–36, *131*
    cardiovascular changes with cirrhosis, 127–29, *129*
    cirrhosis, autonomic dysfunction in, 132
    diagnostic criteria, 127
    differential diagnosis, 127
    end-stage liver disease, 132–33
    hepatopulmonary syndrome, 130–31, *131*
    natural history, 133
    orthotopic liver transplantation, 132
    pathophysiology, 127–33
    portal hypertension, 129–30
    portosystemic shunts, hemodynamic consequences
     of, 130
    presenting manifestations, 126–27
     history, 126
     laboratory evaluation, 127
     physical examination, 127
    treatment, 133
    vasodilatation, hyperdynamic circulation in, *129*
  noncardiac chest pain, 119–26
    diagnostic criteria, 120
    differential diagnosis, 121
    natural history, 124
    pathophysiology, 121–24, *123*
     esophageal motor disorders, 121–22, *122*
     esophagocardiac reflexes, 123–24, *123–24*
     gastroesophageal reflux disease, 121
    presenting manifestations, 119
     history, 119
     laboratory evaluation, 120
     physical examination, 119
    treatment, 125
Glucocorticoid excess, *see* Cushing's syndrome
Guillain-Barré syndrome, 209–13
  cardiac manifestations, 210
  diagnosis, 210–11
  differential diagnosis, 211
  natural history, 211–12
  pathophysiology, 211

  presenting manifestations, 209–10
  treatment, 212

H

Hematology, diseases associated with, 165–90
Hemochromatosis, 173–76
  diagnostic criteria, 174
  differential diagnosis, 174
  history, 173–74
  laboratory evaluation, 174
  natural history, 175
  pathophysiology, 174–75
  physical examination, 174
  presenting manifestations, 173–74
  treatment, 175
Hemodynamic disorders, effect on heart, 89t
Hemoglobinopathy, 177–80, *178*
  diagnostic criteria, 178
  differential diagnosis, 178
  natural history, 179
  pathophysiology, 178–79
  presenting manifestations, 177–78
    history, 177
    laboratory evaluation, 177–78
     sickle cell disease, 177, *178*
     thalassemia, 177–78
    physical examination, 177
  treatment, 179
Human immunodeficiency virus, cardiac manifestations,
  69–76
  arrhythmias, 74
  cardiac malignancies, 74
  cardiomyopathy, 72–73
    etiology, 72–73
    presentation, 72
    treatment, 73
  definition, 69–70
  endocarditis, 73–74
    presentation, 73–74
    treatment, 74
  myocardial disease, 71–72
    differential etiology, 71–72
    presentation, 71
  pericardial disease, 70–71
    diagnosis, 70–71
    differential etiology, 70–71
    natural history, 70
    presentation, 70
    treatment, 71
  presenting manifestations, 69–70
Hyperaldosteronism, 19–21
  diagnostic criteria, 20
  differential diagnosis, 20
  natural history, 21
  pathophysiology, 20
  presenting manifestations, 19–20
    history, 19
    laboratory evaluation, 20
    physical examination, 20
  treatment, 21
    cardiovascular symptoms, management of, 21
    excessive aldosterone secretion, management of, 21
     pharmacotherapy, 21
     surgery, 21
Hyperkalemia, 100–04
  diagnostic criteria, 101
  differential diagnosis, 102, *103*
  ECG findings in, 101
  natural history, 102
  pathophysiology, 102
  presenting manifestations, 101

Hyperkalemia (*contd.*)
history, 101
laboratory evaluation, 101
physical examination, 101
treatment, 103–04
Hypermagnesemia, 117–18
diagnostic criteria, 117
differential diagnosis, 117
natural history, 117
pathophysiology, 118
presenting manifestations, 114
history, 117
laboratory evaluation, 117
physical examination, 117
treatment, 118
Hypertension
pulmonary, primary, 151–57, 154t
diagnostic criteria, 153, 153t
differential diagnosis, 153–54
natural history, 155
pathophysiology, 153, 154t, 155
presenting manifestations, 151–53
history, 151
laboratory evaluation, 152–53
physical examination, 151–52
pulmonary hemodynamics, 153t
treatment, 156
systolic, 192–95, 193t
diagnostic criteria, 193
differential diagnosis, 193, 193t
natural history, 194
pathophysiology, 193
presenting manifestations, 192
treatment, 194
Hyperthyroidism, 10–17
diagnostic criteria, *12,* 12–13
differential diagnosis, 13
natural history, 14
pathophysiology, 13–14
presenting manifestations, 10–11
assessment, thyroid function, thyroid stimulating
hormone assay, *12*
history, 10–11
laboratory evaluation, 11
ocular signs of, *11*
physical examination, 11, *11*
treatment, 14–16
Hypertrophic obstructive cardiomyopathy, pregnancy
and, 227
Hypocalcemia, 110–13
causes of, 111t
diagnostic criteria, 111
differential diagnosis, 111, 111t
natural history, 112
pathophysiology, 112
presenting manifestations, 110–11
history, 110–11
laboratory evaluation, 111
physical examination, 111
treatment, 112–13
Hypokalemia, 104–07
diagnostic criteria, 104
differential diagnosis, 104–05, *105*
natural history, 106
pathophysiology, 105
presenting manifestations, 104
history, 104
laboratory evaluation, 104
physical examination, 104
treatment, 106
Hypomagnesemia, 113–18
causes of, 115t

diagnostic criteria, 114
differential diagnosis, 115, 115t
pathophysiology, 115–16
presenting manifestations, 114
history, 114
laboratory evaluation, 114
physical examination, 114
treatment, 116
Hypotension, orthostatic, 195–96
diagnostic criteria, 195
differential diagnosis, 195–96
natural history, 196
pathophysiology, 196
presenting manifestations, 195
treatment, 196
Hypothyroidism, 4–10
diagnostic criteria, 6
differential diagnosis, 7–8
natural history, 8–9
pathophysiology, 8
presenting manifestations, 4–6
facial appearance, *5*
facial puffiness, *5*
history, 4–5
laboratory evaluation, 6
physical examination, 5, *5*
treatment, 9

I

Infection, diseases related to, 69–87
human immunodeficiency virus, cardiac manifestations, 69–76
arrhythmias, 74
cardiac malignancies, 74
cardiomyopathy, 72–73
etiology, 72–73
presentation, 72
treatment, 73
definition, 69–70
endocarditis, 73–74
presentation, 73–74
treatment, 74
myocardial disease, 71–72
differential etiology, 71–72
presentation, 71
pericardial disease, 70–71
diagnosis, 70–71
differential etiology, 70–71
natural history, 70
presentation, 70
treatment, 71
presenting manifestations, 69–70
sepsis, heart and, 80–87
antimicrobial therapy, in sepsis, 85
cardiac physiology of septic shock, 83–84
clinical presentation, 81–82
definitions, 80–81
diagnosis, 82
differential etiology, 82
experimental therapy, in sepsis, septic shock, 86
pathophysiology, 82–83
supportive therapy, 85–86
treatment, 84
spirochetal disease, heart and, 76–80
diagnostic criteria, 77–78
laboratory evaluation, 77–78
natural history, 78
pathophysiology, 78
presenting manifestations, 76–77
history, 76–77
physical examination, 76–77
treatment, 79

Interstitial lung disease, 146–49
   cardiac complications of, 146–48
      diagnostic criteria, 147
      history, 146–47
      laboratory evaluation, 147
      presenting manifestations, 146
   differential diagnosis, 147
   natural history, 148
   pathophysiology, 147–48
   treatment, 148
Ischemic heart disease, 91–96, *94*
   diagnostic criteria, 93, *94*
   differential diagnosis, 93–94
   natural history, 95
   pathophysiology, 94–95
   presenting manifestations, 92–93
      history, 92
      laboratory evaluation, 92–93
      physical examination, 92
   treatment, 95–96

L

Lightning, being struck by, 232–37
   diagnostic criteria, 235
   differential diagnosis, 235
   natural history, 236
   pathophysiology, 235–36
   presenting manifestations, 232–34
      history, 232–33
      laboratory evaluation, 234
      physical examination, 233–34
   treatment, 236
   ventricular fibrillation, effect of water, 235t
Liver disease, cardiac involvement in, 126–36, *131*
   cardiovascular changes with cirrhosis, 127–29, *129*
   cirrhosis, autonomic dysfunction in, 132
   diagnostic criteria, 127
   differential diagnosis, 127
   end-stage liver disease, conditions affecting cardiovas-
      cular system, 132–33
   hepatopulmonary syndrome, 130–31, *131*
   natural history, 133
   orthotopic liver transplantation, hemodynamic conse-
      quences of, 132
   pathophysiology, 127–33
   portal hypertension, 129–30
   portosystemic shunts, hemodynamic consequences
      of, 130
   presenting manifestations, 126–27
      history, 126
      laboratory evaluation, 127
      physical examination, 127
   treatment, 133
   vasodilatation, hyperdynamic circulation in, *129*
Lupus, systemic, erythematosus, 35–39
   classification of, criteria for, 36t
   diagnostic criteria, 36, 36t
   differential diagnosis, 36
   mitral valve leaflet, rupture, with vegetations, *38*
   natural history, 36–38
      antiphospholipid antibody syndrome, 37
      conduction defects, 38
      coronary artery disease, 37
      myocarditis, 36–37
      pericarditis, 36
      valvular disease, 37, *38*
   pathophysiology, 36
   presenting manifestations, 35
      history, 35
      laboratory evaluation, 35
      physical examination, 35
   treatment, 38–39

M

Magnesium homeostasis, disorders of, 113–18
Marfan's syndrome, 51–54
   aortic root, echocardiography, *53*
   diagnostic criteria, 52, 52t
   differential diagnosis, 52
   natural history, 53–54
   pathophysiology, 53
   pregnancy and, 227
   presenting manifestations, 51–52, 52t, *53*
   treatment, 54
Medications
   diseases related to excess use of, 66–68
      cardiovascular side effects, drugs with, 67t
      diagnostic criteria, 67
      differential diagnosis, 67
      history, 66
      laboratory evaluation, 66
      natural history, 68
      pathophysiology, 67, *67*
      physical examination, 66
      presenting manifestations, 66
      treatment, 68
   excessive use of, diseases related to, 55–68
Metabolic disorders, effect on heart, 89t
Mitochondrial myopathies, 220–23
   cardiac manifestations, 221
   clinical manifestations, 220
   diagnosis, 221
   pathophysiology, 221–22
   prognosis, 222
   treatment, 222
Mitral stenosis, pregnancy and, 226
Mitral valve prolapse, pregnancy and, 226
Multiple myeloma, 180–83
   diagnostic criteria, 182
   differential diagnosis, 182
   natural history, 182
   pathophysiology, 182
      high-output cardiac states, 182
      multiple myeloma, 182
   presenting manifestations, 180–82, *181*
      history, 180
      laboratory evaluation, 180–82
      physical examination, 180, *181*
   treatment, 182
Muscular dystrophy
   Becker's, 207–09
      cardiac disease, 207–08
      diagnosis, 208
      differential diagnosis, 208
      natural history, 208–09
      pathophysiology, 208
      presenting manifestations, 207
      treatment, 209
   Duchenne's, 204–07
      cardiac disease, 205
      diagnosis, 205
      differential diagnosis, 205
      natural history, 206
      pathophysiology, 205–06
      presenting manifestations, 204
      treatment, 206
Myocardial disease, 71–72, *see also* Myocardial
      sarcoidosis
   differential etiology, 71–72
   presentation, 71
Myocardial sarcoidosis, 149–51
   differential diagnosis, 150
   history, 149
   laboratory evaluation, 149–50
      diagnostic criteria, 150

Myocardial sarcoidosis (*contd.*)
  natural history, 150
  pathophysiology, 150
  physical examination, 149
  presenting manifestations, 149
  treatment, 151
Myotonic dystrophy, 201–04
  cardiac disease, 201–02
  diagnosis, 202
  differential diagnosis, 202–03
  natural history, 203
  pathophysiology, 203
  presenting manifestations, 201
  treatment, 203

N

Neuromuscular disease, 199–223
  Becker's muscular dystrophy, 207–09
    cardiac disease, 207–08
    diagnosis, 208
    differential diagnosis, 208
    natural history, 208–09
    pathophysiology, 208
    presenting manifestations, 207
    treatment, 209
  dermatomyositis, 216–20
    cardiac manifestations, 217
    diagnosis, 217
    differential diagnosis, 217
    natural history, 218
    pathophysiology, 218
    presenting manifestations, 216
    treatment, 218–19
  Duchenne's muscular dystrophy, 204–07
    cardiac disease, 205
    diagnosis, 205
    differential diagnosis, 205
    natural history, 206
    pathophysiology, 205–06
    presenting manifestations, 204
    treatment, 206
  epilepsy, 200
  Friedreich's ataxia, 213–16
    cardiac manifestations, 214
    diagnosis, 214
    differential diagnosis, 214
    pathophysiology, 215
    presenting manifestations, 213–14
    prognosis, 215
    treatment, 215
  Guillain-Barré syndrome, 209–13
    cardiac manifestations, 210
    diagnosis, 210–11
    differential diagnosis, 211
    natural history, 211–12
    pathophysiology, 211
    presenting manifestations, 209–10
    treatment, 212
  mitochondrial myopathies, 220–23
    cardiac manifestations, 221
    clinical manifestations, 220
    diagnosis, 221
    pathophysiology, 221–22
    prognosis, 222
    treatment, 222
  myotonic dystrophy, 201–04
    cardiac disease, 201–02
    diagnosis, 202
    differential diagnosis, 202–03
    natural history, 203
    pathophysiology, 203
    presenting manifestations, 201
    treatment, 203

  polymyositis, 216–20
    cardiac manifestations, 217
    diagnosis, 217
    differential diagnosis, 217
    natural history, 218
    pathophysiology, 218
    presenting manifestations, 216
    treatment, 218–19
  stroke, 199–200
Noncardiac chest pain, 119–26
  diagnostic criteria, 120
  differential diagnosis, 121
  natural history, 124
  pathophysiology, 121–24, *123*
    esophageal motor disorders, 121–22, *122*
    esophagocardiac reflexes, 123–24, *123–24*
    gastroesophageal reflux disease, 121
  presenting manifestations, 119
    history, 119
    laboratory evaluation, 120
    physical examination, 119
  treatment, 125
Nutritional conditions, affecting cardiovascular system,
    136–38
  diagnostic criteria, 136
  differential diagnosis, 136
  miscellaneous considerations, 138
  natural history, 137
  pathophysiology, 137
  presenting manifestations, 136
    history, 136
    laboratory evaluation, 136
    physical examination, 136
  treatment, 137

O

Obesity, 25–27
  causes of, 26t
  diagnostic criteria, 25
  differential diagnosis, 25, 26t
  natural history, 26
  pathophysiology, 25–26
  presenting manifestations, 25
    history, 25
      laboratory evaluation, 25
      physical examination, 25
  treatment, 26–27
    behavioral modification, 26
    pharmacotherapy, 26
    surgical therapy, 27
Obstructive pulmonary disease, chronic, 139–43
  diagnostic criteria, 139
  differential diagnosis, 139
  natural history, 141
  pathophysiology, 140–41
  presenting manifestations, 139
  treatment, 141–42
Oncology, diseases associated with, 165–90
Orthostatic hypotension, 195–96
  diagnostic criteria, 195
  differential diagnosis, 195–96
  natural history, 196
  pathophysiology, 196
  presenting manifestations, 195
  treatment, 196
Orthotopic liver transplantation, hemodynamic conse-
    quences of, 132

P

Patent ductus arteriosus, pregnancy and, 227
Pericardial disease, 70–71
  diagnosis, 70–71
  differential etiology, 70–71

natural history, 70
presentation, 70
treatment, 71
Pericarditis, 96–100
  diagnostic criteria, 98
  differential diagnosis, 98
  natural history, 99
  pathophysiology, 98–99
  presenting manifestations, 97–98
    history, 97
    laboratory evaluation, 97–98
    physical examination, 97
  treatment, 99
Peripartum cardiomyopathy, 227
Pheochromocytoma, 27–31
  diagnostic criteria, 29
  differential diagnosis, 29, 29t
  methods of treatment, 30
  natural history, 30
  pathophysiology, 29–30
  presenting manifestations, 27–28
    history, 27–28, 28t
    laboratory evaluation, 28
    physical examination, 28
  symptoms, 28t
Polymyositis, 216–20
  cardiac manifestations, 217
  diagnosis, 217
  differential diagnosis, 217
  natural history, 218
  pathophysiology, 218
  presenting manifestations, 216
  treatment, 218–19
Portal hypertension, 129–30
Potassium balance, disorders of, 100–07
Pregnancy, cardiovascular diseases during, 224–28
  pathophysiology, 225–29
    congenital heart disease, 226–27
      atrial septal defect, 227
      coarctation of aorta, 227
      Eisenmenger's syndrome, 226
      hypertrophic obstructive cardiomyopathy, 227
      Marfan's syndrome, 227
      patent ductus arteriosus, 227
      tetralogy of Fallot, 227
      ventricular septal defect, 227–28
    coronary artery disease, 227–28
    hemodynamics, 225, 225t
    peripartum cardiomyopathy, 227
    valvular disease, 225–26
      aortic regurgitation, 225
      aortic stenosis, 225
      mitral stenosis, 226
      mitral valve prolapse, 226
      pulmonary and tricuspid valve disease, 226
  presenting manifestations, 224–25
    hemodynamic changes, 225t
    history, 224
    laboratory evaluation, 224–25
    physical examination, 224
Prescription medications, diseases related to excess use
  of, 66–68
  cardiovascular side effects, drugs with, 67t
  diagnostic criteria, 67
  differential diagnosis, 67
  history, 66
  laboratory evaluation, 66
  natural history, 68
  pathophysiology, 67, 67
  physical examination, 66
  presenting manifestations, 66
  treatment, 68
Pulmonary, tricuspid valve disease, pregnancy and, 226

Pulmonary disease, cardiac involvement in, 139–64
  chronic obstructive pulmonary disease, 139–43
    diagnostic criteria, 139
    differential diagnosis, 139
    natural history, 141
    pathophysiology, 140–41
    presenting manifestations, 139
    treatment, 141–42
  cystic fibrosis, 143–46
    diagnostic criteria, 144
    differential diagnosis, 144
    natural history, 145
    pathophysiology, 144–45
    presenting manifestations, 143
    treatment, 145–46
  interstitial lung disease, 146–49
    cardiac complications of, 146–48
      diagnostic criteria, 147
      history, 146–47
      laboratory evaluation, 147
      presenting manifestations, 146
    differential diagnosis, 147
    natural history, 148
    pathophysiology, 147–48
    treatment, 148
  myocardial sarcoidosis, 149–51
    differential diagnosis, 150
    history, 149
    laboratory evaluation, 149–50
      diagnostic criteria, 150
    natural history, 150
    pathophysiology, 150
    physical examination, 149
    presenting manifestations, 149
    treatment, 151
  primary pulmonary hypertension, 151–57, 154t
    diagnostic criteria, 153, 153t
    differential diagnosis, 153–54
    natural history, 155
    pathophysiology, 153, 154t, 155
    presenting manifestations, 151–53
      history, 151
      laboratory evaluation, 152–53
      physical examination, 151–52
    pulmonary hemodynamics, 153t
    treatment, 156
  pulmonary embolism, 158–62, *159, 160*
    diagnostic criteria, 160
    differential diagnosis, 160
    natural history, 161
    pathophysiology, 160–61
    presenting manifestations, 158
      history, 158
      laboratory evaluation, 158, *159*
      physical examination, 158
    treatment, 161
  pulmonary vasculitis, 162–64
    diagnostic criteria, 163
    differential diagnosis, 163
    natural history, 164
    pathophysiology, 163
    presenting manifestations, 162–63
    treatment, 164
Pulmonary embolism, 158–62, *159, 160*
  diagnostic criteria, 160
  differential diagnosis, 160
  natural history, 161
  pathophysiology, 160–61
  presenting manifestations, 158
    history, 158
    laboratory evaluation, 158, 159
    physical examination, 158
  treatment, 161

Pulmonary hypertension, primary, 151–57, 154t
  diagnostic criteria, 153, 153t
  differential diagnosis, 153–54
  natural history, 155
  pathophysiology, 153, 154t, 155
  presenting manifestations, 151–53
    history, 151
    laboratory evaluation, 152–53
    physical examination, 151–52
  pulmonary hemodynamics, 153t
  treatment, 156
Pulmonary vasculitis, 162–64
  diagnostic criteria, 163
  differential diagnosis, 163
  natural history, 164
  pathophysiology, 163
  presenting manifestations, 162–63
  treatment, 164

R
Radiation therapy, cardiac complications, 187–90, *188*
  diagnostic criteria, 188, *188*
  differential diagnosis, 189
  natural history, 189
  pathophysiology, 189
  presenting manifestations, 187–88
    history, 187
    laboratory evaluation, 188
    physical examination, 188
  treatment, 189
    radiation shielding, 189
    revascularization, 189
    risk factor modification, 189
Reiter's syndrome, 46–47
  diagnostic criteria, 46
  differential diagnosis, 47
  natural history, 47
  pathophysiology, 47
  presenting manifestations, 46
    history, 46
    laboratory evaluation, 46
    physical examination, 46
  treatment, 47
Renal disease, cardiovascular involvement, 88–118, 89t
  calcium homeostasis, disorders of, 107–10
    diagnostic criteria, 108
    differential diagnosis, 108–09, *109*
    natural history, 109
    pathophysiology, 109
    presenting manifestations, 108
      history, 108
      laboratory evaluation, 108
      physical examination, 108
    treatment, 109–10
  electrolyte disorders, 100–18
    calcium homeostasis, disorders of, 107–13
    hyperkalemia, 100–04
      diagnostic criteria, 101
      differential diagnosis, 102, *103*
      ECG findings in, *101*
      natural history, 103
      pathophysiology, 102
      presenting manifestations, 101
        history, 101
        laboratory evaluation, 101
        physical examination, 101
      treatment, 103–04
    hypokalemia, 104–07
      diagnostic criteria, 104
      differential diagnosis, 104, 105
      natural history, 106
      pathophysiology, 105
      presenting manifestations, 104

        history, 104–05
        laboratory evaluation, 104
        physical examination, 104
      treatment, 106
    potassium balance, disorders of, 100–07
  hemodynamic disorders, effect on heart, 89t
  hypermagnesemia, 117–18
    diagnostic criteria, 117
    differential diagnosis, 117
    natural history, 118
    pathophysiology, 118
    presenting manifestations, 114
      history, 117
      laboratory evaluation, 117
      physical examination, 117
    treatment, 117, 118
  hypocalcemia, 110–13
    causes of, 112t
    diagnostic criteria, 111
    differential diagnosis, 111, 111t
    natural history, 112
    pathophysiology, 112
    presenting manifestations, 110–11
      history, 110–11
      laboratory evaluation, 111
      physical examination, 110
    treatment, 112
  hypomagnesemia, 113–16
    causes of, 115t
    diagnostic criteria, 114
    differential diagnosis, 115, 115t
    pathophysiology, 115–16
    presenting manifestations, 114
      history, 114
      laboratory evaluation, 114
      physical examination, 114
    treatment, 116
  ischemic heart disease, 91, 96, *94*
    diagnostic criteria, 93, *94*
    differential diagnosis, 93
    natural history, 95
    pathophysiology, 94–95
    presenting manifestations, 92–93
      history, 92
      laboratory evaluation, 92–93
      physical examination, 92
    treatment, 95–96
  magnesium homeostasis, disorders of, 113–18
  metabolic disorders, effect on heart, 89t
  pericarditis, 96–100
    diagnostic criteria, 98
    differential diagnosis, 98
    natural history, 99
    pathophysiology, 98–99
    presenting manifestations, 97–98
      history, 97
      laboratory evaluation, 97–98
      physical examination, 97
    treatment, 99–100
  renal failure, 88–100
    diagnostic criteria, 90
    differential diagnosis, 90
    left ventricular dysfunction in, 91
    natural history, 90
    pathophysiology, 90
    presenting manifestations, 91
      history, 88
      laboratory evaluation, 89–90
      physical examination, 88–89
    treatment, 91
Renal failure, 88–100
  diagnostic criteria, 90
  differential diagnosis, 90

left ventricular dysfunction in, 88–91
natural history, 90
pathophysiology, 90
presenting manifestations, 88–91
history, 89
laboratory evaluation, 89
physical examination, 89–90
treatment, 91
Rheumatoid arthritis, 48–51
diagnostic criteria, 48
differential diagnosis, 49
natural history, 50
pathophysiology, 49
presenting manifestations, 48
history, 48
laboratory evaluation, 48
physical examination, 48
treatment, 50

S
Sarcoidosis, myocardial, 149–50
differential diagnosis, 150
history, 149
laboratory evaluation, 149–50
diagnostic criteria, 150
natural history, 150
pathophysiology, 150
physical examination, 149
presenting manifestations, 149
treatment, 151
Sclerosis, systemic, 39–42
diagnostic criteria, 40
differential diagnosis, 40
natural history, 41
pathophysiology, 40
presenting manifestations, 39–40
history, 39–40
laboratory evaluation, 40
physical examination, 40
treatment, 41–42
Sepsis, heart and, 80–87
antimicrobial therapy, in sepsis, 84–85
cardiac physiology of septic shock, 83
clinical presentation, 81
definitions, 80–81
diagnosis, 81–82
differential etiology, 81–82
experimental therapy, in sepsis, septic shock, 86
pathophysiology, 82–83
supportive therapy, 85–86
treatment, 84
Spirochetal disease, heart and, 76–80
diagnostic criteria, 77–78
laboratory evaluation, 77–78
natural history, 78
pathophysiology, 78

presenting manifestations, 76–77
history, 76–77
physical examination, 76–77
treatment, 79
Stroke, 199–200
Systemic lupus erythematosus, 35–39
classification of, criteria for, 36t
diagnostic criteria, 36, 36t
differential diagnosis, 36
mitral valve leaflet, rupture, with vegetations, *38*
natural history, 36–38
antiphospholipid antibody syndrome, 37
conduction defects, 38
coronary artery disease, 37
myocarditis, 36–37
pericarditis, 36
valvular disease, 37, *38*
pathophysiology, 36
presenting manifestations, 35
history, 35
laboratory evaluation, 35
physical examination, 35
treatment, 38–39
Systemic sclerosis, 39–42
diagnostic criteria, 40
differential diagnosis, 40
natural history, 41
pathophysiology, 40
presenting manifestations, 39–40
history, 39–40
laboratory evaluation, 40
physical examination, 40
treatment, 41–42
Systolic hypertension, isolated, 192–95, 193t
diagnostic criteria, 193
differential diagnosis, 193, 193t
natural history, 194
pathophysiology, 193
presenting manifestations, 192
treatment, 194

T
Tetralogy of Fallot, pregnancy and, 227
Tricuspid valve disease, pregnancy and, 226

V
Valvular disease, pregnancy and, 225–26
Vasculitis, pulmonary, 162–64
diagnostic criteria, 163
differential diagnosis, 163
natural history, 164
pathophysiology, 163
presenting manifestations, 162–63
treatment, 164
Ventricular septal defect, pregnancy and, 227–28

ISBN 0-89640-317-3